2578   WD205

HOLTON,J.B.

The inherited metabolic diseases

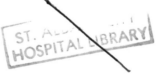

The Inherited Metabolic Diseases

The Inherited Metabolic Diseases

Edited by

John B. Holton BSc PhD ARCS FRCPath

Clinical Biochemist, Southmead Hospital, Bristol;
Recognized Teacher in Biochemistry, University of Bristol;
Visiting Lecturer in Biochemistry, University of Bath

CHURCHILL LIVINGSTONE
EDINBURGH LONDON MELBOURNE AND NEW YORK 1987

CHURCHILL LIVINGSTONE
Medical Division of Longman Group UK Limited

Distributed in the United States of America by
Churchill Livingstone Inc., 1560 Broadway, New York,
N.Y. 10036, and by associated companies, branches
and representatives throughout the world.

First published 1987

ISBN   0-443-03195-9

British Library Cataloguing in Publication Data
The Inherited metabolic diseases.
  1. Metabolism, Inborn errors of
  I. Holton, John B.
  616.3'9042   RC 627.8

Library of Congress Cataloging in Publication Data
The Inherited metabolic diseases.
  Includes index.
  1. Metabolism, Inborn errors of.   I. Holton, J. B.
(John B.) [DNLM: 1. Metabolism, Inborn Errors.
WD 205 I55]
RC627.8.I54   1987   616.3'9042   87–731

Produced by Longman Singapore
Publishers (Pte) Ltd.
Printed in Singapore

Preface

For some time I have felt that there was a need for a book which filled a gap somewhere between the large, multi-author, '*Metabolic Basis of Inherited Disease*' of Stanbury and his colleagues and a variety of short, single author texts on the inherited metabolic diseases. Whilst it is to be hoped that the former will remain the standard reference work for those actively engaged in this field, it is rather daunting for those who are less committed yet still require a fairly comprehensive, accurate and up-to-date account of the subject. On the other hand, the subject has grown to such an extent that a single author can only write authoritatively on a small part of it, or give an overview illustrating general principles and describing representative diseases.

The object of this book is to be concise, but nevertheless comprehensive and accurate. It is hoped that it will be acceptable to the student but, also, with the use of the bibliography to such important practical aspects as diagnosis and treatment, that it will be a valuable alternative source of reference to all those more directly involved with the diseases. Twelve authors have written a chapter each on one of the accepted sub-divisions of the subject. Although none of these authors is likely to have first-hand experience of all the diseases within their chapter, they should be able to write critically in an area in which they are recognised to have a special expertise.

The production of this book has highlighted for me a number of problems which arise from the fact that there is no clear, systematic classification of the inherited metabolic diseases. The sub-divisions I have employed, which are in use widely, are not based on a uniform criterion. Some of the sections are concerned with diseases which all share a well-defined area of metabolism; but, more often, they include a heterogeneous collection of diseases which have in common only that abnormal metabolites which are excreted have similar chemical properties, conveniently linked because they can be investigated by the same analytical techniques. Other sections describe disorders in which the primary defects are in the same tissue, type of cell or subcellular organelle.

The practical difficulties that arise because of the above method of subdividing the inherited metabolic diseases are, firstly, that a disorder may be reasonably classified into two or more sections; secondly, some disorders do not fit conveniently into any section and tend to get omitted; and thirdly, a chapter may cover groups of diseases with very little in common other than, for example, that they are all diagnosed by the use of gas chromatography. In this last situation, in particular, it is extremely difficult to write a concise account of the diseases within such a group. Unfortunately, it seems that alternative methods of classification involve many more subdivisions, or are based on even more arbitrary criteria.

It should be noted that, in common with many other publications in human genetics, throughout the book diseases have been cross-referenced to the 'catalogs of autosomal dominant, autosomal recessive and X-linked phenotypes' of McKusick (McKusick V 1983 *Mendelian Inheritance in Man*, 6th edn. John Hopkins University Press, Baltimore), although there were a few recently described conditions where this was not possible. This has two main purposes. Firstly, it is a further means of identifying and distinguishing a specific disease. This may be useful when several variant or closely related forms exist. Secondly, it gives access to an additional bibliography on each condition. In particular, references to the original descriptions of a disease may usually be found in McKusick.

Finally, I would like to acknowledge a debt of real gratitude to the contributors, who have all had to face the difficult challenge of how to approach their task; what to put in and what to leave out. Finally, I would like to thank Miss Iris Lynn who typed my manuscript and re-typed parts of many others.

Bristol, 1987   J. B. H.

Contributors

G M Addison MA PhD
Consultant Chemical Pathologist, Royal Manchester and Booth Hall Children's Hospitals, Manchester

P J Aggett MSc MRCP
Senior Lecturer, Department of Child Health and Nutrition, University of Aberdeen; Honorary Consultant Paediatrician, Royal Aberdeen Children's Hospital, Aberdeen

C H Bolton BSc PhD
Lecturer in Biochemistry, Department of Medicine, Bristol Royal Infirmary, Bristol

R A Chalmers PhD FRSC MIBiol MRCPath
Senior Member, Scientific Staff, Medical Research Council, Clinical Research Centre, Harrow

D R Dunger MD MRCP DCH
Consultant Paediatrician, John Radcliffe Hospital, Headington, Oxford

G H Elder BA MD FRCPath MRCP
Professor and Head of Department of Medical Biochemistry, University of Wales College of Medicine, Cardiff

A J Grimes BSc PhD FRCPath
Professor of Experimental Haematology, Department of Haematology, United Medical and Dental Schools of Guy's and St Thomas's Hospitals, London

J B Holton BSc PhD ARCS FRCPath
Clinical Biochemist, Southmead Hospital, Bristol; Recognized Teacher in Biochemistry, University of Bristol; Visiting Lecturer in Biochemistry, University of Bath

A C Nicholls BSc PhD
Scientist, Medical Research Council, Clinical Research Centre, Harrow

C A Pennock MD BSc FRCPath
Consultant Paediatric Chemical Pathologist, Bristol and Western Health Authority; Senior Lecturer in Child Health, University of Bristol

R J Pollitt MA PhD MRCPath
External Scientific Staff, Medical Research Staff; Scientist in Charge, Trent Region Neonatal Screening Laboratory, Middlewood Hospital, Sheffield

H A Simmonds MSc PhD
Research Fellow, Purine Research Laboratory, United Medical and Dental Schools of Guy's and St Thomas's Hospitals, London

Contents

Introduction

WHAT ARE INHERITED METABOLIC DISEASES?

There are many divergent views regarding what constitutes an inherited metabolic disease, but this question is rarely of real consequence unless one is concerned with problems like considering what should be included in a book such as this. Everyone agrees that the *inborn errors of metabolism*, described by Garrod in the early part of this century[1], form a major part of the subject. These diseases, that Garrod postulated were due to a block in a metabolic pathway, were shown to arise from an enzyme deficiency which led directly to the disruption of cellular metabolism. However, 40 years after the original description of four *models* of this type of abnormality, it was discovered that one of them, cystinuria, was not due to an enzyme deficiency but to a defect in an amino acid transport system affecting both the intestine and the renal tubule.

Many examples of inherited diseases caused by abnormality of a *transport* process have now been described including those which affect movement of specific metabolites within the vascular compartment, within the cell and across the cell membrane: uptake into the cells may be altered by a defect in a membrane receptor. In addition, there are diseases in which the basic disorder is in other important biological functions; for example, in cell structure, in blood coagulation and in the oxygen carrying capacity of haemoglobin. Many of these disorders lead to a profound metabolic disturbance and, therefore, should be regarded as inherited metabolic diseases.

Numerous examples of metabolic diseases with a non-enzymic basis will be found within this book. Only practical considerations lead to some restrictions in the text. The haemoglobin disorders form a vast subject, and have become a speciality in their own right, but they are dealt with only briefly. Also, conditions like cystic fibrosis and the muscular dystrophies have been omitted because, although they are associated with multiple biochemical abnormalities, and they are usually classified as inherited metabolic diseases, there is no clear understanding of the primary defect at present.

GENETIC MECHANISM OF THE INHERITED METABOLIC DISEASES

Introduction

The common feature of all the kinds of disorder described in the preceding section is that their primary phenotypic abnormality is a qualitative or quantitative change in the synthesis of a *protein* which has enzymic or other functional properties. Elucidation of the precise mechanism of this abnormality has many implications for the diagnosis, treatment and prevention of the diseases which are caused.

The way in which *genes* control the synthesis of proteins is now well established and knowledge of the type of errors which can occur in this process is particularly advanced in the case of disorders in the synthesis of the α and β chains of haemoglobin.[2,3] Similar aberrations in the synthesis of enzymes and other proteins are now being discovered at regular intervals and examples will be found within the chapters of this book.

Normal mechanisms of gene expression

The stages in the expression of a gene are shown in Figure 1.1. The genes, which average about 1000 base pairs of a Watson-Crick double helix, consist of coding regions, often called exons, which will ultimately determine the amino acid sequence of the protein product, interspersed with non-coding regions, which are termed introns, or intervening sequences (IVS). The genome is made up of genes divided up by even larger lengths of spacer, or intergenic, DNA which is not transcribed. The precise function of the intergenic regions is not established: however, it is known that to the left,

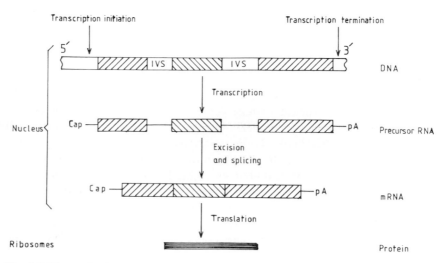

Fig. 1.1 The mechanism of expression of a gene resulting in protein synthesis.

or 'upstream', of the 5' end of the gene there are a number of base sequences which are important in initiating, and determining the rate of, gene transcription. The rate of transcription can be affected by steroid hormones which exert their influence through receptors located in the region just described.

Gene transcription proceeds from left to right, from the 5' to the 3' end of the DNA strand, including both the exons and introns. The first product of gene expression is called precursor RNA and it is made up of ribonucleotide sub-units with a sequence of bases which is complementary to that of the original DNA of the gene. The other regular features of RNA are introduced at this stage. A 7-methylguanosine group is joined to the 5' terminal nucleotide through a 5'–5' pyrophosphate link. This grouping, called the Cap, is thought to enhance the efficiency of translation and it is part of all mammalian RNA molecules. Also, most RNAs have a tail of adenine molecules (pA) attached to the 3' terminal nucleotide, but the significance of this addition to the post translational region of the RNA molecule is unclear.

In the next stage, known as processing, the sequences of nucleotides corresponding to non-coding regions of the gene are excised from the precursor RNA and the remaining, coding, portions are spliced together in a continuous sequence to yield processed, or messenger, RNA (mRNA). The portions of RNA which are removed during the processing are indicated by specific nucleotide sequences which will be coded originally at the beginning and end of the IVS.

In the final step of gene expression, mRNA is transported from the cell nucleus to the ribosomes where the RNA code is translated into the amino acid sequence of a unique polypeptide chain.

Disorders of gene expression

Disorders of protein synthesis underlying the inherited metabolic diseases may be classified into three types with varying causes at the gene level. The fundamental changes which occur in the genome are 'deletions' involving just one nucleotide up to those involving many hundreds of nucleotides. Similarly, there may be 'additions' of one or more nucleotides. Finally, 'substitutions' may arise in which there is a change in one or more nucleotides in the DNA sequence without a difference in the actual number.

Those in which no protein is synthesised. This situation may arise if an mRNA is produced which cannot sustain protein synthesis at the polysomes; for example, if it contains a change in the nucleotide sequence such that chain termination is signalled prematurely and the resulting shortened polypeptide is very unstable. Alternatively, it can occur if no translatable mRNA reaches the polysomes. This may happen for a number of reasons. In some mutations a massive deletion of the DNA of the genome has been found, so that the gene is completely missing. In other cases, a small mutation in a DNA sequence in a critical area controlling gene transcription or RNA processing may cause a failure of mRNA synthesis, although the coding region of the gene may be intact.

Reduced synthesis of protein of normal structure occurs. This can arise when a small deletion, addition or substitution in the nucleotide sequence, usually in the intergenic region of the genome or in the IVS, causes a reduction in the rate of transcription or processing to mRNA, although the messenger is normal in structure. It is also possible for a small substitution in a nucleotide triplet in the coding portion of a gene to cause reduced rate of synthesis of normal protein. If the triplet changes to one which codes for precisely the same amino acid the mutation is said to be synonymous. Although, in these circumstances, an identical polypeptide chain is produced, the different nucleotide sequence may make transcription or translation less efficent, thus reducing the rate of protein synthesis.

Synthesis of a protein with abnormal structure. Mutations in the genome may cause an mRNA to be produced which is short of considerable numbers of nucleotides or, conversely, one which has inserted, or added, extra nucleotides. These extra nucleotides may correspond to regions of IVS or intergenic DNA which have been transcribed in error. On translation this may lead to the synthesis of an abnormal polypeptide chain of shorter, or longer, length respectively. However, by far the most common form of structural abnormality is one in which there is a substitution of just one nucleotide for another in the coding portion of the gene. This, in turn, causes a similar, isolated substitution in mRNA and the coding of one amino acid wrongly in the polypeptide chain. This type of change is called a 'point' mutation.

As mentioned above, point mutations are the most frequent cause of structural disorders, and they are almost certainly the most common of all types of protein synthesis disorders. For example, it can be calculated that for the β chain of haemoglobin, a polypeptide of 146 amino acids, there are 960 possible point mutations or one amino acid substitution. Of these about a third, or 320, would confer a charge difference on the haemoglobin molecule and these abnormal haemoglobins should be detected by electrophoresis. About one third to a half of these abnormal haemoglobins have been discovered. There is no reason to believe that other proteins are any less likely to possess these many mutant forms.

Direct and indirect demonstration of a mutant gene

The inherited metabolic diseases result from a mutation in the gene determining one specific functional polypeptide unit and are often described as monogenic disorders to distinguish them from diseases which are associated with a gross abnormality of chromosome morphology, called polygenic. In some monogenic disorders the complete nucleotide sequence of normal and mutant genes have been determined so that the precise abnormality in the latter becomes apparent. This process is very time consuming and is unnecessary if all that is required is to demonstrate the presence, or absence, of the mutant gene, as is the case for most diagnostic purposes.

In direct analysis an actual difference in the DNA sequence of the gene, or polymorphism, is demonstrated for normal and variant alleles. Indirect analysis seeks to show the presence of the normal or the mutant gene by examining other inherited characteristics which are known to be determined by genes closely linked to either of the genes under investigation, or by demonstrating nucleotide polymorphisms within chromosomal DNA which are linked to the normal or abnormal gene but not within the sequences of the genes themselves. It is clear that for completely accurate analysis and diagnosis this linkage, either to genetic characteristics or to DNA polymorphisms, must remain absolute during meiosis.

The technique for demonstrating the presence of DNA polymorphism, either for direct or indirect gene analysis, involves the use of restriction endonucleases. These enzymes, of which there are several hundred, split the DNA molecule at specific points which are determined by a characteristic nucleotide sequence. For example, EcoR1 splits guanine from adenine when they occur in sequence GAATTC (G, A, T and C are guanine, adenine, thymine and cytosine respectively). The double stranded DNA molecule is split thus by the enzyme:

$$\begin{array}{ccc} \text{G} & \quad\lrcorner & \text{AATTC} \\ \text{CTTAA} & \ulcorner\quad & \text{G} \end{array}$$

Several cleavage points, or restriction sites, will occur within a given DNA molecule for each endonuclease, and it will be split into a number of fragments of varying length which will be a characteristic of the molecule. The object of direct analysis is to find an endonuclease which has a different pattern of restriction sites in the normal and mutant genes, due to polymorphism in their nucleotide structure, thus producing a different size and/or number of fragments with the DNA from each allele. The polymorphisms within the gene which are so demonstrated are called *restriction fragment length polymorphisms* (RFLPs). Emery[4] describes the techniques involved in selecting DNA fragments coming exclusively from the gene of interest and in studying the pattern of these fragments by electrophoresis.

Indirect gene analysis was first practiced using phenotypic characteristics linked to the genetic abnormality under investigation. For example, antigens of the HLA system are determined by genes located on the same chromosome as the defective enzyme in adreno-genital syndrome, 21-hycroxylase (p. 345). Analysis of the complex HLA types segregating within a family can reveal some which are linked to the normal 21-hydroxylase gene and those linked to the mutant gene. A study of HLA types may enable the prediction of a persons status with respect to 21-hydroxylase deficiency when this could not be achieved directly, for example for prenatal diagnosis. More recently, however, and of much wider application, linked DNA polymorphisms have been used as the means of indirect analysis. This indirect method is sometimes referred to as gene tracking. The techniques of identifying and studying the DNA fragments are essentially similar to those used for direct analysis.

INVESTIGATION OF A PROTEIN ABNORMALITY

At the present time few inherited metabolic disorders are investigated primarily at the gene locus, but most are looked at from the aspect of the functional properties of the abnormal protein; for example, enzyme activity, or transport characteristics in the case of a transport defect. Table 1.1 summarises the observations that may be made and the possible causes.

Table 1.1 Possible protein abnormalities in inherited metabolic disorders approached by the study of functional and physical properties

Observation	Possible causes
1. No detectable functional properties characteristic of the protein	a. The specific protein is not synthesised b. A structurally altered protein is synthesised but it lacks completely the functional sites of the normal protein, or it is extremely unstable.
2. Functional properties of the protein are partially detected	a. There is a reduced rate of synthesis of structurally normal protein b. There is a normal rate of synthesis of a structurally altered protein which has partly modified functional sites, or has normal function but moderately increased instability.

Further elucidation of the problem when there is a complete absence of functional activity is rather difficult. The commonest approach has been by often complex studies using an antibody raised to the corresponding purified normal protein. The presence of cross reacting material (CRM) to the normal protein in a patient suggests that alternative 1(b) (Table 1.1) is the probable cause of the defect. However, much work has been done with antibodies of doubtful specificity and, therefore, the above conclusion may not always be valid. The absence of any CRM (or a so-called CRM negative patient) would suggest that 1(a) is the cause, but it is possible that a protein has been synthesised which has lost completely all the antigenic determinants to the antibody.

Although it can be seen that the investigation of CRM has limitations it is, nevertheless, a useful technique in demonstrating genetic heterogeneity within a metabolic disorder. Patients showing varying degrees of CRM to the same antibody may be assumed to have different types of molecular defects.

Disorders showing some functional activity are much easier to study because the residual activity can be characterised. For example, in the case of an enzyme defect, the Km for substrate and cofactor, the substrate specificity, the effects of inhibitors and the stability under various conditions of the variant form can be compared with normal. Similar studies can be done in the case of a defective transport mechanism. If all the properties of a protein appear normal it would be presumed that there was a reduced rate of synthesis of a structurally normal protein. If some of the properties were abnormal a structural abnormality would be indicated. The structurally altered protein may, or may not, have a different charge. Electrophoresis is a useful tool to investigate the former group, particularly if the residual functional properties can be exploited to show up the protein on, or within, the electrophoretic supporting medium.

INHERITANCE

The modes of inheritance of the inherited metabolic diseases are usually described in classical Mendelian terms.[5] It will be seen, however, that the original simple concepts need to be extended in the light of further knowledge of the biochemical disorders.

Autosomal genes

The majority of inherited metabolic diseases are determined by genes on the autosomes and most of them are said to have recessive inheritance; that is the clinical disease is manifest only in homozygotes for a variant allele. Both mother and father are heterozygous for the variant allele and such couples have a 1 in 4 chance of producing an affected child (Fig. 1.2). It has been pointed out earlier that it is probable that hundreds of variant alleles exist for a given protein. It is likely, therefore, that mother and

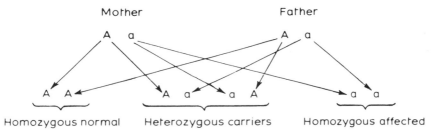

Fig. 1.2 Possible genotype of offspring in autosomal recessive inheritance: A, normal gene for a given characteristic; a, mutant, allelic, form of the gene. Random association of the genes at conception results in three possible genotypes—AA, Aa and aa—the probability of each occurring being in the ratio 1:2:1 respectively.

father each possess different variant alleles and, strictly speaking, the affected offspring is not homozygous, but is heterozygous for these two alleles. This situation has been confirmed in families with several different diseases, but unless heterogeneous alleles have been specifically demonstrated we shall usually refer to the affected patient as a homozygote. A patient is likely to be a true homozygote for the same allele if there is consanguinity in the family.

Assuming independent expression of each gene, it would be anticipated that the level of functional activity found in a heterozygote for normal and variant alleles would be midway between that found in homozygous subjects for the two alleles. This expectation is called 'simple gene dosage' and it applies in most families for most disorders: in others it is found that heterozygotes have rather more, or less, than the predicted functional activity. Variations from simple gene dosage in which heterozygotes have less activity than expected have been described in homocystinuria and histidinaemia, enzyme disorders affecting cystathionine-β-synthetase and L-histidine ammonia lyase respectively (see p. 112 & 131). On the other hand, heterozygotes for acatalasia in Swiss families have much more enzyme activity than expected; although in Japanese families with the same enzyme defect simple gene dosage operates. Various reasons for the deviation from simple gene dosage have been suggested[6].

It will be seen from the preceding paragraphs that the primary phenotypic change of the disease, i.e. the protein defect, is expressed in the heterozygote to a greater or lesser extent and this may lead to secondary metabolic abnormalities: in other words, the disease is incompletely recessive for the biochemical disorder. When the full spectrum of biochemical abnormalities, and the disease itself, is expressed in the heterozygote the condition becomes an 'autosomal dominant'. Usually only one parent is an affected heterozygote in autosomal dominantly inherited conditions and the chance of producing similar offspring is shown in Figure 1.3.

From theoretical considerations one might expect dominant inheritance

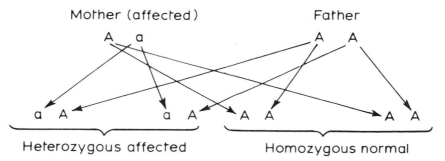

Fig. 1.3 Possible genotype of offspring in autosomal dominant inheritance. The symbols for the genes are the same as in Fig. 1.2. At conception there is an equal probability of aA, affected, and AA, unaffected, individuals occurring.

to occur either in disorders in which simple gene dosage does not operate and heterozygotes have very low functional concentration of the affected protein, or in those which involve key processes in which more than 50% functional activity is required for normal health. Most enzymes are present in very great excess, as little as 1% of their normal activity being adequate to maintain operation of the metabolic pathway in some cases. However, this may not be true for some key enzymes.

Autosomal dominantly inherited diseases are uncommon and the finding of homozygotes for them is rare. This may be because they do involve enzymes in key biochemical pathways, the complete absence of which is incompatible with life.

X-linked genes

Diseases determined by genes located on the X chromosome affect the male predominantly. A variant allele for a gene locus on the single X chromosome which the male possesses is always dominant. In the female heterozygote the variant allele is usually recessive for the clinical disorder and the homozygous female, who is affected with the disease, is relatively uncommon. The pattern of inheritance in these so-called X-linked recessive conditions is shown in Figure 1.4.

Some X-linked diseases may be expressed in the heterozygous female, although she is rarely as badly affected as the male; see, for example, ornithine transcarbamylase (OTC) deficiency (p. 120). In these circumstances the female probably has a particularly low enzyme activity. There may be a number of reasons for this, but one important factor is the operation of the *Lyon hypothesis*. This hypothesis is that in any cell of the female body only one X chromosome is actively expressed. It is postulated that at a stage in early embryological development random inactivation of one X chromosome occurs in each of the existing cells; either that chro-

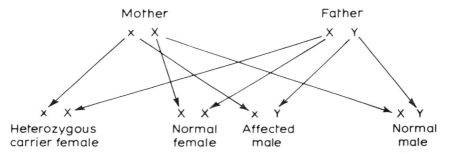

Fig. 1.4 Possible genotypes of the offspring in X-linked inheritance. X and Y represent the normal sex chromosomes and x is an abnormal X chromosome containing a mutant gene. Random association of the genes at conception results in the genotypes shown. There is an overall chance of 1 in 4 of producing an affected male (xY) and the same probability of producing a heterozygous female who may, or may not, be affected (see text).

mosome originating from the mother or that from the father. Clones of cells derived subsequently from each of these cells of the embryo perpetuate the type of X inactivation in the parent cell. The hypothesis explains why males and females have equivalent levels of most enzymes determined by genes on the X chromosome although there are some exceptions to this; steroid, or placental, sulphatase, for example. It appears that a few gene loci escape inactivation.

Most females who are heterozygous for a variant allele of a gene which determines synthesis of an enzyme on part of the X chromosome which is inactivated, will be expected to have, on average, enzyme activity which is midway between normal and that of the affected male; but throughout the body there will be two distinct populations of cells, those which express only the normal allele and those which express the variant allele. There will be a mosaic of cells possessing normal and low enzyme activity respectively. However, some heterozygous females may have a preponderance of cells in which the normal allele is inactivated and will have generally low enzyme activity. What is more likely is that particular organs, the liver for example, have unequal proportions of cells having the normal or variant allele inactivated. Thus a disease like OTC deficiency, involving an enzyme which is of particular significance in the liver, will be expressed in heterozygous females whose liver contains a high proportion of cells with the normal allele inactivated and generally low enzyme activity.

METABOLIC AND PATHOLOGICAL CONSEQUENCES OF A PROTEIN DEFECT

About one quarter of the known inherited metabolic disorders involve 'non-catalytic' proteins. The functions of these proteins is extremely varied and, therefore, it is difficult to rationalise the types of secondary metabolic consequences which they cause. Specific examples of non-catalytic protein defects will be found in the appropriate chapters: for example, on apolipoproteins in Chapter 10 and on amino acid transport defects in Chapter 4. It is possible, however, to approach the metabolic and pathological consequences of the 'catalytic' protein, or enzyme, defects more systematically.

Garrod[1] pointed out the salient features of an enzyme block in a metabolic pathway; notably, a deficiency of metabolites distal to, and an accumulation of metabolites proximal to, the defective enzyme. It is now appreciated that, in addition, an accumulation of metabolites in the pathway is frequently associated with the production of significant amounts of unusual metabolites. This sequence of changes is shown in Figure 1.5.

The end product

Numerous disorders can be cited in which the shortage of the end product

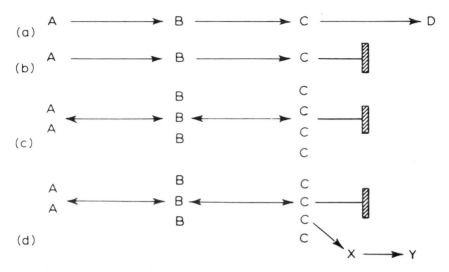

Fig. 1.5 The consequences of a metabolic block shown in a hypothetical pathway synthesising D from A through intermediates B and C(a). The block between C and D may lead to a failure to form the end product (b), with a possible accumulation of precursors prior to the block (c) and the formation of unusual metabolites (d).

of a metabolic pathway leads directly to some, or all, of its clinical symptoms. For example, the failure to synthesise melanins is responsible for lack of pigmentation in albinism[6] in Glycogen Storage Disease type 1, hypoglycaemia is an end result of an inability to release glucose from glucose-6-phosphate (p. 22) and in the inherited thyroid disorders, cretinism is a direct consequence of enzyme blocks in the synthetic pathway for thyroxin[6]. A rather interesting example is afforded by I-cell disease (p. 90), in which the enzyme defect leads to many lysosomal enzymes lacking their identity marker which normally targets them to their particular sub-cellular organelle. This produces a distribution abnormality with a deficiency of numerous hydrolases in the lysosomes and a complicated storage disease.

It is pertinent to mention here that some variant enzymes have increased catalytic activity and this may, in very rare circumstances, result in an over-production of the end product of a pathway. A variant of phosphoribosyl-pyrophosphate synthetase is super-active: individuals with the defect produce the end product of purine metabolism—uric acid—in excess and this causes them to have gout (p. 232).

End product deficiency is not an invariable result of a low activity enzyme variant. For example, in the case of a structurally altered, high Km, variant accumulation of precursor may then increase the reaction rate and restore the end product level to normal. The result is simply a different equilibrium between precursor and product. This situation is sometimes referred to as a *leaky mutation*. Alternatively, the end product may be synthesised by a different metabolic pathway which can make up the deficit from the usual route.

Occasionally an end product may be synthesised in amounts which are adequate to fulfil normal requirements, but not to respond to extreme demands. In glucose-6-phosphate dehydrogenase deficiency (p. 432), one end product of glucose-6-phosphate metabolism, reduced glutathione, is adequate for its function of maintaining the integrity of the red cell membrane, even though the level of erythrocyte enzyme is some 15% of normal. When certain oxidising drugs, like quinine or sulphonamides, also make demands on the limited capacity to generate reduced glutathione, haemolysis occurs.

Precursor accumulation

Precursor accumulation is often the most notable secondary feature of an enzyme defect and is the commonest factor in the discovery and diagnosis of inherited metabolic diseases. It must be recognised that, in the absence of the necessary nutritional or metabolic source of the precursor, accumulation may not occur. Accumulation may not be seen either in the fetus, because the precursor may pass to the maternal circulation. A build-up may then proceed slowly after birth. These factors may lead to missed prenatal and early postnatal diagnoses.

Precursor accumulation is supposed to be the cause of the pathology of many disorders and sometimes this is obviously the case, as in the porphyrias where deposition of porphyrins in the skin results in the sensitivity to sunlight (Ch. 7). However, there is surprisingly little evidence to support other commonly held hypotheses—for example, that phenylalanine is the cause of mental retardation in phenylketonuria (p. 100), that accumulated macro-molecules are responsible for cellular damage in the storage diseases (Ch. 3) or that the hexose phosphates have a directly toxic effect in galactosaemia and hereditary fructose intolerance (Ch. 2). In all these cases it would appear that excess precursor levels coincide with the active pathological process, but it is not necessarily true that the precursor is a direct cause of the pathology.

Unusual metabolites

The formation of abnormal amounts of unusual metabolites may be a useful diagnostic feature of a disease but may not be found in every patient. This was a problem when screening for phenylketonuria was instituted by testing for increased phenylpyruvic acid. It was found that some infants gave false negative results because they had a transient deficiency of the liver transaminase which converts excess phenylalanine to phenylpyruvic acid. This situation is common in the first weeks, or months, of life.

It is probable that the unusual metabolite is a link in the pathogenesis of some disorders. In primary oxaluria type 1 (p. 208), for example, the

excess urinary oxalate is a by-product of the normal metabolism of glyoxylate. In most cases, however, the involvement of unusual metabolites in
pathological processes is pure conjecture.

Pathways involving negative feedback control

The normal metabolic patterns of an enzyme deficiency may be magnified
if the end product exerts negative feedback control on a preceding enzyme
in the pathway. In this case accumulation of precursors may be greater.
This is depicted in Fig. 1.6.

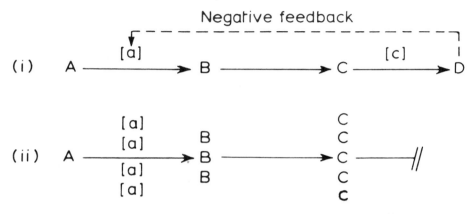

Fig. 1.6 Exaggeration of the consequences of an enzyme defect by an effect on a
controlling step in a metabolic pathway. In (i) the metabolic pathway is controlled by the
end product D exerting negative feedback and inhibiting the rate limiting enzyme [a].
When the end product is no longer formed due to a defect in enzyme [c], negative
feedback inhibition on [a] no longer occurs and its increased activity causes B and C to
accumulate in very large, uncontrolled, amounts; see (ii).

Acute intermittent porphyria (AIP, p. 267) is an interesting example of
this phenomenon. It is inherited as an autosomal dominant, affected
heterozygotes having about 50% normal activity of porphobilinogen (PBG)
deaminase which is on the haem synthetic pathway. An earlier enzyme in
this pathway, δ-aminolaevulinic acid (ALA) synthetase is rate limiting and
is controlled by negative feedback which is related to the size of the free
haem pool. In AIP adequate haem synthesis is usually maintained but
certain circumstances, for example administration of barbiturates or oestrogens, make demands on the free haem pool for synthesis of cytochrome
P450 which is used to metabolise the drugs. Haem depletion leads to
marked stimulation of ALA synthetase and the increased flux of metabolites
through the pathway is more than the reduced PBG deaminase can accom-
modate and, ALA and PBG, in particular, now accumulate. This excess of
ALA and PBG is linked with the appearance of the acute symptoms of the
disease.

HETEROGENEITY OF THE INHERITED METABOLIC DISEASES

One of the principal factors which has made the inherited metabolic diseases much more clinically relevant, and interesting, in recent years— apart from the increasing number that are being discovered—is the realisation of the wide variety of ways in which a disorder can present. From a situation in which it was supposed that all patients with a particular disorder had a rather uniform and characteristic disease spectrum, presenting within a fairly narrow time window, it now appears that the signs and symptoms can vary greatly—both in overall severity and in their relative significance—from one patient to another. It should be appreciated, also, that the presentation of the same acute disease may occur from the neonatal period to somewhere in the second decade of life, possibly being almost as devastating and life-threatening whenever it first appears. Thus our concept of which patients could have an inherited metabolic disease has expanded.

There are many reasons for the clinical heterogeneity:

Heterogeneity in the enzyme defect

What is superficially, from the pattern of secondary metabolic abnormality, the same disorder, may arise from very many different genetic mutations. These may be broadly classified as being caused by multiple alleles or multiple loci.

Multiple allelism was alluded to earlier when it was stated that numerous point mutations may exist for each kind of polypeptide. Each variant polypeptide should have slightly different functional or physical activities. It has been shown that minute changes in the residual activity of an enzyme, perhaps too small to detect analytically in some cases, can alter the degree of metabolic abnormality; thus perhaps altering overall severity. Moreover each variant may have different relative functional activities in the environment which different kinds of cells provide. This could explain the variation in emphasis of the signs and symptoms of a disease for different families.

Multiple locus, or non-allelic, variants may arise in a number of ways. A protein may be composed of two, or more, subunits, determined by separate gene loci, possibly located on different chromosomes. Mutations at any of these loci may lead to synthesis of an abnormal protein. In addition, the same secondary metabolic error can be caused by quite different protein variants. For example, methylmalonic aciduria (p. 176) is caused by defects in the activity of the methylmalonyl CoA mutase. A number of allelic variants in the mutase apo-enzyme are known which can be differentiated by their activity and their cross reactions with an antibody to normal apo-enzyme. However, seven mutants are known in which the defect is in the availability of the co-enzyme adenosylcobalamin. Three of these are due to a transport defect, affecting the absorption of Vitamin B_{12}, hydroxycobalamin, from the intestine. The other four are due to abnormalities in the synthesis of active co-enzyme from the vitamin precursor[7].

Variations of expression in different cells

All nucleated cells, that is every type of cell apart from the erythrocyte, contain the genetic information to code for every protein synthesised in the body; but, of course, not all genes are expressed in every kind of cell, or tissue. It would appear likely, however, that all cells that were capable of expressing a particular gene would be equally affected by a mutation coding for a variant protein. In fact this is not the case, and there are basically three reasons why this is not so:

1. What may appear to be identical proteins with the same function may be determined by different genes in different types of cells. The enzyme phosphorylase is genetically distinct in liver and muscle. Hence two quite distinct diseases are known, one affecting the phosphorylase of liver, the other muscle (p. 24 and 32).

2. Many proteins are composed of more than one polypeptide subunit which may be of different structure and determined by separate gene loci. It is also possible that the functionally similar proteins from different kinds of cells have varying proportions of the different subunits in their structure. When there is a variant of one of these subunits produced the effect may differ between different cell types.

An example of this is phosphofructokinase (PFK) which usually exists as a tetramer composed of three kinds of subunit: namely M, muscle type; L, liver type; and F, found in fibroblasts, brain, platelets, lymphocytes and kidney.

Muscle synthesises only M subunits and its PFK has the structure M_4. Erythrocytes synthesise approximately equal amounts of M and L subunits and contains the five PFK isoenzymes which you would expect from the random association of M and L—M_4, M_3L, M_2L_2, ML_3 and L_4. These isoenzymes can be separated by chromatographic techniques.

Two PFK deficiency diseases exist. The most common affects both muscle and red cells which can have enzyme levels of zero and 50% of normal respectively (p. 33). In this form there is a genetic defect in the M subunit. Only the L_4 isoenzyme is found in the erythrocytes in this condition. The rare form affects only erythrocytes which, again, have about half normal activity (p. 424). In this type there is, presumably, a defect in L subunit synthesis.

3. The possibility that structural variants may have differing effects in various cell types was suggested earlier. It is well established that a structural modification which principally alters protein stability affects the erythrocyte in particular. This is because the erythrocyte has a very long life span of 120 days and the mature cell cannot synthesise new protein to compensate for the abnormality. If the protein involved is very important in eryth-

rocyte metabolism and function the disorder will be clinically significant. For example, the unstable variants of glucose-6-phosphate dehydrogenase (p. 432) cause haemolytic anaemia under certain circumstances. On the other hand, an unstable form of uridine diphosphate galactose-4-epimerase which causes low erythrocyte levels of the enzyme, is of no particular consequence. The liver, the main site of galactose metabolism, has relatively normal amounts of epimerase activity (p. 38).

Other factors determining the severity and timing of clinical presentation in the inherited metabolic disorder

Most of the considerations of the preceding sections have been about factors which are genetically determined and should remain relatively constant with time. There are other factors which can affect the overall severity and the timing of presentation which vary both between and within individuals. One of these is the hormonal state of a person. It is well recognised that the signs and symptoms of some diseases regress whilst others become more severe at puberty: still more diseases present for the first time at this period of life. Unfortunately the reasons for such observations are often unclear. The effects of two more factors, namely diet and infection, are more obvious.

The secondary biochemical changes and pathological consequences of many inherited metabolic disorders arise through the metabolism of normal dietary components. Defects occur in the metabolic pathways of amino acids, fats and the carbohydrates, galactose and fructose. The metabolic abnormality in these disorders will vary depending on the amount of protein, fats, or offending carbohydrate in the diet and this may be reflected in the clinical severity of the disease. In some cases, disorders which may present in an acute and life threatening form in the neonatal period are not manifest for many years because of unusual dietary habits.

Many patients with an inherited metabolic disease present for the first time, or have recurring attacks, when they have an infection. This may stress a patient's metabolism in many ways—in particular, it is known to have a tremendous catabolic effect. A big increase in protein catabolism may precipitate a crisis in the disorders of amino acid metabolism or of the urea cycle.

REFERENCES

1 Garrod A E 1923 Inborn errors of metabolism. Oxford University Press, London
2 Higgs D R, Weatherall D J 1983 Alpha-thalassaemia. Current Topics in Haematology 4: 37–97
3 Orkin S H, Antonarakis S E, Kazazian H H 1983 Polymorphism and molecular pathology of the human beta-globin gene. Progress in Haematology 13: 49–73
4 Emery A E H 1984 Introduction to recombinant DNA. John Wiley and Sons, Chichester, p 35–57

5 McKusick V 1983 Mendelian inheritance in man, 6th edn. Johns Hopkins University Press, Baltimore
6 Holton J B 1985 An introduction to inherited metabolic diseases. Chapman and Hall, London, New York
7 Rosenberg L E 1982 Vitamin responsive inherited metabolic disorders: propionic acidaemia and methylmalonic acidaemia. In: Cockburn F, Gitzelmann R (eds) Inborn errors of metabolism in humans. MTP Press, Lancaster p 37–52

Disorders of carbohydrate metabolism

INTRODUCTION

The major dietary carbohydrates, starch, sucrose, and lactose are hydrolytically degraded in the gut. The free monosaccharides glucose, fructose and galactose are absorbed and reach the liver via the portal circulation, where they are rapidly utilised. Glucose is phosphorylated within the hepatocyte to glucose-6-phosphate by glucokinase. The hexose sugars, fructose and galactose are also taken up by the hepatocyte and enter the pathways of carbohydrate metabolism as triose sugars and glucose-1-phosphate respectively (Fig. 2.1).

Carbohydrate metabolism in the liver is primarily concerned with the maintenance of plasma glucose homeostasis. Glucose may be generated by the breakdown of stored glycogen, the uptake and metabolism of dietary carbohydrate, and gluconeogenesis whereby amino acids, glycerol and lactate are metabolised via a reversal of the Embden-Meyerhof sequence.

Glucose-6-phosphate occupies a central position in carbohydrate metabolism, for there are five direct pathways for its metabolism:
1. synthesis of glycogen
2. glycolysis to yield either lactic acid or through acetyl CoA and the Krebs cycle to yield CO_2
3. release as free glucose
4. via the pentose cycle with production of NADPH and CO_2
5. glucuronate formation.

Curiously the first defect of carbohydrate metabolism to be identified, pentosuria, which is the result of an enzyme defect affecting the last of these pathways, glucuronate formation, proved to be the least clinically important. Essential pentosuria (McKusick 26080) first described by Salkowski and Jashrowitz in 1892,[1] is the result of a defect in the glucuronic acid oxidation pathway. It has an incidence of 1:40 000, and occurs primarily in those of Jewish race, being inherited as an autosomal recessive. Apart from the diagnostic confusion with diabetes mellitus it has no clinical significance.

Since that early description, inborn errors involving all of the major path-

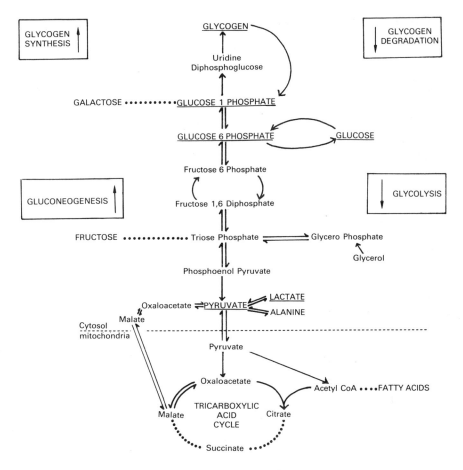

Fig. 2.1 The major pathways of carbohydrate metabolism.

ways of carbohydrate metabolism have been discovered and these will be surveyed in the following chapter.

DISORDERS OF GLYCOGEN METABOLISM

The first description of a child with an apparent defect of glycogen mobilisation appeared in 1928 and the hepatic form of glycogen storage disease (GSD) was identified by Von Gierke the following year. Four years later Pompe described a patient where the glycogen accumulation was principally in the heart, and in 1951 McArdle reported a condition presenting in adult life with excess glycogen deposition in skeletal muscle. Hepatic glucose-6-phosphatase deficiency (Von Gierke's disease) was the first enzyme defect to be identified and there followed identification of many other defects of glycogen metabolism.

Normal glycogen metabolism

Glycogen is a high molecular weight polysaccharide which occurs in many cells but is principally found in the liver and muscle. It has a multitiered structure being composed of glucose residues linked by (1–4) bonds to form long chains, which are branched every 12–18 residues by the inclusion of a (1–6) linkage (Fig. 2.2). The precursor for glycogen synthesis is glucose-1-phosphate which is in equilibrium with glucose-6-phosphate (Fig. 2.1). Glucose-1-phosphate is converted to uridine diphosphoglucose (UDPglc) by a specific pyrophosphorylase. In a second reaction catalysed by glycogen synthetase (EC 2.4.1.21) the glucose residue from UDPglc is attached to a glycogen primer through a (1–4) bond, lengthening the glucose chain. The branch points of the glycogen molecule are incorporated by the action of the enzyme amylo (1–4), (1–6) transglucosidase (1,4-α-glucan branching enzyme, EC 2.4.1.18).

Glycogen degradation is mediated through two enzyme systems: phosphorylase and the debrancher (amylo-(1-6)-glucosidase). The enzyme phosphorylase (EC 2.4.1.1) exists in two forms, one active and the other inactive. The activation of phosphorylase is complex and involves several steps. It is initiated by glucagon and adrenaline which cause the release of a second messenger, cyclic (3′5′)-adenosine monophosphate, from the cell membrane. This in turn activates a series of enzymes including a specific phosphorylase kinase (EC 2.7.1.38) which result in the conversion of phosphorylase from its inactive to its active form (Fig. 2.3). Once activated phosphorylase cleaves the (1–4) bonds of glycogen releasing glucose-1-phosphate but it does not hydrolyse the (1–6) bonds and stops along the straight chains four glucose residues from the branch points. The debrancher enzyme (EC 3.2.1.33, transferase 2.4.1.25) is necessary for glycogen breakdown to proceed. Three glucose residues are transferred from the side chain

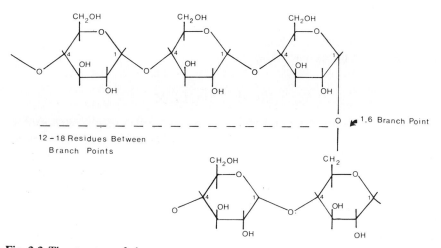

Fig. 2.2 The structure of glycogen.

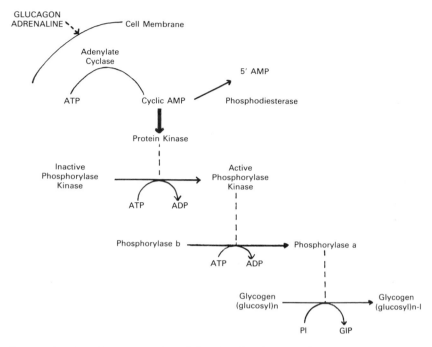

Fig. 2.3 A schematic representation of the phosphorylase cascade.

to the main chain by the transferase that forms part of the debrancher enzyme, leaving one glucose residue which is linked by a (1–6) bond. This is then hydrolysed by the debrancher, amylo-(1–6)-glucosidase. Sequential degradation of glycogen results in the production of about 8–12% free glucose and 90% glucose-1-phosphate. The glucose-1-phosphate formed on glycogen degradation is converted to glucose-6-phosphate via the action of phosphoglucomutase (EC 5.4.2.2). Further glucose is released through the hydrolysis of glucose-6-phosphate. This reaction is catalysed by the enzyme glucose-6-phosphatase (EC 3.1.3.9) which is found only in the liver, kidney and intestinal mucosa. Hepatic glycogen functions as a reserve of glucose which can be rapidly utilised during fasting to maintain normoglycaemia.

In contrast muscle glycogen functions solely as a fuel reserve for ATP generation during muscle contraction and does not contribute to maintaining plasma glucose homeostasis. Glycogen synthesis and degradation in muscle involve the same enzymes as those found in liver. The activation of phosphorylase is controlled by changes in the concentrations of ATP and AMP and by adrenaline. Generally muscle glycogen is oxidised when supplies of glucose and fatty acids are low, to provide additional energy, but under conditions where oxygen is lacking glycogen can be degraded to lactate by glycolysis. Phosphofructokinase (EC 2.7.1.11), the enzyme which catalyses the conversion of fructose-6-phosphate to fructose 1:6-diphosphate, is important in the regulation of glycolysis in muscle.

Classification of the glycogen storage disorders

Unfortunately a single classification of the glycogen storage diseases is not accepted by all. The classification shown in Table 2.1 is based on specific enzyme defects but it also takes into account the tissues that are affected. Type VIII has been excluded because as yet no enzyme deficiency has been demonstrated in these children who have cerebral deposition of glycogen.[2] Discussion of Type II (Pompe's disease) where the defect is one of lysosomal glucosidase is probably more appropriately reserved for the chapter on lysosomal disorders (Ch. 3).

Although several of these conditions affect both hepatic and muscle glycogen, it is convenient to distinguish those disorders where the liver is principally affected from those where the primary defect is in muscle glycogen metabolism.

Table 2.1 Classification of the glycogen storage diseases

Type	Alternative name	Principal tissues involved	Enzyme	Tissues or cells for diagnosis
O		Liver	Glycogen synthetase	Liver
I	Von Gierke	Liver, intestine, kidney	Glucose-6-phosphatase	Liver, intestinal mucosa
Ib	Pseudo Type I	Liver, kidney intestine	Defective glucose-6-phosphate transport	Liver
II	Pompe	Heart, liver, skeletal muscle	Lysosomal glucosidase	WBC, fibroblasts
III	Cori	Liver, muscle	Amylo-(1–6)-glucosidase (debrancher)	WBC, liver
IV	Amylopectinosis	Liver	Branching enzyme	Liver
V	McArdle	Muscle	Phosphorylase	Muscle
VI	Hers	Liver, muscle	Phosphorylase	Liver, WBC
VII		Muscle	Phosphofructokinase	Muscle, RBC
IX		Liver, Muscle	Phosphorylase kinase	Liver, red cells

The hepatic glycogen storage disorders

The overall frequency of the hepatic glycogen storage diseases is approximately 1:60 000 live births. Type I with an incidence of 1:200 000 was thought to be the most common form, but the defects of phosphorylase kinase (Type IX) which are often asymptomatic may be more frequent than was previously suspected.

Glucose-6-phosphatase (Type I)

Glucose-6-phosphatase deficiency, or Von Gierke's disease (McKusick 23220), classically presents in early infancy with hepatomegaly, fasting hypoglycaemia and recurrent acidosis. However there is enormous variation in the severity of the clinical presentation. In its most severe form it may present within the first few days of life with profound hypoglycaemia and acidosis. On the other hand it may present in later childhood with short stature and hepatomegaly. Abnormal bleeding, usually epistaxis may occur and gastro-intestinal symptoms such as intermittent diarrhoea, vomiting and failure to thrive are surprisingly common.

The infants are short, with decreased muscle mass, and a protuberant abdomen due to massive hepatomegaly. Adipose tissue around the face may be increased: the so called 'doll like' facies. There is no splenomegaly and there are no signs of cirrhosis. Renal enlargement may be noted on ultrasound examination. Xanthomata and lipaemia retinalis may be present.

Untreated, children with Type I may die during infancy or later from intercurrent infections complicated by hypoglycaemia or acidosis. However there is considerable variation. Survival beyond adolescence is said to be associated with adaption to the disease and amelioration of the symptoms. Severe growth delay usually occurs and sexual maturation is delayed. Successful pregnancies in patients with Type I have been reported. Gout and uric acid nephropathy may develop and there have been an increasing number of reports of hepatic adenomata formation. Furthermore there have been reports of hepatocellular carcinoma developing in patients thought to have benign adenomata.

Glucose-6-phosphatase deficiency can be confirmed in the liver, kidney and intestinal mucosa. Deficiency of the enzyme is inherited as an autosomal recessive, and heterozygotes have significantly decreased intestinal enzyme activity.[3]

In the past children have been described who are clinically and biochemically indistinguishable from Type I but have normal glucose-6-phosphatase activity in the liver.[4] These children were classified as Type IB (McKusick 23222). Recent work has shown that in Type IB glucose-6-phosphatase activity may be normal in liver biopsy material which has been frozen, athough it is reduced in fresh tissue. It appears that the hitherto normal activity detected was the result of freezing which disrupts the membrane structure within the hepatocyte. Glucose-6-phosphatase activity is located on the luminal surface of the microsomes and there is a specific mechanism which shuttles glucose-6-phosphate from the cytoplasm. It seems likely that this transport mechanism is defective in Type IB.

In most respects patients with Type IB are indistinguishable from those with Type I although they do tend to present with a severe form of the disease. Abnormalities of neutrophil mobility and neutropenia, leading to recurrent bacterial infections, have been described in Type IB but not in Type I. Vitamin D resistant rickets and a Fanconi syndrome have also been reported, again, only in Type IB.

Amylo-(1-6)-glucosidase, the debranching enzyme (Type III)

The majority of children with deficiency of amylo-(1–6)-glucosidase

(McKusick 23240), the debranching enzyme, present within the first year of life with fasting hypoglycaemic convulsions and hepatomegaly, although a few will be diagnosed in later childhood when they are investigated for short stature, the protuberant abdomen and hepatomegaly are noted. As in Type I, vomiting and diarrhoea are common symptoms at presentation.

The outcome of Type III is generally milder and survival into adulthood is common. With adolescence the hepatomegaly becomes less pronounced and catch-up growth occurs, although sexual maturation is delayed. The associated myopathy is generally mild, but occasionally it may be severe and there may be cardiac involvement. Rarely, cirrhosis requiring portal diversion or milder degrees of hepatic fibrosis may develop.

Deficiency of amylo-(1–6)-glucosidase can be detected in the liver and white blood cells. The glycogen content of red cells is markedly increased.[5] Type III is inherited as an autosomal recessive.

Hepatic phosphorylase and phosphorylase kinase (Type VI and IX)

Low activity of phosphorylase in the liver was first reported in 1959 but the deficiency was not complete and it was not possible to decide whether the primary defect was of the phosphorylase or the kinase. Improved methodology has enabled recognition of several enzyme defects of the phosphorylase complex.[6]

Clinically, these patients have a very mild disease. Hypoglycaemia is rare and hepatomegaly develops slowly and may only be noted as an incidental finding. Muscular hypotonia may be present. Although growth delay may be evident at diagnosis, catch-up occurs during childhood. There has been one report of two children with Type IX who developed nodular cirrhosis with portal hypertension in later childhood.[6]

Type IX is by far the commonest defect of the phosphorylase cascade and it is inherited as an X-linked recessive (Type IXB, McKusick 30600), or more rarely as an autosomal recessive (Type IXA, McKusick 26175). The enzyme, a specific phosphorylase kinase, can be detected in the liver and red blood cells.

Type VI, a defect of the hepatic phosphorylase (McKusick 23270), can be diagnosed in liver and white blood cells, and has been reported in two brothers and one girl. It is probably inherited as an autosomal recessive. Partial phosphorylase deficiency in red cells has been reported with normal activity of phosphorylase in the liver and there remains a number of patients with reduced activity of enzymes of the phosphorylase complex who are difficult to classify.[6]

Glycogen synthetase deficiency (Type O)

Children with glycogen synthetase deficiency (McKusick 24060) present during the first year with hypoglycaemic convulsions after fasting. Ketosis is evident but the patients do not have hepatomegaly or any of the other features characteristic of the hepatic glycogen storage disorders. True deficiency of this enzyme is probably rare. The difficulty is in distinguishing these cases from others presenting with ketotic hypoglycaemia. The diagnosis has to be made on liver biopsy material. Insulin is a regulator of glycogen synthetase activity and when insulin levels are low the enzyme activity may also be reduced making interpretation of the results difficult. Type O has been reported in twins and an unrelated girl, and is probably inherited as an autosomal recessive.

Amylo-(1–4),(1–6)-transglucosidase, the branching enzyme (Type IV)

Type IV is probably the rarest form of hepatic glycogen storage disease (McKusick 23250). Infants with the condition are normal at birth, but develop failure to thrive, hepatomegaly and splenomegaly within a few months. Hypotonia, muscular atrophy and absent reflexes may be noted. Cirrhosis and portal hypertension follow, and death usually occurs within two years. Heart dilatation with polysaccharide accumulation has been reported and death can occur from tamponade and cardiac failure. The diagnosis can be made by examination of leucocytes which contain an abnormal polysaccharide, or at liver biopsy. The enzyme defect is inherited as an autosomal recessive.

Pathophysiology

The pathogenesis of the various types of GSD can be predicted in part from the site of the enzyme defects.

Glucose-6-phosphatase activity is essential for the normal release of hepatic glucose, irrespective of whether it is the product of glycogenolysis or gluconeogenesis. Further, the metabolism of the other hexose sugars, fructose and galactose will not result in the release of free glucose; thus in *Type I* fasting hypoglycaemia is a common finding. During fasting, the humoral response to hypoglycaemia (glucagon and adrenaline release) results in activation of phosphorylase and hepatic glycogenolysis. The resulting glucose-6-phosphate is metabolised via glycolysis to lactate. Gluconeogenic activity is also increased and there is recycling between lactate and glycogen; however, overall there is net production of lactate by the liver and an increase in blood lactate concentrations.[7]

The increase in glycerol, acetyl CoA and NADH generated by the increased flux of the glycolytic pathway contributes to an increased rate of triglyceride and cholesterol synthesis and serum cholesterol concentrations are elevated in *Type I*. Hypoglycaemia will also lead to an increase in the mobilisation of peripheral lipid stores with a rise in circulating free fatty acids. Clearance of chylomicra and VLDL is also impaired because of reduced activities of hepatic and extrahepatic lipoprotein lipase.

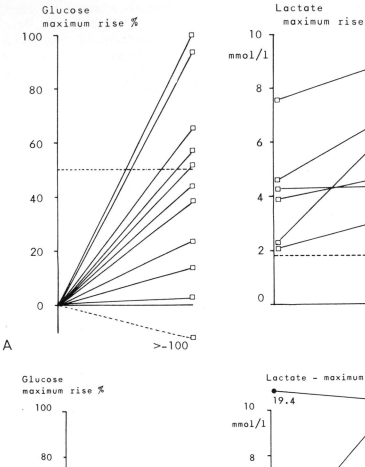

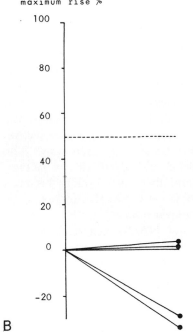

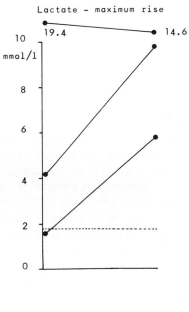

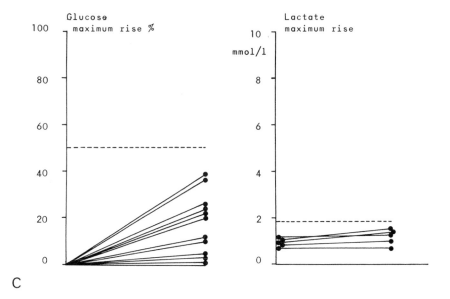

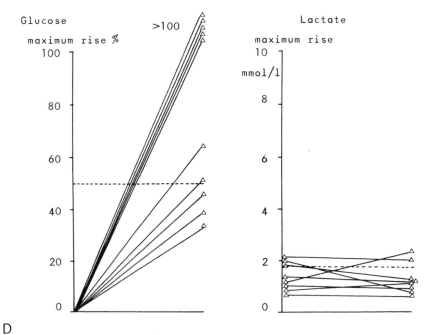

Fig. 2.4 Maximum change in blood glucose and lactate during fasting glucagon tests in patients with (A) Type I (B) Type Ib (C) Type III and (D) Type IX hepatic glycogen storage disease.

Plasma urate levels are elevated in *Type I*. This was originally attributed to competitive inhibition of urate excretion by lactate, however an increased rate of purine synthesis is probably a more important contributory factor. The mechanisms leading to increased purine synthesis are not clear, but raised levels of glutamine and depletion of hepatic nucleotides[8] may be important in this respect and similar metabolic abnormalities in other carbohydrate disorders will be described in later sections of this chapter.

The abnormal bleeding in *Type I* is thought to be due to a defect of platelet adhesiveness secondary to hypoglycaemia. The gastrointestinal symptoms are only partially understood. There does not appear to be any intolerance to mono- or disaccharides or to fat, but impaired glucose absorption has been demonstrated which might contribute to the pathogenesis of the diarrhoea. The vomiting and failure to thrive are probably related to recurrent acidosis.

The enzyme defects in the other two major forms of hepatic GSD (*Type III* and *defects of the phosphorylase cascade*) might be expected to impair glucose release from glycogen, but do not interfere with glucose release from gluconeogenesis. This is undoubtedly one explanation for the mild clinical presentation of these conditions. Fasting lactate concentrations are generally normal in *Type III* although they may be raised after a carbohydrate meal. Fasting lactate in *Type IX* may be normal or only very slightly raised. Ketonuria is a common finding in both conditions and fasting ketone concentrations in the plasma are elevated whereas they are normal in *Type I*. Concentrations of urate and cholesterol may be slightly elevated in *Type III*, but they are frequently normal in disorders of the phosphorylase complex.

The growth delay which occurs in the hepatic glycogen storage diseases is not completely understood. A number of endocrine abnormalities have been described including low levels of insulin and somatomedin, together with normal or elevated growth hormone, and raised cortisol concentrations. It has been suggested that growth delay may be part of an hormonal adaption to the failure to maintain normal glucose homeostasis,[9] although chronic acidosis and disordered calcium metabolism may also be important.

Diagnosis

A diagnosis of hepatic glycogen storage disease is usually suggested by the finding of hypoglycaemia and hepatomegaly. The standard fasting glucagon test (20 μg/kg i.m.) is useful in this situation although it is important to remember that there may be considerable variation in the response (Fig. 2.4). A normal test response is defined as a rise in blood glucose of more than 2 mmol/l or 50% over the fasting level. Some children with *Type I* will have a normal response to glucagon, but lactate levels are invariably elevated during the test.

The glucagon test should not be carried out in children with very low fasting glucose concentrations or severe lactic acidaemia, and alone it will not necessarily differentiate between the various types of hepatic glycogen storage disease.

The type of glycogen storage disease may be evident from clinical history alone, but there are a few additional biochemical pointers which may be of help. Whereas lactate concentrations may be slightly elevated in *Type IX* they are normal, except after a carbohydrate meal, in *Type III*, and significant lactic acidaemia either fasting or during the glucagon test always points to *Type I* or *IB*. The only other differential diagnoses are the disorders of gluconeogenesis. High plasma concentrations of urate and blood lipids usually indicate *Type I* but cholesterol concentrations may be

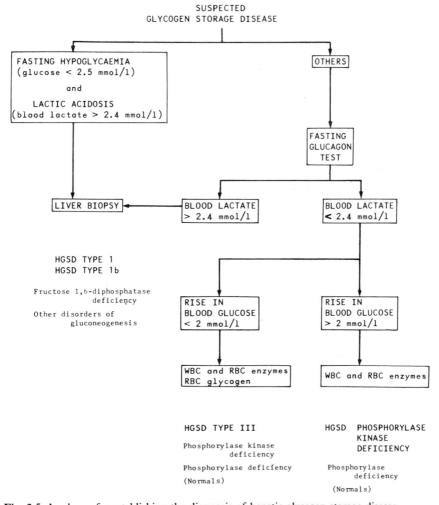

Fig. 2.5 A scheme for establishing the diagnosis of hepatic glycogen storage disease.

quite high in *Type III*. Transaminases may be elevated in *Type I* but the highest values are seen in *Type III*. Finally where it is possible to measure red cell glycogen concentrations these are highest in *Type III*.

Further differentiation of the various types of hepatic glycogen storage disease may be possible with a variety of loading tests. These include: the oral glucose tolerance combined with a post prandial glucagon test;[10] intravenous galactose[11] or fructose tolerance tests; and glycerol loading tests.[12] However, these tests may be technically difficult and distressing in young infants and do not always give clear results. Ultimately the diagnosis must be established by enzymology, and for *Type III, VI* and *IX*, this is possible by examination of peripheral blood cells. The approach outlined in Figure 2.5 offers a simple and reliable guide to the diagnosis of the common forms of hepatic glycogen storage disease.

The diagnosis of *Type IV* and *O* are based on liver biopsy. Their presentation is so unlike the other hepatic forms that differentiation is rarely a problem. The fasting glucagon test is usually abnormal in glycogen synthetase deficiency but may be normal if it is repeated after a meal. Glucose intolerance may be noted during a standard oral glucose tolerance test. There is little information regarding the investigation of *Type IV*. Transaminases may be elevated and the glucagon response is variable, but the diagnosis may only be reliably made at liver biopsy.

Treatment

Frequent carbohydrate feeds are often instituted in *Type I* in order to prevent hypoglycaemia but they do not correct the acidosis, hyperlipidaemia, hyperuricaemia and growth delay which also contribute to the morbidity. Diazoxide[13] may be of help in the young infant with intractable hypoglycaemia but none of the other drugs—which have been tried—glucagon, corticosteroids and anabolic steroids, have proved to be consistently useful. Portocaval anastamosis which acts by diverting glucose from the liver to the tissues may be of help,[14] however, not all patients show lasting benefit.[15] Continuous intravenous glucose, not only prevents hypoglycaemia but also leads to a dramatic improvement in many of the biochemical abnormalities (Fig. 2.6).

Clearly this form of treatment, although useful for stabilising patients during intercurrent infections or prior to surgery, is not suitable in the long term.

Frequent glucose drinks by day with nasogastric tube feeds of glucose at night have proved an effective alternative and this is the optimal treatment for *Type I* and *Type IB*.[16,17] The glucose is usually given in the form of the polymer Caloreen and in quantities which equal or even exceed the normal hepatic glucose production rate (0.25–0.5 g/kg/hr). Some degree of galactose and fructose exclusion is usually recommended as neither can be converted to free glucose and instead they will lead to increased lactate

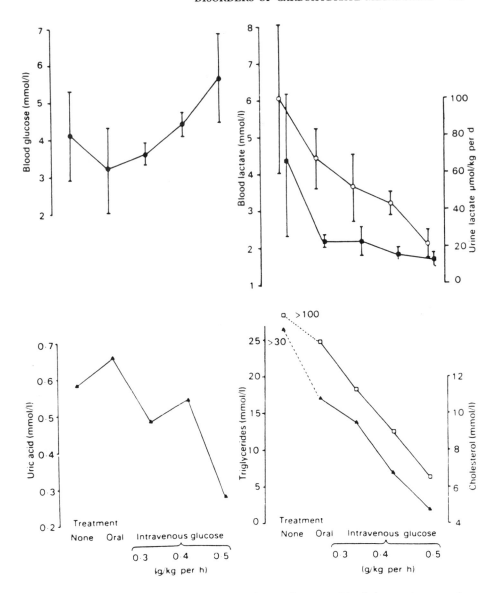

Fig. 2.6 The effects of oral and intravenous glucose therapy on blood glucose, lactate, uric acid, total cholesterol and triglycerides and on urinary lactate excretion in a patient with Type I glycogen storage disease. Each graph represents five consecutive weekly periods: week 1 no treatment, week 2 oral treatment with glucose drinks 2 hourly by day and 3 hourly by night (0.5 g/kg/hr), week 3, 4, 5 intravenous treatment with glucose 0.3, 0.4 and 0.5 g/kg/hr respectively. Top left: Blood glucose ●, levels represent the mean and SD of 6 values taken at 4 hourly intervals over a 24 hour period. Top right: Blood lactate ○, levels represent the mean and SD in samples taken as above. Urine lactate ■ values are mean and SD of seven 24 hour collections. Bottom left: Blood uric acid ▲, single values taken at end of each treatment period. Bottom right: Blood cholesterol ▲ and triglyceride □, single values taken at end of each treatment period.

production. The results from this form of treatment indicate that improvements in growth, a reduction in liver size and correction of the metabolic abnormalities can be expected and hepatic adenoma formation may be prevented.[18] Treatment is not without complication however. Untreated children with *Type I* may have remarkable tolerance of hypoglycaemia, which is thought to be due, in part, to their ability to utilise lactate as an alternative substrate to glucose in the brain. With treatment intolerance of hypoglycaemia returns, and if interruption of the night feeds occurs the consequent hypoglycaemia will be symptomatic and may be severe.[19]

Intensive treatment may not improve all of the biochemical abnormalities. Urate levels may remain elevated and treatment with allopurinol may have to be tried. High glucose infusion rates may actually increase blood lactate concentrations[20] and optimal rates are still to be determined.

Various food compositions for nocturnal feeds have been investigated[21] and dextrimaltose and starch have been recommended to delay absorption. Starch feeds alone may be a satisfactory alternative to nasogastric night feeds in some children with mild forms of *Type I*.[22] The starch is given as a suspension in water, 1–2 g/kg/dose every eight hours. Some children cannot tolerate it and it can cause diarrhoea and flatulence. Starch feeds have proved to be very useful in young adults, where growth is complete and intensive treatment is no longer needed.

Treatment of *Type III* is usually dietary. Fructose and galactose are not excluded from the diet and, further, in order to promote gluconeogenesis from amino acids the protein intake is increased to approximately twice the normal intake for age. A late night feed, high in protein, should be given and there is rarely any need for continuous night feeds.

Children with *disorders of the phosphorylase complex* rarely need treatment. In those who are symptomatic, or growth is seriously impaired, measures such as those used in Type III may be effective. Reports of the beneficial effects of D-thyroxin have not been confirmed.[23]

The muscle glycogen storage diseases

The muscles are affected in the previously described Types III, VI and IX GSD and the resulting myopathy may be quite severe in Type III. There are two conditions, Type V (McArdles) which is a defect of muscle phosphorylase and Type VII where the enzyme phosphofructokinase is deficient, which primarily affect skeletal muscle.

Muscle phosphorylase deficiency (Type V)

McArdles disease (McKusick 23260) usually presents in adult life and symptoms in childhood are rare. During the teenage years the only symptom is muscle fatigue particularly after strenuous exercise. With early adult life progressive weakness develops associated with cramping pains, and myoglobinuria may occur. No muscle wasting is noted until the 4th or 5th decade. Hepatomegaly is absent and the cardiovascular system is normal. Fasting hypoglycaemia does not occur. The diagnosis can be confirmed by muscle biopsy. The activity of phosphorylase is reduced and the glycogen content is either elevated or at the upper limit of normal. Muscle phosphorylase deficiency is inherited as an autosomal recessive.

Phosphofructokinase deficiency Type VII

The clinical presentation of this disease (McKusick 23280) is identical to that seen in McArdles disease although one child has been described who presented in infancy and died, aged 6 months, of respiratory failure.

Muscle phosphofructokinase is a different iso-enzyme to that found in the liver. Erythrocytes have approximately half of each form and in affected individuals levels are reduced by 50%. Absence of the muscle iso-enzyme may be confirmed in muscle biopsy specimens.

Pathophysiology

Resting muscle derives its energy mainly from the oxidation of glucose and fatty acids. The requirement for ATP may increase 100 fold during strenuous exercise and the demand exceeds the supply of substrates from the blood despite increases in blood flow. Glycogenolysis occurs under these circumstances, supplying substrate for oxidation or anaerobic metabolism to lactate.

Deficiency of the phosphorylase results in an inability to degrade glycogen, limiting the availability of this important source of substrate. The phenomenon of second wind is often described in *McArdles*, where continued exercise actually leads to a lessening of symptoms. It has been suggested that this results from changes in blood flow and increased availability of alternative substrates such as free fatty acids.

Diagnosis

Ischaemic exercise in patients with *Type V* and *VII* fails to produce a rise in blood lactate. During attacks myglobinuria may be noted and lactate dehydrogenase, aldolase and creatinine kinase levels may be elevated in the blood. The reduced tolerance of exercise can be demonstrated by getting the patient to squeeze a rubber ball while a blood pressure cuff is inflated to above systolic. This test can be very painful. Nuclear magnetic resonance may offer an alternative aid to diagnosis. Phosphorus nuclear magnetic resonance (^{31}P NMR) permits non-invasive measurements of intracellular pH, ATP and phosphocreatine. *McArdles* patients differ from normal in having no fall in intramuscular pH and an excessive reduction in phosphocreatine in response to exercise.[24]

Treatment

Avoidance of strenuous exercise is usually the only recommended treatment. Improving the availability of substrates with dietary glucose and fructose supplementation has been attempted and drugs which increase blood flow to the muscles have been tried but have not proved to be consistently effective.

DISORDERS OF GALACTOSE METABOLISM

Patients who had galactosuria, and presumably had a disorder of galactose metabolism, were recognised almost eighty years ago. Three separate enzyme defects have now been described, each associated with galactosaemia, galactosuria and some clinical abnormality.

Normal galactose metabolism

Galactose is a constituent of many functionally important macro-molecules. However, dietary galactose does not appear to be essential for the synthesis of these galactosides. It is believed that uridine diphosphate galactose (UDPgal), the galactosyl donor for their synthesis, can be made from glucose-1-phosphate (glc-1-P) by the pathway shown in Figure 2.7. The pathway may extend beyond UDPgal, to galactose-1-phosphate (gal-1-P) by a reversal of the pyrophosphorylase reaction, because the enzyme also catalyses the interconversion of the corresponding galactose compounds. This ability to generate gal-1-P from glc-1-P may complicate the treatment of some galactose disorders, as discussed later.

The succession of reactions in Figure 2.7 form what is known as the pyrophosphorylase pathway of galactose metabolism. The key enzymes, pyrophosphorylase and epimerase, are widespread and relatively active in

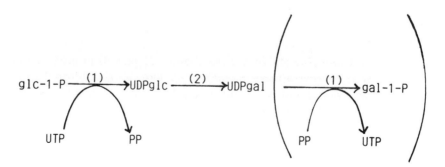

Fig. 2.7 The pyrophosphorylase pathway for the synthesis of UDPgal from glc-1-P. The possible generation of gal-1-P is important in classical galactosaemia. Enzymes: (1) pyrophosphorylase, (2) uridine diphosphate galactose-4-epimerase.

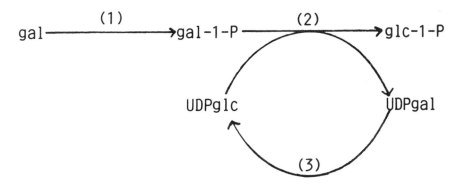

Fig. 2.8 The Leloir, or main, pathway of galactose metabolism to glc-1-P. Enzymes: (1) galactokinase, (2) galactose-1-phosphate uridyl transferase, (3) uridine diphosphate galactose-4-epimerase.

many body tissues. The pathway was thought originally to be most important in the reverse direction to that shown, being capable of metabolising galactose to glc-1-P after phosphorylation to gal-1-P. Its significance in this respect is not well established.

Galactose has to be diverted into the pathways of glucose metabolism in order to function as an energy source. This occurs by the Leloir pathway (Fig. 2.8) and predominantly in the liver, although the enzymes involved are present in other cells, including the erythrocytes. The pathway is particularly important in infancy when galactose usually constitutes about half the dietary carbohydrate.

In the Leloir, or main, pathway of galactose metabolism, the hexose is first phosphorylated to gal-1-P by a specific galactokinase. The gal-1-P then takes part in a transferase reaction involving UDPglc to generate glc-1-P and UDPgal. At this point there has been no net conversion of the galactose to a glucose moiety. This occurs through the action of the third enzyme, epimerase, which inverts the H and OH groups at position C_4 of the galactosyl group of UDPgal. Thus, UDPglc is regenerated and the net effect is the production of 1 molecule of glucose-1-phosphate for each molecule of galactose, with the expenditure of 1 molecule of ATP. It is possible that in some circumstances the transferase reaction is primed by UDPglc synthesised by pyrophosphorylase, particularly at the initial influx of a galactose load.

Two other minor routes of galactose metabolism may become important in situations in which galactose accumulates. First, it may be reduced by a non-specific aldose reductase to galactitol (Fig. 2.9). This reaction is implicated in the formation of cataracts associated with galactosaemia. Secondly, increased urinary excretion of galactonic acid, an oxidative product of galactose (Fig. 2.9), is also found in galactosaemia. This may not be of any particular significance.

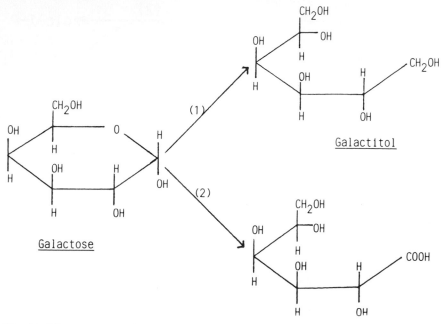

Fig. 2.9 Minor pathways of galactose metabolism by non-specific aldose reductase (1) to galactitol and by aldehyde dehydrogenase (2) to galactonic acid.

Enzyme defects

Galactose-1-phosphate uridyl transferase

Deficiency of transferase (EC 2.7.7.10), or classical galactosaemia (McKusick 23040), was the first recognised disorder of galactose metabolism and seems to be the most widely occurring. Affected infants appear normal at birth but, typically, become ill in the second week of life. The first symptoms, which include feeding difficulties, vomiting, lethargy, hypoglycaemia and diarrhoea, are by no means specific for the disease. The severe illness is frequently associated with sepsis, which is often interpreted as the primary cause of the problems, but it is probable that galactosaemia predisposes the infant to the infection. Death may ensue without the real diagnosis being recognised. If the more characteristic picture of classical galactosaemia develops, with jaundice, ascites, hepatomegaly, cataracts, glycosuria and amino aciduria, the diagnosis becomes more clear. Nevertheless, in one large series 40% of the patients were not diagnosed until they were more than 1 month of age, and many of them were more than 4 months old before successful diagnosis. Mental retardation of varying severity is a later recognised effect of the disorder.

Transferase deficiency is inherited as an autosomal recessive condition, affected individuals being homozygous for a so-called galactosaemia allele.

The activity of transferase in all tissues examined is zero, or only a few per cent of the level in normal subjects. Estimates of the incidence of the disease have varied widely, from 1:35 000 to 1:200 000, but this probably reflects the inaccuracy of using a small sample population in studying a rare disease. A mean incidence of 1:62 000, based on newborn screening of 6 million infants in parts of North America, Europe and Asia, probably represents a close approximation of the true incidence in these populations.

A number of other mutant alleles exist which code for variant transferases with characteristic activities varying from zero to 140% of that of the normal enzyme. The enzyme variants may be distinguished by their activity, electrophoretic mobility and stability. Individuals who are homozygous for some of the variant alleles, and some who are compound heterozygotes for a variant and the galactosaemia allele, have clinical symptoms of galactosaemia. The variants, and their characteristics, are summarised in Table 2.2. The most common variant enzyme is determined by the Duarte allele. It is estimated that 8–13% of the population are carriers for the allele, a frequency about 10 times higher than the galactosaemia allele.

Table 2.2 Variant alleles of the transferase gene and their effect

Variant allele	Homozygote transferase activity as percentage of normal mean*	Clinical symptoms	
		Homozygotes	Compound heterozygotes with galactosaemia allele
Galactosaemia	0 to few (also in liver, slightly higher in fibroblasts)	Yes	—
Negro	0 (up to 10 in liver)	Yes	Yes
Duarte	About 50	No	Possibly in neonates
Rennes	7 to 10	Yes	Yes
Indiana	0 to 40	?	Yes
Münster	About 30	Yes	Yes
Berne	About 40	?	?
Chicago	About 25 (also in fibroblasts)	?	Yes
Los Angeles	100 to 140	No	No

* Enzyme activities measured in erythrocytes except where stated

Galactokinase (EC 2.7.1.6)

The salient feature of complete galactokinase deficiency (McKusick 23020) is nuclear cataracts which usually develop in early infancy. It is probable that no other clinical features are directly related to the biochemical defect. Retarded development in some earlier cases is explained by the handicap of their total blindness.

The enzyme deficiency may be easily demonstrated in red cells or skin fibroblasts, but probably involves all galactose metabolising tissues. It is inherited as an autosomal recessive condition. The incidence in Switzerland has been calculated from the heterozygote frequency to be 1:40 000, but the cases detected in newborn screening programmes have been only a third to a quarter of the number expected from this figure. The reason for the discrepancy is not apparent. Very few cases have been recorded in other populations. Negro variant enzymes have been reported which have about 30% less activity in red cells than the usual form.

Uridine diphosphate galactose-4-epimerase (EC 5.1.3.2)

Defects of epimerase (McKusick 23035) were the most recent of the galactose disorders to be described and it has emerged that there are two quite distinct forms. In 1971 infants were discovered to have positive results in a galactosaemia screening method which was sensitive to increased concentrations of galactose and galactose-1-phosphate. The transferase activity was normal but they were shown to have a deficiency of red cell epimerase. Subsequent studies indicated that the overall ability to metabolise galactose was little affected and that the abnormality was consistent with normal health. The red cell abnormality did not cause any change in cell morphology or function.

Further investigation showed that the variant epimerase was relatively unstable and that it had a high Km for its cofactor, NAD^+. It was presumed that the long life span of the red cell, combined possibly with an unfavourable $NAD^+/NADH$ ratio, leads to the decline of its epimerase activity. Apart possibly from circulating lymphocytes, other cells, notably liver and skin fibroblasts, had relatively normal epimerase activity.

The second form of epimerase deficiency was discovered in 1981 when a newborn infant presented with a similar clinical picture to that of the transferase defect, that is jaundice, weight loss, vomiting, hypotonia, hepatomegaly, generalised amino aciduria and marked galactosuria. Transferase deficiency was excluded, but the infant was found to have no erythrocyte epimerase activity. Moreover, enzyme activity was absent from liver and skin fibroblasts, also. A few other cases of this complete deficiency variant are now thought to exist.

Evidence suggests that both types of epimerase defect are autosomal recessive in their inheritance. The incidence of the benign form in a newborn screening programme covering eastern Switzerland and Liechtenstein was 1:46 000. Cases have not been reported from other areas carrying out galactosaemia screening, but it is possible that moderate increases in red cell galactose and galactose-1-phosphate may be missed. The incidence of the severe, or complete, defect appears to be low, although these cases may also have been missed since most laboratories only exclude transferase deficiency in ill children with galactosuria and galactosaemia.

Pathophysiology of the enzyme defects

Biochemistry

The accumulation of precursor compounds and the excretion of abnormal metabolites in the three enzyme defects of galactose metabolism can be predicted from the position and extent of the block in the Leloir pathway.

In *galactokinase* deficiency it appears that there is an almost total inability to metabolise galactose. This suggests that the enzyme block is almost complete in all tissues which normally metabolise galactose. On a normal galactose intake, cases of galactokinase deficiency have a pronounced galactosaemia and galactosuria and an increased galactitol excretion. Galactitol will accumulate intracellularly within body fluid compartments, particularly within the eye lens where it is believed to play an important role in cataract formation. As mentioned earlier, the metabolism of galactose through the Leloir pathway may not be essential for the synthesis of UDPgal and the galactosides. In galactokinase deficiency it is likely that UDPgal synthesis could occur through the pyrophosphorylase pathway.

Transferase deficiency is also widespread throughout the body tissues leading to an inability to metabolise galactose. In patients with galactose in the diet there is an accumulation of galactose and galactose-1-phosphate and increased synthesis of galactitol. Galactose is distributed throughout intra and extracellular fluid and is readily excreted, whereas Gal-1-P accumulates intracellularly and its loss from the cell is slow. Newly diagnosed galactosaemic children put on a galactose free diet have high red cell gal-1-P levels persisting for 10–15 days. When older galactosaemic children who are on a well controlled restricted diet are given a small dose of galactose, higher red cell gal-1-P concentrations are found in the following 5–24 hours. The increased galactitol is distributed and excreted as in galactokinase deficiency.

The build up of abnormal metabolites in transferase deficiency has been shown to occur in the fetus as early as 21 weeks gestation (Table 2.3). The concentration of erythrocyte gal-1-P was equivalent to those in children diagnosed a few weeks after birth and the liver concentrations of galactose, galactose-1-phosphate and galactitol were 20–50% of the levels in infants dying of galactosaemia. High gal-1-P concentrations have also been found in cord blood of transferase deficient infants.

When transferase deficient subjects are given a galactose restricted diet red cell gal-1-P levels fall from very high pre-treatment levels but remain elevated above normal indefinitely. Also, the infants of mothers who have

Table 2.3 Concentration of galactose and its metabolites in liver and erythrocytes of a fetus with transferase deficiency

Subjects	Liver*			Erythrocytes**
	Galactose	Galactose-1-phosphate	Galactitol	Galactose-1-phosphate
Transferase deficient	277	115	247	990
Controls (2)	0	0	0	0

* Concentrations in μmol/kg wet tissue
** Concentrations in μmol/l packed erythrocytes

been on a galactose free diet during the pregnancy still have high cord blood gal-1-P concentrations. This has led to the belief that gal-1-P can be produced endogenously from sources other than galactose. The likelihood of this was even more conclusively demonstrated in a transferase deficient infant who was given only intravenous glucose for the first 24 hours of life. In spite of this the erythrocyte red cell level increased steadily between 5 and 24 hours of age. It has been concluded that the endogenous source of gal-1-P is from glc-1-P, via the pyrophosphorylase pathway, as previously described.

In the benign form of *epimerase* deficiency erythrocyte gal-1-P levels are increased but, as was mentioned earlier, the overall body capacity to metabolise galactose is probably little effected by the isolated red cell defect and galactosaemia and galactosuria is not a feature.

In the more complete form of epimerase deficiency galactose accumulates when milk is consumed and there is a marked galactosaemia and galactosuria similar to the other generalised forms of enzyme defect. These signs disappear on removal of galactose from the diet.

Although erythrocyte gal-1-P levels have been shown to be increased in a patient with complete epimerase defect, as in transferase deficiency, there was a difference since in the former condition gal-1-P could not be detected once galactose was removed from the diet. This supports the concept that the persisting erythrocyte gal-1-P in galactose restricted transferase deficient patients is synthesised endogenously from glc-1-P, via the pyrophosphorylase pathway, because epimerase is essential for the biogenesis of galactose by this means. A further consequence of the block in the pyrophosphorylase pathway in epimerase deficiency is an inability to synthesise UDPgal without a dietary source of galactose. Hence, galactoside synthesis and normal growth and development would seem to be at risk unless some galactose is contained in the diet.

Figure 2.10 shows that in the complete epimerase defect erythrocyte gal-1-P rises linearly with daily galactose intake over a limited range. It shows, also, that epimerase deficiency is unique in that UDPgal accumulates, rising rapidly and reaching a plateau concentration on a galactose intake of only 1g/24h. The possible explanation for these findings is that at the very low galactose intakes the gal-1-P formed can be metabolised to UDPgal by transferase, utilising newly synthesised UDPglc as cofactor. Hence mainly UDPgal accumulates at this point. As the flux of the galactose entering the Leloir pathway increases the supply of UDPglc becomes limiting, particularly as the UDPgal cannot be shuttled back to UDPglc by epimerase. At this stage the transferase reaction is impaired and gal-1-P accumulates.

Pathogenesis

The main organs involved in the diseases of galactose metabolism are the lens, liver, kidney and brain. It is generally considered that the cause of

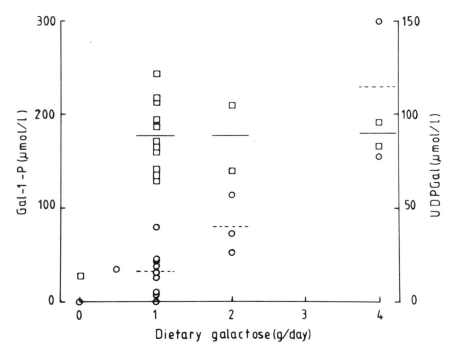

Fig. 2.10 Accumulation of galactose metabolites in a child with uridine diphosphate galactose-4-epimerase defect on varying galactose intakes.
o   Level of gal-1-P in packed red cells
- -   Mean level of gal-1-P for samples taken when galactose intake was identical
□   Level of UDPgal in packed red cells
—   Mean level of UDPgal for samples taken when galactose intake was identical

the cataracts which occur in all the clinically important enzyme deficiencies is an accumulation of galactitol. It is suggested that there is a characteristic degree of risk of cataract formation for homozygotes, heterozygotes and compound heterozygotes for the galactokinase and transferase variant alleles and this is related to the extent of impairment of galactose metabolism.[25] The lens may be particularly vulnerable since it contains a high concentration of aldose reductase.

The increased galactitol levels result in osmotic swelling of the lens and many other secondary biochemical changes have been found. Experimental evidence for this hypothesis is based on observations that cataract formation can be retarded by inhibition of aldose reductase, and hence galactitol synthesis, or by direct prevention of the osmotic swelling.

Although galactitol accumulates to varying degrees throughout numerous body tissues in all the galactose disorders, it is not thought to be part of the pathogenesis of the disease processes other than cataract formation. This is because liver, kidney and brain pathology is a feature only of transferase and epimerase deficiencies. Since gal-1-P is increased in these two disorders with similar widespread clinical features, its formation is thought to have an essential role in their pathogenesis.

Two hypotheses have been put forward to explain the role of the gal-1-P in the pathology of transferase and epimerase deficiency. The first is based on in vitro observations that gal-1-P inhibits a number of enzymes including phosphoglucomutase, glucose-6-phosphate dehydrogenase and phosphorylase. This could cause a reduction in glucose metabolism through the glycolytic and pentose phosphate pathways and a consequent reduction in energy supply. It could also explain the hypoglycaemia found occasionally in transferase deficiency. However, there is no evidence for significant inhibition of the enzymes in vivo. The second hypothesis is that the trapping of ATP in gal-1-P causes a general depletion of inorganic phosphate and uridyl compounds in the cells. Reduced liver ATP levels have been reported in transferase deficiency and lowered UTP concentrations in erythrocytes. The oral administration of galactose to patients causes an increase in serum urate suggesting an increased breakdown of adenine nucleotides. Experimental work on galactose toxicity suggests that there is causal relationship between reduced uridyl compounds and liver damage.[26] All specific effects, like hypoglycaemia, would be secondary to the generalised liver damage.

On the basis of the second hypothesis above it might be expected that a patient with the severe form of epimerase deficiency would be more sensitive to galactose than one with the transferase defect. This is because on a low galactose intake it is UDPgal which accumulates in epimerase deficiency and, for each molecule of UDPgal which is formed, one molecule of UDPglc is used. The overall reaction, from galactose to UDPgal, is very costly in its requirement for ATP.

Treatment

The treatment for all the clinically important galactose disorders is to exclude this carbohydrate from the diet. In the case of *galactokinase* and *transferase* deficiencies it is generally agreed that this restriction should be as complete as possible since, as previously discussed, it is assumed that it will not affect the availability of UDPgal for synthesis of the galactosides. The diet must exclude lactose, that is milk and all products made with milk. Uncertainty has existed about the need to exclude galactose in α-linked galactosides, for example in offal, soya and vegetables. The available evidence suggests that this galactose is not absorbed in man, although it has been proposed that, as a precaution, these foods should be excluded in early life.[27]

The galactose restricted diet prevents galactosuria and excess galactitol excretion but, in the case of transferase deficiency, erythrocyte gal-1-P levels remain above normal, which is zero, though very much reduced from pre-treatment levels. It has been suggested from empirical reasoning that gal-1-P should be kept below 150 μmol/l packed red cells for good diet control. Occasional patients exceed these levels in spite of careful attention to galactose restriction particularly in the first months or years of life. It is postulated that in these cases there is a more rapid generation of gal-1-P from glc-1-P.

In *epimerase* deficiency it would appear that some galactose should remain in the diet in order to allow UDPgal synthesis, but restriction is nevertheless essential to reduce the toxic symptoms. Gal-1-P and UDPgal levels can be monitored in erythrocytes,[28] but it is not clear what indicates good dietary control in this disorder.

The restriction of dietary galactose usually reverses, quickly and dramatically, the cataracts and early acute symptoms and signs of the galactose disorders providing it is started in the first few months of life. However, it is clearly established in transferase deficient galactosaemia that long-term mental development is impaired in at least half the early treated cases. Other neurological signs, particularly tremor and ataxia, have been described in a few cases.[29] The neurological problems may be ascribed to damage occurring in utero, to self toxicity with gal-1-P or to the effects of galactose restriction itself. Unfortunately it is impossible to say which of these factors is most significant. Although maternal restriction of lactose is often recommended to prevent prenatal damage in pregnancies known to be at risk of producing a galactosaemic fetus, it is not established that this is effective.

Primary ovarian failure has been found very recently in patients with transferase deficiency who have mostly been treated from early infancy.[30] Signs of the disorder have first appeared from a few months of age to the late teens. There is some suggestion that delays in starting treatment might be a factor in the cause of ovarian failure, but the main indications point to prenatal gonadal damage. It remains to be seen whether any of these children require hormone replacement therapy in order to undergo a normal puberty.

Biochemical diagnosis

The primary investigation in all galactose disorders is the urine total reducing substances and if this is abnormally increased the demonstration that galactose is responsible, by using chromatographic methods. A number of mistakes may be encountered with these simple methods. Firstly, babies presenting with the acute forms of galactose disorders may not be taking in and excreting galactose once milk feeding has precipitated the initial severe illness. If there is a suspicion that this might be the case it is important to use an enzyme test for diagnosis. Even infants with less severe symptoms, who appear to be feeding fairly normally, may not give a positive test for galactose in urine collected some hours following the last milk intake. Secondly, it is recognised that non-laboratory staff may use a

method which measures urine glucose specifically (Clinistix) instead of a
total reducing substance method (Clinitest). Obviously the former will give
a negative result even in the presence of definite galactosaemia. Thirdly,
the urine of normal neonates may contain small amounts of galactose,

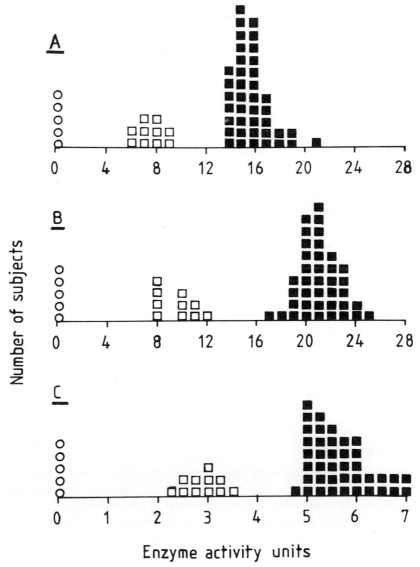

Fig. 2.11 Distribution of red cell activity of galactose-1-phosphate uridyl transferase
expressed as μmol substrate converted per hour per g protein in A, per g haemoglobin in B
and per ml packed red cells in C.
The genotypes are: ○   transferase deficient homozygotes
                   □   Normal/transferase deficient heterozygotes
                   ■   Normal homozygotes.

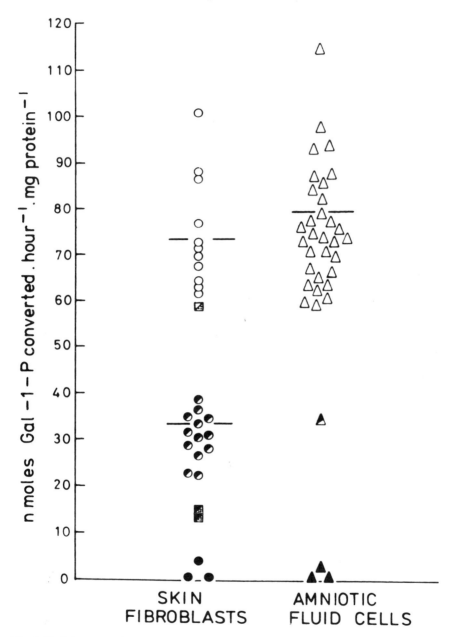

Fig. 2.12 Galactose-1-phosphate uridyl transferase activity in cultured skin fibroblasts and amniotic fluid cells.

○△   Normal homozygotes
◑▲   Normal/transferase deficient heterozygotes
●▲   Transferase deficient homozygotes
▨   Normal/Duarte heterozygotes
▦   Transferase deficient/Duarte heterozygotes.

usually associated with lactose. Inexperienced persons may report this as a positive result, but this is not a serious concern providing further tests are done to confirm the diagnosis.

A baby should not remain on a galactose free diet for a long period based only on the result of a screening test. A diagnosis should be confirmed by one of the enzyme tests which is available for all three defects using either red cells or skin fibroblasts. For the most commonly occurring disorder, *transferase* deficiency, the very simple Beutler enzyme screening test may first be used.[31] In this method red cells are incubated with gal-1-P substrate, UDPglc and NADP$^+$. In the presence of normal transferase glc-1-P is generated and converted sequentially to glc-6-P and 6-phosphogluconate using the red cells' phosphoglucomutase and glucose-6-phosphate dehydrogenase respectively. The last reaction in the sequence is accompanied by reduction of NADP$^+$ to NADPH, and the formation of this end product is detected by its fluorescence under u.v. after the reaction mixture is spotted onto filter paper. The absence of transferase prevents the whole series of reactions and NADPH is not formed.

Quantitative measurement of transferase in erythrocytes distinguishes homozygous abnormal and heterozygotous carriers for the condition (Fig. 2.11). These genotypes may also be differentiated using skin fibroblasts or amniotic fluid cells (Fig. 2.12) and the latter technique can be used to do a prenatal diagnosis. Prenatal diagnosis by amniotic fluid cell enzyme assay is possible for all three galactose disorders, although it is questionable whether they warrant this approach, particularly in the case of galactokinase deficiency.

Newborn screening is carried out in some places, using either the Beutler enzyme method or a microbiological assay which detects galactose and gal-1-P.[32] The latter seems to be preferred because it gives few false positive results and it should be capable of detecting all three defects. However, the case for screening the galactose disorders is not universally accepted. Although it should ensure the complete detection of all affected patients it has been found that the positive screening test is frequently found post mortem. In some instances the test is performed on cord blood to obtain the earliest possible diagnosis, but this requires separate, quite difficult, organisation from other screening programmes. Other contra-indications are the low frequency of the disease and the uncertain benefit of early treatment with respect to long term prognosis.

DISORDERS OF FRUCTOSE METABOLISM AND RELATED PATHWAYS

There are two disorders on the specific pathway which converts fructose to metabolites which can be utilised for glycolysis or gluconeogenesis. The first of these, known as essential fructosuria, was described as early as 1876, although it is a completely benign condition. Less than 30 years ago, the second, a clinically significant defect, was discovered and was called hereditary fructose intolerance.

This section deals also with fructose 1:6-diphosphatase deficiency. This enzyme is not essential for fructose metabolism, but is a key enzyme in the gluconeogenesis pathway. In common with other defects of the gluconeogenesis pathway there is an unfavourable response to fructose ingestion and there may be some diagnostic confusion with hereditary fructose intolerance. In addition there is a brief mention of a recently described disorder of sorbitol dehydrogenase, an enzyme which can generate fructose from sorbitol. This may be a cause of congenital cataracts.

Normal fructose metabolism

A normal diet may contain free fructose but the monosaccharide is derived mainly from sucrose and some from sorbitol (Fig. 2.13). Apart from a small amount which may be converted to glucose in the intestine, most absorbed fructose is metabolised in the liver. A small part of it may reach the periphery where it can be handled by muscle or adipose tissue.

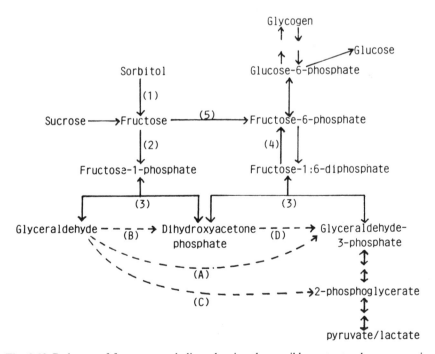

Fig. 2.13 Pathways of fructose metabolism showing the possible routes to gluconeogenesis or to glycolysis. In liver the main pathway is to fructose-1-phosphate and the smaller amount of fructose metabolised in muscle is via fructose-6-phosphate. (Note that release of glucose from glucose-6-phosphate only occurs in liver.) The key enzymes shown are: (1) sorbitol dehydrogenase, (2) fructokinase (ketohexokinase), (3) fructaldolase, (4) fructose-1:6-diphosphatase, (5) hexokinase.

In liver, fructose is rapidly converted to fructose-1-phosphate by a specific ketohexokinase, often referred to as fructokinase (Fig. 2.13). The hexose phosphate is then split by fructaldolase B to glyceraldehyde and dihydroxyacetone. In vivo the predominant pathway for the former metabolite is a simple phosphorylation to glyceraldehyde phosphate which is catalysed by triokinase, but other possible fates are shown in Figure 2.14. The glyceraldeyde phosphate may then be metabolised to pyruvate or may be condensed with dihydroxyacetone phosphate to fructose 1:6-diphosphate, by a reversal of fructaldolase, and thence to glucose and glycogen. As mentioned earlier, the enzyme fructose 1:6-diphosphatase plays a key role in determining the flux of metabolites in the direction of gluconeogenesis. Dihydroxyacetone phosphate, the second product of fructose metabolism, may, therefore, be disposed of by gluconeogenesis, but may also be converted to glyceraldehyde phosphate and thereby to pyruvate (Fig. 2.13.).

It will be seen that the products of fructose degradation may be diverted into gluconeogenesis and glycogen synthesis, or into glycolysis and the Krebs cycle, depending on the prevailing metabolic needs. It has been calculated that in man, under normal nutritional circumstances, an average of 20% of fructose can be accounted for as lactate production.

A small amount of fructose which is metabolised in muscle or adipose tissue is phosphorylated slowly by hexokinase to fructose-6-phosphate. The hexose phosphate may be converted to glycogen, via glucose-6-phosphate, or to fructose 1:6-diphosphate by phosphofructokinase (Fig. 2.13). The aldolase of muscle (fructaldolase A) splits the fructose 1:6-diphosphate to triose phosphates which enter the glycolysis and Krebs cycle pathways.

Fructaldolase plays an important role in fructose metabolism and it is relevant to an understanding of the enzyme defects and their diagnosis that it exists in three isoenzyme forms, designated A, B and C. These are the predominant, but not the exclusive, forms in muscle, liver and brain respec-

(A)   glyceraldehyde —(1)→ glyceraldehyde-3-phosphate

(B)   glyceraldehyde —(2)→ glycerate —(3)→ 2-phosphoglycerate

(C)   glyceraldehyde —(4)→ glycerol —(5)→ glycerol-3-phosphate —(6)→ dihydroxyacetone phosphate

(D)   dihydroxyacetone phosphate —(7)→ glyceraldehyde phosphate

Fig. 2.14 Pathways of glyceraldehyde and dihydroxyacetone-phosphate metabolism. Pathways A, B, C and D are the same as shown in the general plan of fructose metabolism (Fig. 2.13). A is the principal route for glyceraldehyde. Enzymes shown are: (1) triokinase, (2) aldehyde dehydrogenase, (3) glycerate kinase, (4) alcohol dehydrogenase, (5) glycerol kinase, (6) α-glycerophosphate dehydrogenase, (7) triose phosphate isomerase.

Table 2.4 The three isoenzyme forms of fructaldolase, their tissue distribution and activity ratios

Type	Tissue	Activity ratio*
A	Muscle	50
B	Liver	1
C	Brain	5–10

* Rate with fructose-1:6-diphosphate compared with rate with fructose-1-phosphate

tively. The isoenzymes may be distinguished by the relative activities, or activity ratios, with fructose 1:6-diphosphate and fructose-1-phosphate (Table 2.4). All the isoenzymes contain four identical sub-units, but the type of sub-unit differs from one form of enzyme to the other. The form of fructaldolase appears to change during development however; human fetal liver having a higher activity ratio than is typical of adult liver fructaldolase B.[33]

Enzyme defects

Fructokinase (EC 2.7.1.4)

Fructokinase deficiency was first described in 1876 as essential fructosuria (McKusick 22980). The most important site of the enzyme is liver and the absence of activity in this organ has been demonstrated by direct assay. It is likely that in affected individuals fructokinase is deficient also in intestine and kidney cortex, the other tissues in which it is normally to be found.

Fructokinase deficiency appears not to cause any clinical symptoms and is usually found incidentally when urine is tested for reducing substances as a screen for diabetes. A clinical history and more specific laboratory tests should reveal the correct diagnosis. The disorder is rare and only an approximate idea of the incidence is available. The best estimate is 1:130 000 of the population. The significance of a preponderance of Jews in some larger published series is unclear. The inheritance is autosomal recessive.

Fructaldolase (EC 2.1.2.13)

Fructaldolase deficiency, or hereditary fructose intolerance (HFI) is the most important disorder of fructose metabolism (McKusick 22960). The enzyme deficiency has been demonstrated in liver, kidney cortex and intestinal mucosa, the tissues in which fructaldolase B usually predominates. However, the liver is the main site of fructose metabolism. The activity of the liver enzyme with fructose-1-phosphate is reduced to 15%, or less, of normal. Studies using immunological cross reacting methods, antibody activation and heat inactivation point to very considerable heterogeneity in the residual enzyme activity and the nature of the enzyme defect in different families.[34]

The appearance of clinical symptoms in HFI is dependent entirely on the ingestion of fructose and, therefore, will be delayed so long as the infant is breast fed and is given no sucrose. The condition tends to be more severe the earlier the exposure to fructose. The clinical picture includes both acute episodes, which follow immediate exposure to large amounts of fructose, and a chronic course, which develops as the result of protracted feeding of more moderate quantities of the monosaccharide. The former are characterised by sweating, trembling, nausea, vomiting, lethargy and coma, symptoms attributable to hypoglycaemia. They may end in death. The most frequent features of the longer-term presentation are poor feeding, vomiting, failure to thrive and, less commonly, drowsiness, crying, jaundice, haemorrhages, abdominal distension, irritability and diarrhoea. Clinical examination nearly always shows trembling jerks, shock and hepatomegaly and a renal tubular syndrome; ascites, splenomegaly and oliguria are frequent findings. A blood picture suggesting disseminating intravascular coagulation has been found in about half the children in one large series.[35]

It is interesting that the clinical course may be modified in many cases of HFI because the patients, or their parents, realise that certain foods are harmful and, thus, to be avoided. In patients displaying minimal symptoms of the condition there is a total lack of dental caries, due to the avoidance of sucrose containing foods. Diagnosis may arise through a dental examination, so remarkable is the finding. The heterogeneity of the residual liver aldolase in patients from different families, previously described, could explain some of the variation in clinical severity.

HFI is an autosomal recessive condition. The majority of published cases have been found in Europe and North America. In Switzerland, where there is much interest in the disease, an incidence of 1:20 000 has been estimated. However, it is probable that many cases have died without diagnosis or escape medical attention because of the intuitive restriction of fructose.

Fructose 1:6-diphosphatase (EC 3.1.3.11)

Fructose 1:6-diphosphatase deficiency was described in 1970 (McKusick 22970). Prior to that, patients with the disorder may have been confused with other metabolic defects, including HFI. However, in the more recently delineated condition there is not usually a marked dietary history suggesting fructose intolerance. The enzyme has been shown to be deficient in liver, jejunum and kidney cortex. Muscle is unaffected because its fructose 1:6-diphosphatase is under different genetic control.

In the acute presentation, the main features comprise metabolic acidosis and hypoglycaemia, together with hyperventilation, shock apnoea, trembling, lethargy, convulsions and loss of consciousness. The metabolic acidosis is due to the accumulation of lactic acid, compounded by effects of ketosis. These episodes tend to occur on fasting. Accumulated data from the literature indicates that half the cases are known to have had their first symptoms in the neonatal period. The presentation of the remainder was delayed in some cases to more than six months. In many of the later presenting patients an acute episode appeared to have been precipitated by infection. Between crises the most frequent abnormality was hyperventilation and lactic acidosis. Hepatomegaly and muscular hypotonia are persistent findings on examination and these signs may continue through childhood.

From the number of cases reported it would appear that the condition is relatively rare, although the possibility of diagnostic failures exist. The inheritance is autosomal recessive.

Sorbitol dehydrogenase (EC 1.1.1.14)

Investigation of patients with congenital cataracts has revealed two families in which both cataracts and a red cell sorbitol dehydrogenase deficiency occur. Deficient individuals had 20 to 25% of mean normal enzyme activity, with other family members being affected to a lesser extent. The mode of inheritance of the abnormal red cell enzyme levels was not clearly established.

It was postulated that coexisting sorbitol dehydrogenase deficiency in the lens could cause sorbitol accumulation and cataract, the osmotic effect of increased lens sorbitol being one explanation for cataract formation in diabetes mellitus. Unfortunately, within one of the families reported,[36] there was not an exact concurrence between the presence of cataracts and reduced enzyme activity. Therefore, there must be some doubt about a direct causal relationship between sorbitol dehydrogenase deficiency and cataract formation.

Pathophysiology of the enzyme defects

The administration of fructose may cause symptoms and marked metabolic derangement even in normal subjects. Extensive studies of these effects in humans and in animals have helped the study of the disorders of fructose metabolism, both in providing normal data against which the patients' investigations may be compared and in understanding the causes of metabolic defects.

The immediate effect of fructose utilisation by the normal cell is a fall in inorganic phosphate (Pi) and ATP concentration because of its rapid conversion to fructose-1-phosphate. The intracellular drop in Pi is reflected in a corresponding fall in its concentration extracellularly, and the loss of ATP leads to a transfer of magnesium from the cell because the metal ion is normally chelated by the nucleotide. The decrease in intra-cellular levels of Pi and ATP cause a rapid degradation of adenine nucleotides through an enhancement of 5-nucleotidase and adenosine deaminase activities, these enzymes usually being inhibited by Pi and ATP. This breakdown of nucleotides is again shown by a rise of plasma uric acid. The ultimate metabolism of fructose via the gluconeogenesis and glycolysis pathways causes rises in plasma glucose and lactate although, as will be seen later, there may occasionally be a hypoglycaemic response.

Accumulation of fructose-1-phosphate occurs when fructose is metabolised rapidly by normal subjects, although the exact reason for this is controversial. However, this accumulation does have considerable secondary consequences. Fructose-1-phosphate inhibits fructokinase which explains fructose accumulation. It inhibits enzymes in the gluconeogenesis pathway and the formation of active phosphorylase. Thus, fructose-1-phosphate accumulation can potentially cause the hypoglycaemia which sometimes occurs when fructose is given to normal people.

In *essential fructosuria*, a fructose load is followed by a much increased and sustained rise in blood fructose concentration compared to normal. However, there is no subsequent metabolic response to fructose—that is no rise in blood glucose, uric acid or lactic acid—since the fructose is not converted to fructose-1-phosphate. The lack of metabolic response is in line with the absence of clinical effect in the disorder.

The situation in HFI is usually considered to be an exaggeration of the normal response to fructose, presumably due to the completely futile synthesis of fructose-1-phoshate and its accumulation which has been demonstrated in those tissues usually having a high concentration of fructaldolase B. Relative inhibition of fructokinase can explain the findings of fructosaemia and fructosuria when the monosaccharide is being fed.

Following an intravenous load in patients with HFI there is a decrease in serum Pi and increases in uric acid and magnesium which are all greater than in normal subjects. There is a rapid fall in blood glucose to hypoglycaemic levels, the minimum value usually occurring about 40 minutes after the load. The predominant cause of this is considered to be the inhibition of glycogenolysis. In spite of the block in the normal route of fructose metabolism less than 20% of an administered load is excreted unchanged in HFI. It is presumed that the remainder is utilised in tissues, like muscle and adipose tissue, which are usually of minor importance in fructose metabolism.

The main clinical consequences of HFI are the acute hypoglycaemic episodes which occur when fructose is fed and a derangement of liver and renal tubular function. The probable mechanisms of hypoglycaemia secondary to fructose-1-phosphate accumulation have already been discussed. It is postulated that the cause of the liver and kidney dysfunction is a consequence of the adenine nucleotide breakdown and a shortage of high energy compounds for energy requiring processes in these tissues. There are obvious similarities to the situation in classical galactosaemia (see p. 42).

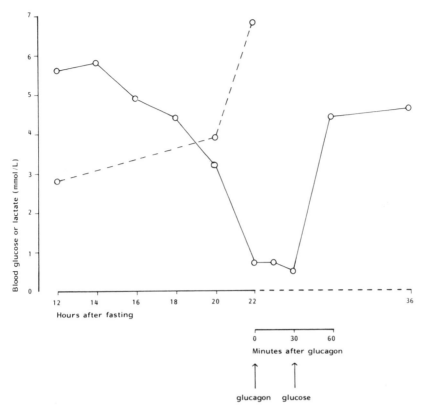

Fig. 2.15 Effect of prolonged fasting on blood glucose and lactate concentrations in a 17-month-old boy with fructose 1:6-diphosphatase deficiency.[37] Glucagon was given after 22 hours. o——o, glucose o----o lactate.

The predominant effect of *fructose 1:6-diphosphatase deficiency* is the block in gluconeogenesis with an inability to maintain blood glucose levels on prolonged fasting when glycogen stores are depleted (Fig. 2.15). Lactic acidosis and ketosis develop. As expected from the position of the metabolic block, the hypoglycaemia is relieved by glucose or galactose, but not by fructose, glycerol, alanine or dihydroxyacetone. The main effect of the administration of 'gluconeogenesis' substrates is to cause more lactic acidosis and a depression of plasma bicarbonate.

Although there is no particular clinical history of fructose intolerance in patients with fructose 1:6-diphosphatase deficiency, ingestion of large amounts of fructose may precipitate a crisis. A fructose load, although cleared at normal rates from the blood, causes a significant fall in blood glucose. The hypoglycaemic response is not as severe as in HFI, however. The cause of the fall in blood glucose is not entirely clear. It may be seen as an exaggeration of normal responses to fructose due to a possible enhanced accumulation of fructose-1-phosphate and other phosphate esters, and to the permanent block in gluconeogenesis.

Diagnosis

Fructosaemia and fructosuria in a patient in whom fructose intolerance has been excluded is indicative of *essential fructosuria*. The diagnosis may be supported by performing a fructose load test, the monosaccharide being given orally at a dose of 1 g/kg body weight up to a maximum of 50 g. As mentioned earlier, there is a large and prolonged rise in blood fructose in this condition but no response in blood glucose, or in the levels of other compounds normally affected by fructose administration.

HFI is usually suspected because of its clinical presentation, by a dietary history and by a favourable response to removal of fructose from the diet. The findings of fructosuria and fructosaemia is confirmation of the diagnosis, but it should be remembered that the blood level of fructose, and its excretion, may be normal if some hours have elapsed between the last ingestion of fructose and obtaining the sample. In an ill child who is vomiting it may be difficult to be certain when significant amounts of fructose were last taken. It is important, of course, to confirm the excretion of fructose by TLC methods, and not to assume that a positive test for reducing substances is due to fructose.

Unless the facts point clearly to HFI it is necessary to consider that many other conditions can have a similar clinical presentation. These include: tyrosinosis, some glycogeneses, galactosaemia, hepatitis, liver cirrhosis and tumours, pyloric stenosis, septicaemia and intrauterine infections.

Further confirmation of the diagnosis may be obtained with a fructose load test or tissue biopsy for enzyme assay. The former should be done only when the patient is in a stable condition and, because of untoward effects of oral fructose administration in HFI, the load should be given intravenously with a dose of no more than 200 mg/kg. Blood fructose and glucose, and serum Pi, urate and magnesium are the main measurements made and the abnormal responses in these substances have been described in the previous section. Some typical results found in children are shown in Figure 2.16.

Tissue aldolase assays are usually performed on liver biopsy, although the successful use of intestinal biopsies make this an attractive alternative tissue.[39] It is usual to use both fructose 1:6-diphosphate and fructose-1-phosphate as substrates in the assay. In HFI there is a reduction in activity with both substrates but the finding of an activity ratio greater than 1, the normal for fructaldolase B (Table 2.4), is additional confirmation of the defect. It should be noted that diagnostic confusion is possible with some liver diseases, when fructaldolase assays are performed on liver biopsies, and with malabsorption states, when intestinal biopsies are used.[39] Unfortunately, although leukocytes and skin fibroblasts have fructaldolase activity it is not of the B form and is not reduced in HFI patients.[33]

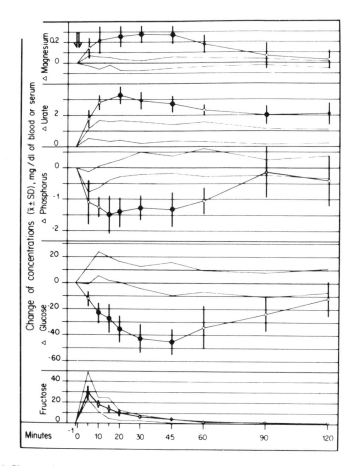

Fig. 2.16 Changes in blood concentration of fructose, glucose, phosphorus, urate and magnesium following an intravenous fructose load (200 mg/kg body weight) in 10 children with HFI and 16 control children.[38] The area between the faint lines represent the ± 1 SD limits for the control children. The vertical bars represent the mean ± 1 SD of the patient sample. Patient means indicated as a large solid circle indicate that there is a significant difference from the control group. To convert to S. I. units (mmol/l) multiply by the following factors: glucose and fructose, 0.06; phosphorus, 0.32; urate, 0.06; magnesium, 0.41.

Fructose 1:6-diphosphatase deficiency should be considered in a child with hypoglycaemia and lactic acidosis but a very similar presentation may be associated with glucose-6-phosphatase deficiency (see p. 22), or the disorders of pyruvate metabolism (p. 204). A fasting test (Fig. 2.15), and the lack of glycaemia response to fructose, glycerol, alanine and dihydroxy-acetone, may help to support the diagnosis.[40] The enzyme may be assayed in liver or jenunal biopsies.[41] Contradictory claims have been made regarding the use of leukocytes for diagnosis, which seem to be due to the low activity of enzyme in these cells.

Treatment

The essential treatment for HFI is immediate and life long removal of all sources of fructose from the diet. All signs and symptoms should go rapidly on this regime apart from hepatomegaly which, for an unknown reason, may remain for months, or years. A severely ill child may require additional supportive measures in the early days, including the infusion of fresh frozen plasma, or exchange transfusion. However, death is not always prevented by this treatment, particularly when liver failure is well advanced before diagnosis.

The importance of maintaining very strict dietary control throughout childhood is apparent from a report of growth retardation in some children with HFI who showed no other symptoms or signs of chronic fructose intolerance.[42] More rigorous fructose restriction led to dramatic acceleration of growth.

The management of crises in fructose 1:6-disphosphatase deficiency requires the administration of glucose and bicarbonate in order to correct the hypoglycaemia and acidosis. The most important features of longer term management are frequent meals and avoidance of long fasts. This is very necessary at times when the patient has a febrile illness. In addition, sources of fructose should be restricted, because crises may be brought on by significant amounts of this sugar, and a low fat diet has been recommended.[43]

REFERENCES

1 Hiatt H H 1978 Pentosuria. In: Stanbury J B, Wyngaarden J B and Fredrickson D S (eds) The metabolic basis of inherited disease, 8th edn. McGraw Hill, New York, ch 5
2 Hug G, Garancil J C, Schubert W K, Kaplan S 1966 Glycogen storage diseases, Types II, III, VII and IX. American Journal of Diseases of Children 111: 457–474
3 Sidbury J B 1965 The genetics of the glycogen storage diseases. Progress in Medical Genetics 4: 32–58
4 Spencer Peet J, Norman M E, Lake B D, McNamara J, Patrick A D 1971 Hepatic glycogen storage disease: clinical and laboratory findings in 23 cases. Quarterly Journal of Medicine 40: 95–114
5 Sidbury J B, Cornblath M, Fisher J, House E 1961 Glycogen in erythrocytes of patients with glycogen storage disease. Pediatrics 27: 103–111
6 De Barsy Th, Lederer B 1980 Type VI glycogenosis: identification of subgroups. In: Burman D, Holton J B, Pennock C A (eds) Inherited disorders of carbohydrate metabolism. MTP Press, Lancaster, ch 19, p 369–380
7 Sadeghi-Nejad A, Presente E, Binkiewicz A, Senior B 1974 Studies in Type I glycogenosis of the liver: the genesis and disposition of lactate. Journal of Pediatrics 85: 49–54
8 Greene H L, Wilson F A, Hefferan P et al 1978 ATP depletion a possible role in the pathogenesis of hyperuricaemia in glycogen storage disease Type I. Journal of Clinical Investigation 62: 321–328
9 Dunger D B, Holder A T, Leonard J V, Okae J, Preece M A 1982 Growth and endocrine changes in the hepatic glycogenoses. European Journal of Pediatrics 138: 226–230
10 Fernandes J, Koster J F, Grose W F A, Sogedrager N 1974 Hepatic phosphorylase

deficiency. Its differentiation from other hepatic glycogenoses. Archives of Diseases in Childhood 49: 186–191

11 Schwartz R, Ashmore J, Rendold A E 1957 Galactose tolerance in glycogen storage disease. Pediatrics 19:585

12 Senior B, Loridan L 1968 Studies of liver glycogenosis with particular reference to the metabolism of intravenously administered glycerol. New England Journal of Medicine 279: 958–965

13 Rennert O M, Mukhopadhyay D 1968 Diazoxide in von Gierkes disease. Archives of Diseases in Childhood 43: 358–361

14 Starzl T E, Putnam C W, Porter K A et al 1973 Portal diversion for the treatment of glycogen storage disease in humans. Annals of Surgery 178: 525–539

15 Burr I M, O'Neal J, Karzon D T, Howard L J, Greene H L 1974 Comparison of the effects of total parenteral nutrition, continuous intragastric feeding and portocaval shunt in a patient with Type I glycogen storage disease. Journal of Pediatrics 85: 792–795

16 Greene H L, Slonim A E, O'Neill J A Jr, Burr I M 1976 Continuous nocturnal intragastric feeding for the management of Type I glycogen storage disease. New England Journal of Medicine 294: 423–425

17 Fernandes J, Jansen H, Jansen T C 1979 Nocturnal gastric feeding in glucose-6-phosphatase deficient children. Pediatric Research 13: 225–229

18 Roe T F, Kogut M D, Buckingham B A, Miller J H, Gates G F, Landing B H 1979 Hepatic tumours in glycogen storage disease Type I. Pediatric Research 13:481

19 Leonard J V, Dunger D B 1978 Hypoglycaemia complicating feeding regimens for glycogen storage disease. Lancet ii: 1203–1204

20 Stanley C A, Mills J L, Baker L 1981 Intragastric feeding in Type I glycogen storage disease. Factors affecting the control of lactic acidaemia. Pediatric Research 15: 1504–1508

21 Slonim A E, Terry A B, Moran R, Benke P, Greene H L, Burr I M 1978 Differing food composition for nocturnal intragastric therapy in Types I and III glycogen storage disease. Pediatric Research 12:512

22 Chen Y, Cornblath M, Sidbury J B 1984 Cornstarch therapy in Type I glycogen storage disease. New England Journal of Medicine 310:171–175

23 Lonsdale D, Hug G 1976 Normalisation of hepatic phosphorylase kinase activity and glycogen concentration in glycogen storage disease Type IX during treatment with sodium dextro-thyroxine. Pediatric Research 10:368

24 Ross B D, Radda G K, Gadian D G, Rocker G, Esiri M, Falconer-Smith J 1981 Examination of a case of suspected McArdle's syndrome by ^{31}P nuclear magnetic resonance. New England Journal of Medicine 304: 1338–1342

25 Winder A F 1982 Galactose intolerance and the risk of cataract. British Journal of Ophthalmology 66: 438–441

26 Keppler D 1975 Consequences of uridine triphosphate deficiency in liver and hepatoma cells. In: Keppler D (ed) Pathogenesis and mechanisms of liver cell necrosis. MTP Press, Lancaster, ch 9, p 87–101

27 Clothier C M, Davidson D C 1983 Galactosaemia workshop. Human Nutrition: Applied Nutrition 37A: 483–490

28 Henderson M J, Holton J B, MacFaul R 1983 Further observations in a case of uridine diphosphate galactose-4-epimerase deficiency with a severe clinical presentation. Journal of Inherited Metabolic Disease 6: 17–20

29 Lo W, Packman S, Nash S et al 1984 Curious neurologic sequelae in galactosaemia. Pediatrics 73: 309–312

30 Kaufman F R, Kogut M D, Donnell G N, Goebelsmann U, March C, Koch R 1981 Hypergonadotropic hypogonadism in female patients with galactosaemia. New England Journal of Medicine 304: 994–998

31 Beutler E, Baluda M 1966 A simple spot screening test for galactosaemia. Journal of Laboratory and Clinical Medicine 68: 137–141

32 Paigen K, Pacholec F, Levy H L 1982 A new method of screening for inherited disorders of galactose metabolism. Journal of Laboratory and Clinical Medicine 99: 895–906

33 Shin Y S, Rimböck H, Endres W 1982 Fructose-1-phosphate aldolase activity in human fetal and adult tissues as well as leukocytes and cultured fibroblasts in hereditary fructose intolerance. Journal of Inherited Metabolic Disease 5, Suppl 1: 45–46

34 Gregori C, Schapira F, Kahn A, Delpech M, Dreyfus J C 1982 Molecular studies of liver aldolase B in hereditary fructose intolerance using blotting and immunological techniques. Annals of Human Genetics 46: 218–292
35 Maggiori G, Borgna-Pignatti C 1982 Disseminated intravascular coagulopathy associated with hereditary fructose intolerance. American Journal of Diseases of Children 136: 169–170
36 Vaca G, Ibarra B, Bracamontes M et al 1982 Red cell sorbitol dehydrogenase in a family with cataracts. Human Genetics 61: 338–341
37 Baerlocher K, Gitzelmann R, Nussli R, Dumermuth G 1971 Infantile lactic acidosis due to hereditary fructose 1,6-diphosphatase deficiency. Helvetia Paediatrica Acta 26: 489–506
38 Steinmann B, Gitzelmann R 1981 The diagnosis of hereditary fructose intolerance. Helvetia Paediatrica Acta 36: 297–316
39 Streb H, Posselt H G, Wolter K, Bender S W 1981 Aldolase activities of the small intestinal mucosa in malabsorption states and in hereditary fructose intolerance. European Journal of Pediatrics 137: 5–10
40 Baerlocher K, Gitzelmann R, Steinmann B 1980 Clinical and genetic studies in fructose metabolism. In: Burman D, Holton J, Pennock C A (eds) Inherited Disorders of carbohydrate metabolism. MTP Press, Lancaster, ch 10, p 163–190
41 Gitzelmann R 1974 Enzymes of fructose and galactose metabolism. In: Curtius H Ch, Roth M (eds) Clinical biochemistry, principles and methods. de Gruyter, Berlin, New York, p 1236–1251
42 Mock D M, Perman J A, Thaler M M, Morris R C 1983 Chronic fructose intolerance after infancy in children with hereditary fructose intolerance. A cause of growth retardation. New England Journal of Medicine 309: 764–770
43 Pagliara A S, Karl I E, Keating J P, Brown B J, Kipnis D M 1972 Hepatic 1,6-diphosphatase deficiency. A cause of lactic acidosis and hypoglycaemia in infancy. Journal of Clinical Investigation 51: 2115–2123

Lysosomal storage disorders

INTRODUCTION

Lysosomes are intracellular cytoplasmic particles containing many acid hydrolases able to digest a wide range of macromolecules[1]. These enzymes are retained within a tripartite impermeable membrane in most primary lysosomes (those which are not actively digesting macromolecular material). These primary lysosomes are formed from endocytic vesicles which become true lysosomes when enzymes are incorporated. There is considerable evidence now that the enzymes are transferred to the lysosomes and taken up by adsorptive pinocytosis and some of these hydrolases are identified by the presence of mannose-6-phosphate which is attached to the enzyme and acts as a recognition marker[2]. A disease entity is known in which there is failure of this uptake, resulting in abnormal catabolism of several different types of macromolecule due to multiple hydrolase deficiency. The condition is known as inclusion cell (I-cell) disease and will be discussed later. Lysosomes which have taken up their enzymes and macromolecules are usually called secondary lysosomes.

The material digested by lysosomes is either exogenous material taken up by endocytosis or is endogenous material separated from other intracellular materials by autophagy. Sometimes lysosomal hydrolases are excreted by exocytosis to degrade extracellular molecules. It has long been known that lysosomes degrade chondromucoprotein and the proteoglycans of cartilage in this way. The wide range of hydrolases in normal lysosomes provides great opportunity for genetic abnormality which can lead to the accumulation or storage of macromolecules which have not been appropriately digested by an inadequate or absent enzyme.[3]

There are many ways in which a lysosomal storage disease may occur. The commonest of these is failure of a gene to produce adequate levels of an active enzyme or the production of an enzyme showing only partial activity due to altered kinetics. Other possibilities include failure to incorporate the enzyme into the lysosome because of failure of lysosomal transport. This might arise because the enzyme recognition marker has not been synthesised or has not been exposed by a specific enzymatic process as well as a primary defect in the receptor protein. It is also possible for an enzyme to undergo premature proteolysis before adequate lysosomal uptake can occur. Alternatively, there may be a mutation of the primary enzyme which, while not affecting its potential activity, affects that portion of the molecule which identifies it as an enzyme destined for lysosomal uptake and thus a substrate for the phosphorylating enzyme. An example of the latter has already been noted as a rare form of GM_2 gangliosidosis (Tay Sachs Disease).

Observation and investigation of the lysosomal storage disorders has, in a relatively short space of time, taken us through almost all of the phases in our understanding of inherited metabolic disease as outlined by O'Brien.[4] Careful clinical delineation and classification has been followed by absolute identity of the mode of inheritance and, in some instances, discovery of information about the chromosome on which the abnormal gene is located. Chemical analysis of accumulated or excreted metabolites has suggested the possible metabolic block which has been confirmed sometimes in a most elegant fashion using complementation studies in tissue culture. The actual enzyme involved in most of these disorders has been identified and in many cases its physical characteristics have been described. Such has been the progress in our understanding of this group of disorders that we are now able to offer sound genetic advice, carrier detection and prenatal diagnosis of the affected fetus in most of these rare, but sadly progressive, afflictions of the human body and mind. More exciting possibilities of enzyme replacement, also organ and marrow transplantation, are currently being tried to alleviate the suffering of affected individuals.[5,6,7]

All that is not to say that much remains to be done. Classification of these disorders (discussed later) in many ways remains cumbersome, not least because some enzyme defects may result in accumulation of more than one type of macromolecule. The latter also leads to problems of differential diagnosis based on clinical presentation which is made worse by the considerable genetic heterogeneity of phenotypic expression seen throughout the lysosomal storage diseases. O'Brien's concept of one gene–one enzyme–many substrates model for metabolic disorders is amply illustrated.[4]

Their rarity means that most physicians will not have seen enough of them to enable them to suggest a possible clinical diagnosis with ease and the chemist will be confronted with a multitude of problems of methodology which precludes a wide ranging screening approach to assist the clinician. Prenatal diagnosis and termination of affected pregnancies is not necessarily an ethically acceptable approach to either treatment or abnormal gene irradication and errors of diagnosis can still be made with ease by the unwary or inexperienced. Current attempts at treatment are fraught with difficulty, either because the diagnosis has been made too late to reverse some of the handicap or because possible treatment regimes are potentially lethal in their own right.

DEFECTS IN THE LYSOSOMAL STORAGE DISEASES

The majority of the currently known lysosomal storage diseases have now been shown to arise from defects in enzymes which are sugar hydrolases responsible for degradation of complex carbohydrate sequences attached to glycoproteins, glycosaminoglycans and glycolipids.

Glycoproteins, as the term implies, are proteins with carbohydrates attached. Strictly speaking, the glycosaminoglycans involved in lysosomal disorders are also glycoproteins in the sense that they are carbohydrate polymers usually attached to protein and usually called proteoglycans. The old term mucopolysaccharide is only retained in the description of the disease affecting such polymers — mucopolysaccharidoses. The term glycolipid, replacing older terms which include mucolipid, designates molecules with carbohydrate attached to a lipid moiety such as ceramide. Thus all of these compounds have one thing in common—a carbohydrate portion attached to protein or lipid—and they may be classified under the general term of glycoconjugates.

There has been a dramatic increase in our knowledge of complex carbohydrate (glycoconjugate) synthesis and catabolism[8] and it is inevitable that many other inheritable disorders affecting metabolism of these macromolecules will be described in the years ahead. Of the many possible glycoconjugate structures already known, some relatively common examples are illustrated in the following classification.

Glycolipids

Galactosyl or glucosyl linkage to ceramide is common to the sphingolipids, globosides, gangliosides and lipid sulphates all of which may be regarded as glycolipids. Degradation of these substances ultimately results in release of individual sugars and ceramide along the lines shown in the simplistic overview in Figure 3.1 which also identifies the site of the defect for lysosomal glycolipid disorders described later in this chapter.

The lipid moiety is a long chain amino-alcohol base to which one of a variety of carboxylic acids of variable chain length (C_{16}–C_{26}) is attached via an amide bond. The trivial name of ceramide has been used for structures of this type in Figure 3.1 but represents a gross oversimplification. Other glycoceramides and cholesteryl esters involved in lipid metabolism may be involved in lysosomal storage disease.

Glycosaminoglycans

Glycosaminoglycans (GAG or mucopolysaccharides) are the major polymers of the ground substance of connective tissue and are high molecular weight polymers of repeating dimers of an amino sugar usually linked to a hexuronic acid.[9] The amino sugar is usually glucosamine or galactosamine both of which are usually acetylated or sulphated at the amino group and both

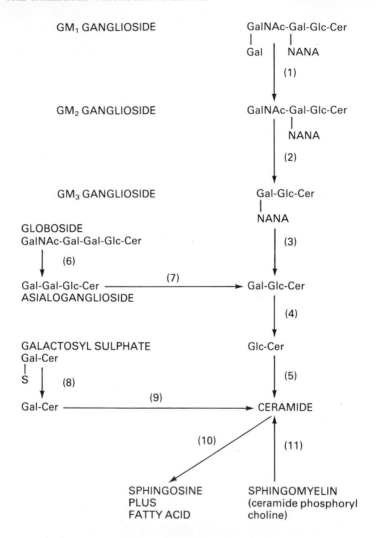

Fig. 3.1 Simplified view of the interrelationships of ceramide glycoconjugates and lysosomal storage disease. Gal = galactose Glc = glucose GalNAc = NAcetylgalactosamine NANA = NAcetyl neuraminic acid Cer = ceramide S = sulphate.

Enzyme	*Deficiency disorder*
1. β Galactosidase	GM_1 gangliosidosis
2. Hexosaminidase	GM_2 gangliosidosis
3. Neuraminidase	GM_3 gangliosidosis?
4. β Galactosidase	?
5. Glucucerebrosidase	Gaucher
6. N Acetylgalactosaminidase	?
7. α Galactosidase	Fabry
8. Arylsulphatase A	Metachromatic leukodystrophy
9. Galactocerebrosidase	Krabbe
10. Ceramidase	Farber
11. Spingomyelinase	Niemann-Pick

Table 3.1 Structure and nomenclature of glycosaminoglycans (GAG)—formerly called acid mucopolysaccharides (MPS)

Current nomenclature	Previous nomenclature	Abbreviation	Hexuronic acid	Hexosamine	Sulphate link	Sulphate
Hyaluronic acid	Hyaluronic acid	HA	GlcA	GlcNAc	O	C–6 GlcNAc
Chondroitin-4-sulphate	Chondroitin sulphate A	C4S	GlcA	GalNAc	O	C–4 GalNAc
Chondroitin-6-sulphate	Chondroitin sulphate C	C6S	GlcA	GalNAc	O	C–6 GalNAc
Dermatan sulphate	Chondroitin sulphate B	DS	IdA and GlcA	GalNAc	O	C–4 GalNAc
Keratan sulphate	Keratosulphate	KS	None—Gal instead	GlcNAC	O	C–6 GlcNAc
Heparin	Heparin	Hep }	IdA and GlcA	GlcNAc	O and N	C–2 IdA
Heparan sulphate	Heparitin sulphate	HS }		GlcNS		C–6 GlcNAc N–S GlcN

GlcA = glucuronic acid   IdA = iduronic acid   Gal = galactose   GlcNS = N-sulphated glucosamine   GlcN = glucosamine   GlcNAc = N-acetylglucosamine   GalNac = N-acetylgalactosamine of which may be sulphated at either carbon 4 or 6 of the hexose ring. The hexuronic acid is either glucuronic acid or its C-5 epimer, iduronic acid. These may also be sulphated at their carboxyl group in the most complex of these compounds. GAG molecules, with the exception of hyaluronic acid, are usually linked in a comb-like structure to a protein core through a short neutral carbohydrate region (usually galactosyl-galactosyl-xylose) linked to serine or threonine. Keratan sulphate is unusual in having galactose instead of a hexuronic acid and it may also contain small amounts of fucose and mannose. The principal features of these structures are summarised in Table 3.1. Heparan and dermatan sulphate figure prominently as accumulated molecules in the group of disorders called mucopolysaccharidoses while keratan sulphate accumulates in only one of these conditions although it may also be found in some other lysosomal disorders.

Glycoproteins

The sugar fraction of glycoproteins may represent anything from 1% to 85% of a molecule with N-acetyl-D-glucosamine, D-galactose, N-acetyl-D-galactosamine, D-mannose, L-fucose and sialic acid as the principle sugars present.[8] N-acetyl glucosamine linked to the amide nitrogen of asparagine is the most common linkage of carbohydrate to protein in serum glycoproteins, N-acetyl-galactosamine linked to the hydroxyl group of serine or threonine in proteoglycans, blood group substances and mucins and galactose linked to hydroxylysine in collagen.

Lysosomal degradation of glycoprotein occurs in three stages, with the protein core being digested by proteases to leave a glycopeptide from which the oligosaccharide is released by the action of N-aspartyl-β-glucosaminidase before further degradation into the constituent sugars by exoglycosidases which sequentially remove single monosaccharides from the non-reducing end of the chain. These lysosomal enzymes are synthesised in the form of pro-enzymes which are phosphorylated before transfer to the lysosome by which they are taken up by specific receptors in the lysosomal membrane which recognises mannose-6-phosphate as the enzyme marker. Some enzymes may be produced in a high molecular weight form which undergoes partial proteolytic digestion after incorporation into the lysosome thus releasing its active form.

Three principle groups of carbohydrate structure are found in glycoproteins:[8]

1. High mannose structures

```
                          M-M-M              Asn   = asparagine
                            |                GlcNAc = N-Acetyl
e.g. Asn-GlcNAc-GlcNAc — M                            glucosamine
                            |                  M   = mannose
                          M-M-M
                            |
                          M-M
```

The above structure, often referred to as M9, has been isolated from Chinese hampster ovary. Variants with 5–9 mannose residues are widespread and the majority of the lysosomal enzymes are also glycoproteins of the high mannose type in which some of the mannose residues are phosphorylated to create a recognition marker which enables them to be targeted to the lysosome.

2. Intermediate structures

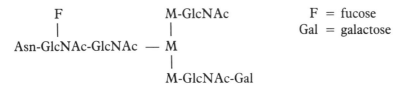

```
F                         M-GlcNAc                F  = fucose
|                         |                       Gal = galactose
Asn-GlcNAc-GlcNAc — M
                          |
                          M-GlcNAc-Gal
```

These are found in human immunoglobulin IgG. Note that several lysosomal enzymes are required for degradation, namely a galactosidase, glucosaminidase, mannosidase, fucosidase and aspartylglucosaminidase. The outer ends of the chain may also be sialylated and a sialidase will be required for degradation. All of these enzymes have been implicated in lysosomal storage disease and a hypothetical model of such a glycoprotein is shown in Figure 3.2 to illustrate these possible disorders.

3. Complex structures—in these the intermediate structure, or variants of it are identifiable in which the carbohydrate chain is complex, usually mannose-free and linked to the protein core through N-acetylgalactosamine α linked to serine or threonine. Many anomalous sequences have also been identified which are not consistent with our current knowledge of complex carbohydrate synthesis. Others are specific to certain types of macromolecule such as the Ser-Xyl-Gal-Gal-GlcNAc linkage sequence found in proteoglycans, and the hydroxyproline-galactose portions of collagen.

In addition to these, mucin sequences are identifiable in which the carbohydrate chain is complex, usually mannose-free and linked to the protein core through N-acetylgalactosamine α linked to serine or threonine.

CLASSIFICATION OF LYSOSOMAL DISEASE

Classification of the lysosomal storage disorders is somewhat confused. Some attempts have been made to overcome these problems[10] but we are still left with a strange mixture of titles sometimes eponymous, sometimes based on the enzyme that is absent and sometimes, as in the case of mucopolysaccharidoses, numerical. None of these approaches is perfect and the difficulties are compounded by the heterogeneity of the phenotypic expression of what appears to be the same enzyme defect. Such heterogeneity may even occur within the same family. Disorders of β-galactosidase activity, for example, range from an infantile generalised ganglioside storage disorder with late infantile and adult forms of milder presentation through to a bone dysplasia of the Morquio type. Deficiencies of β-galactosidase may thus be

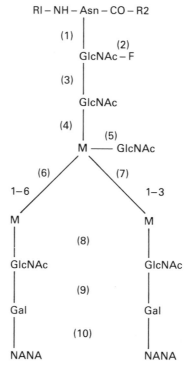

Fig. 3.2 Hypothetical degradation of a complex glycoprotein. Asn = asparagine; GlcNAc = N acetyl-glucosamine; F = fucose; M = mannose; Gal = galactose; NANA = N-acetylneuraminic acid. Lysosomal storage diseases are known which affect each of the sugar hydrolases shown: (1) β aspartylglucosaminidase; (2) α 1–6 fucosidase; (3) β 1–4 endohexosaminidase; (4) β 1–4 mannosidase; (5) β 1–4 hexosaminidase; (6) α 1–6 mannosidase; (7) α 1–3 mannosidase; (8) β 1–2 hexosaminidase; (9) β 1–4 galactosidase; (10) α 2–6 neuraminidase (sialidase).

classified as gangliosidoses, oligosaccharidoses, or mucopolysaccharidoses dependent on the major stored or excreted metabolite.[11] In the following account lysosomal disorders are assigned to groups which seem most appropriate in the light of our current knowledge but will change as our understanding evolves. Only the more common conditions in each group are discussed in detail and description of the rare conditions such as I-cell disease is only made where it introduces new concepts or aids our understanding of the more common problems.

Glycogenosis II and cystinosis have been singled out because they do not fit neatly into any classification. The term mucolipidosis has not been used since a mucolipid is not a defined chemical compound and in many of these disorders storage of mucopolysaccharide or lipid does not occur. Some have been classified as oligosaccharidoses as proposed by Leroy in 1982.[11] The same argument has been applied to the so called glycoproteinoses[12] where the defect affects the carbohydrate portion rather than the protein moiety resulting in oligosaccharide accumulation and excretion. These have also been grouped under oligosaccharidoses. The currently known lysosomal disorders are summarised in Table 3.2.

GENETICS

All of the lysosomal storage disorders are inherited in an autosomal recessive fashion with the exception of Hunter syndrome and Fabry disease which are X-linked disorders.[13] The majority are rare with less than 50 patients having been described in the current medical literature. Some have a predilection for certain ethnic groups. Glycolipid disorders are relatively common among Aschkenazic Jews of whom about 4% are carriers for Tay Sachs disease, 1% carriers for Niemann-Pick disease (Type A) and 0.04% for Gaucher disease. The majority of patients with aspartylglucosaminuria have been found in Finland, although the incidence is still rare. In some conditions, such as Maroteaux-Lamy syndrome, the incidence is unknown while in others failure of biochemical recognition and diagnosis may produce a falsely low apparent incidence. Incorrect diagnostic ascertainment is especially a problem in Morquio disease which may be readily confused with a wide range of other hereditary bone dysplasias, especially in adults where urinary excretion of keratan sulphate, a glycosaminoglycan which accumulates and is excreted in younger patients with the disease, may be undetectable.

The most likely conditions to be seen in Europe and North America have a pan-ethnic distribution and a birth incidence of one in one hundred thousand or less and include Hurler and Sanfilippo syndrome and the metachromatic leukodystrophies. The commonest of these, Sanfilippo syndrome, may be specially difficult to diagnose[14] since affected individuals may appear to be physically normal, the skeletal defects of the disease may be minimal and progression of the mental handicap may be slow. Families may have had more than one affected child before a diagnosis is made and it may be too late to give genetic advice.

Consistent with the possession of half the normal gene dose, the other half being the abnormal gene, the majority of heterozygous or hemizygous carriers of these conditions exhibit half the enzyme activity in selected tissues especially peripheral blood leucocytes, cultured skin fibroblasts and even blood serum. This feature has been used to detect carriers in high risk populations such as Aschkenazic Jews in whom Tay Sachs disease is so common.

LYSOSOMAL STORAGE DISEASES

Glycogenosis II (Pompe)

This condition has a special place in the study of lysosomal storage dis-

Table 3.2 Lysosomal storage disorders

Disorder	Synonym or eponym	McKusick number[13]	Enzyme defect	Principal storage material	Other comments
Glycogenosis I	Pompe disease	23230	α 1–4 glucosidase (acid maltase)	glycogen α 1–4 linked oligosaccharides	Infantile childhood and adult forms exist
Gaucher disease					
Type I	Non cerebral juvenile Gaucher	23080	glucocerebrosidase	glucosylceramide	Lipid laden Gaucher cells are found in bone marrow.
Type II	Infantile cerebral Gaucher	23090			A possible dominant inheritance has been described (McKusick 13730)
Type III	Juvenile or Adult Gaucher	23100			
Sphingomyelin lipidosis	Niemann-Pick disease. Types A, B and C	25720	sphingomyelinase	sphingomyelin	Typical lipid laden foam cells are found in the marrow.
Sphingomyelin lipidosis	Niemann-Pick Type D (Nova Scotia NP)	25725	Not known	sphingomyelin	

Table 3.2 Lysosomal storage disorders (*contd*)

Disorder	Synonym or eponym	McKusick number	Enzyme defect	Principle storage material	Other comments
Galactosyl-ceramide lipidosis	Krabbe disease Globoid cell leukodystrophy	24520	galactocerebroside-β-galactosidase	galactocerebroside and its derivatives	
α-Galactosidase deficiency	Fabry disease Angiokeratoma corporis diffusum	30150	α-galactosidase	globosides	sex linked inheritance
GM$_1$ gangliosidosis					
Type I	Generalized	23050	β-galactosidase	GM$_1$ gangliosides *keratan sulphate *galactosyl-oligosaccharides	see also MPS IVB
Type II	Juvenile	23060			
Type III	Adult	23065			
GM$_2$ gangliosidosis					
Type I	Tay Sachs	27280	β-D-N acetyl hexosaminidase A	GM$_2$ ganglioside	
Type II	Sandhoff disease	26880	β-D-N acetyl hexosaminidase A and B	GM$_2$ ganglioside	
Type III	Juvenile Tay Sachs	23070	β-D-N acetyl hexosaminidase	GM$_2$ ganglioside	
Type IV	Adult (chronic)	23073	β-D-N acetyl hexosaminidase activator peptide	GM$_2$ ganglioside	
Type V	Activator deficient Tay Sachs			GM$_2$ ganglioside	

Table 3.2 Lysosomal storage disorders (contd)

Disorder	Synonym or eponym	McKusick number	Enzyme defect	Principle storage material	Other comments
Metachromatic leukodystrophy	Sulphatidosis MLD		arylsulphatase A	*sulphatides	
Late Infantile		25010			
Juvenile		25020			
Adult		25000			
Multiple sulphatase deficiency	MLD juvenile Austin type	27220	multiple sulphatase	sulphatides *glycosaminoglycans	Excrete abnormal urinary GAG
Wolman disease		27800	acid lipase	cholesteryl esters	
Cholesteryl ester storage disease			acid lipase	cholesteryl esters	
Ceramidase deficiency	Farber lipogranulomatosis	22800	ceramidase	ceramide	
Mucopolysaccharidosis MPS I H	Hurler	25280	α-L-iduronidase	*heparan and *dermatan sulphates	
MPS I S	Scheie	25310	α-L-iduronidase		
MPS I H/S	Hurler/Scheie compound		α-L-iduronidase		
MPS II	Hunter syndrome (mild and severe forms)	30990	iduronate-2-sulphate sulphatase	*heparan and dermatan sulphates	Autosomal form also exists (McKusick 25285)

Table 3.2 Lysosomal storage disorders (*contd*)

Disorder	Synonym or eponym	McKusick number	Enzyme defect	Principle storage material	Other comments
MPS III A	Sanfilippo disease	25290	heparan-N-sulphamidase	*heparan sulphate	
B		25292	N-acetyl-α-D-glucosamini-dase	*heparan sulphate	
C		25293	acetyl CoA: α-glucosaminide transferase	*heparan sulphate	
D		25294	N-acetyl-α-D-glucosamine-6-sulphate sulphatase	*heparan sulphate	
MPS IV A	Morquio disease	25300	N-acetyl galactosamine-6-sulphate sulphatase	*keratan sulphate	
IV B	Morquio disease	25301	β galactosidase	*keratan sulphate	
MPS V	Scheie disease	—	—	—	Redesignated MPS IS
MPS VI	Maroteaux Lamy disease (mild and severe forms)	25320	N-acetyl-galactosamine-4-sulphate sulphatase	*dermatan sulphate	
MPS VII	Sly disease	25322	β-glucuronidase	Not clearly defined	May excrete excess GAG
MPS VIII	DiFerrante disease	25323	glucosamine-6-sulphate sulphatase	*heparan and keratan sulphates	
Sialidosis	Mucolipidosis I (MLI) (normosomatic type or cherry red spot myoclonus syndrome and dysmorphic type	25240	sialidase (neuraminidase)	*sialyloligosaccharides saccharides with α 2-6 linkage	This was the original MLI

Table 3.2 Lysosomal storage disorders (*contd*)

Disorder	Synonym or eponym	McKusick number	Enzyme	Principle storage material	Other comments
Mannosidosis		24850	mannosidase	*mannose-rich oligosaccharides	
Fucosidosis		23000	fucosidase	*fucosyl oligosaccharides	A genetic variant with low plasma fucosidase exists. McKusick 22995
Aspartylglucos-aminuria		20840	aspartamido β N acetyl glucosamine amidohydrolase	*aspartylglucosamine asparagines	
I cell disease	Mucolipidosis II (ML II)	25250	UDP-N acetyl glucosamine glycoprotein phosphotransferase	*GAG especially heparan sulphate *oligosaccharides glycolipids	
Pseudo-Hurler polydystrophy	ML III	25260			Partial enzyme defect in ML III
Cystinosis (several types)		22770 22000 21975 21980 21990	unknown—possible transport defect	free cystine	Nephropathic and benign forms exist with much heterogeneity

* detectable in urine

orders being the first disease to be recognised as such by Hers who demonstrated that the stored material was enclosed in membrane bound vesicles. The other glycogenoses (see Ch. 2) are due to defects in cytoplasmic enzymes. Although cytoplasmic glycogen accumulation can be demonstrated in Pompe disease it is readily dispersed by giving glucagon or adrenaline to stimulate the normal glycogenolytic pathway. Furthermore, the enzyme now known to be deficient, acid maltase (α1–4 glucosidase) sediments in normal cells in the lysosomal cell fraction unlike the enzymes involved in the other glycogenoses.

This disease also illustrates the genetic heterogeneity so common in the lysosomal disorders with infantile, early childhood and adult forms. In the latte , glycogen does not accumulate probably due to a small amount of residual enzyme activity. Pompe disease may also be regarded as an oligosaccharidosis in that oligosaccharides with frequent α1–4 linkages appear in the urine.

Heterozygote detection is difficult because a renal α1–4 glucosidase isoenzyme is present in serum as well as a neutral maltase which may interfere with assays on cellular microsomes. Diagnosis of the condition may be difficult for precisely the same reason and it is important to use two different types of assay or to remove the renal isoenzyme by isoelectric focussing. Since the renal isoenzyme appears in urine it is not possible to make a prenatal diagnosis on the direct examination of amniotic fluid and diagnosis requires culture of amniotic cells.

Although at least three different presentations of this condition exist they do not usually occur within the same family, unlike the pleomorphic presentation sometimes seen in GM_1 gangliosidosis (see p. 76). The infantile form of Pompe disease presents sometime between birth and 6 months of age with severe hypotonia and muscle weakness associated with cardiac hypertrophy and culminating in early death, usually within the first year of life, from cardiorespiratory failure. Unlike the other glycogenoses, the liver is not enlarged (except later on due to cardiac congestion) and abnormalities of glucose homeostasis and lactate metabolism are not found, although the author has seen one patient with episodes of profound unexplained hypoglycaemia. The tongue is often enlarged and this is associated with feeding difficulties. This clinical feature, with hypotonia, may occur in hypothyroidism, a diagnosis which can be easily excluded by measurement of serum thyroxine.

The later infantile and early childhood form of the disease is mainly associated with muscle weakness and a relatively slower progression without cardiac abnormalities and may be similar in presentation to the muscular dystrophies. Death in this group of patients is usually due to respiratory failure sometime before adulthood. The adult form of the disease usually presents over the age of 30 but careful questioning reveals that they have had muscular weakness for many years associated with a respiratory problem prior to their presentation. There is progression of these two clinical features throughout adult life and the diagnosis is probably frequently missed since the condition mimics so many other chronic myopathies with little evidence of cardiac disease. The diagnosis may be established in all of these conditions by the demonstration of increased glycogen in muscle tissue and a deficiency of acid maltase in leucocytes, bearing in mind the possible influence of other isoenzymes.

Glycolipidoses

Gaucher disease

This is the most common of the glycolipidoses and, like Tay Sachs disease, is prominent among Aschkenazic Jews with an incidence of 1:2500 (Type I) with another two clinical types (II and III) seen in non Jewish populations. Type I is a chronic non-neuropathic disease principally seen in adults, although the clinical story probably starts in childhood. Patients present with splenomegaly, thrombocytopenia, leukopenia and anaemia. The liver also becomes involved and increased serum liver enzymes are associated with developing hepatomegaly. Asceptic necrosis of the femoral heads and areas of diminished bone density in both ends of the long bones are seen radiologically and are often associated with intermittent episodes of severe bone pain and hyperpyrexia. The most severely affected patients have lung disease with cor pulmonale, pulmonary hypertension and frequent episodes of bronchopneumonia. The condition is slowly progressive. In Type II the presentation is very early, in the first few months of life, with hepatosplenomegaly and neurological complications typified by affected cranial nerves, poor feeding and misdirection of food due to abnormal function of the pharyngeal musculature. Progressive spasticity develops and death occurs within a couple of years of birth. Type III is a milder condition with some of the features of both of the other types.

Hepatomegaly and neurological changes are also seen in Niemann-Pick disease, GM_1 gangliosidosis and Wolmans disease but in Niemann-Pick disease the child is usually hypotonic and has cherry red maculae. Infants with GM_1 gangliosidosis often show coarse facial features and radiological changes more akin to those seen in the mucopolysaccharidoses while patients with the very rare Wolmans disease have calcified adrenals detectable radiologically.

In all three types of Gaucher disease large lipid laden foam cells derived from splenic histiocytes are to be found throughout the reticulo-endothelial system. Identification of the so-called Gaucher cells in marrow is virtually diagnostic even though foam cells are seen in other lipidoses. Gaucher cells are strongly positive for acid phosphatase activity (the activity of tartrate labile/formol stable acid phosphatase is also markedly increased in serum) and have rod-like inclusions in the cytoplasm thought to be due to glycolipid aggregating with protein to form tubular inclusion bodies.

The glycolipids accumulating have been shown to be glucosylceramide (glucocerebroside) but the view that most of the clinical features result from physical damage due to accumulation is difficult to reconcile with the fact that clinical severity does not correlate with the number of Gaucher cells or the density of inclusions and this problem remains to be resolved. Activity of several lysosomal acid hydrolases is increased but in all three types there is a deficiency of lysosomal glucocerebrosidase which cleaves glucose from glucosylceramide. It seems likely that uptake of glucosylceramide by macrophage lysosomes results in release of other enzymes and macrophage products which damage nearby tissues and account for the progressive destructive nature of the disorder. The major source of the glucosylceramide appears to be the turnover of the erythrocytes, leucocytes and platelets as well as the small contribution made by the slower turnover of other cell membranes.

The presence of several other β-glucosidases in peripheral blood leucocytes has, in the past, precluded the use of an artificial methylumbelliferyl glucopyranoside substrate for enzyme assay for confirmation of the diagnosis. Radioactively labelled glucocerebroside has been the substrate of choice although recent use of detergents or sodium taurocholate has improved specificity of the assay using less expensive artificial substrate. The labelled substrate is preferred for heterozygote detection and is essential for prenatal diagnosis.

Sphingomyelinase deficiency (Niemann-Pick disease)

There are at least four types of Niemann-Pick disease designated A, B, C and D in which sphingomyelin may accumulate in the brain and viscera. A fifth type seen occasionally in adults and not showing any clearly defined genetic pattern is sometimes called Type E. Types A, B, C are allelic disorders in which sphingomyelinase activity is deficient. In Type D, which occurs in Nova Scotia, sphingomyelinase activity is within normal limits and the disorder is not regarded as Niemann-Pick disease by some authorities. The clinical presentation is similar to Type C with normal early development followed by gradual loss of speech associated with epilepsy. There is a mild hepatosplenomegaly and death occurs in late childhood.

The commonest form of Niemann-Pick disease, although still rare, is found mainly among Ashkenazic Jews and usually presents with hepatosplenomegaly, feeding difficulties and cachexia appearing in the first few months of life. Rapid neurological degeneration occurs and a cherry red spot can be observed within the macula in some patients. The skin takes on a brownish hue and death occurs within three years. Type B is a chronic non-neuropathic form with splenomegaly while Type C is a chronic neuropathic form without visceral involvement.

Diagnosis of Niemann-Pick disease is based on the demonstration of typical large lipid-laden foam cells in the marrow (which are quite different from those seen in Gaucher disease when examined by electronmicroscopy) and is confirmed by demonstration of diminished sphingomyelinase activity in peripheral leucocytes using a chromogenic analogue of sphingomyelin which is water soluble. Identification of heterozygotes and prenatal detection of an affected fetus are feasible for Type-A but not reliable in the other types of Niemann-Pick diseases.

Galactosylceramide lipidosis (Krabbe disease)

Krabbe disease, also known as globoid cell leukodystrophy, is an exceedingly rare inherited defect in galactocerebroside β-galactosidase activity leading to a generalised accumulation of galactoceramide and its derivatives. Interestingly, early accumulation inhibits myelin formation so that there is no overall increase of galactocerebroside in brain. The condition is untreatable and is usually fatal in the first few months of life with very rapid neurological degeneration and flaccid paralysis associated with blindness and deafness.

α-Galactosidase deficiency (Fabry disease)

This is a rare sex linked disorder inherited in an X-linked manner in which glycosphingolipids of the globoside type accumulate due to deficiency of α-galactosidase. Deposition is generalised and associated with widespread pain and parasthesiae (often accompanied by severe pyrexia) and the development of angiokeratomata in skin and mucous membranes throughout childhood. Death is usually due to renal failure.

Carrier females are also known to exhibit the full clinical picture usually seen in hemizygous males. Time of presentation in both sexes is very variable and treatment has been directed largely at the relief of severe pain although some success has been obtained by replacement of the defective enzyme, α-galactosidase. Only quite a low percentage of normal activity has to be replaced to normalise metabolism (about 5%). Fetal liver transplantation has also been tried with limited success.

Gangliosidoses

GM$_1$ gangliosidosis

Many different subtypes of this disorder may be seen ranging from a rapidly fatal infantile form with severe neurological degeneration and dysostosis multiplex to an adult form with chronic neurological disease.[15] Another type resembles mucopolysaccharidosis IV (Morquio disease) with which it is usually classified since ganglioside metabolism does not seem to be impaired, at least in nervous tissue. The infantile form usually presents as a hypotonic inactive infant with gargoyle-like facies and dysostosis multiplex. A cherry red macular spot is seen in over half of the patients, hepatosplenomegaly and corneal opacities rapidly develop and the condition may be mistaken for an early Hurler syndrome, I-cell disease or pseudo Hurler polydystrophy. The milder juvenile type presents later, often with seizures, and the facial features are usually normal, although progressive neurological degeneration occurs at an exponential pace. The late adult form usually presents with cerebellar dysarthria starting as a young adult and associated with a progressive spastic ataxia.

In all patients the disorder is due to a greater or lesser diminution of the activity of lysosomal β-galactosidase which cleaves galactose from GM_1 ganglioside, keratan sulphate and many galactose containing oligosaccharides. The enzyme exists as either a monomer, dimer or polymer and its pleiotrophic effects have been explained by the one gene–one enzyme–many substrates model of O'Brien.[4] Residual activity of the enzyme to a selected substrate influences the type and relative amount of substrate which accumulates. This would explain how the biochemical defect in Morquio B is almost confined to a block in keratan sulphate catabolism. Some patients with β-galactosidase defects may be Km mutants and may be difficult to diagnose if reliance is placed on enzyme assay of a single point, single substrate concentration type usually used to diagnose lysosomal enzyme defects.

GM_1 gangliosidosis may present with very similar features to Hurler syndrome or other mucopolysaccharidoses but the latter may be distinguished by a distinctive pattern of urinary mucopolysaccharide (glycosaminoglycan) excretion. A cherry red macula is also seen in children with Tay Sachs disease but they do not have hepatomegaly.

GM_2 gangliosidosis (Tay Sachs and Sandhoff diseases)

GM_2 gangliosidosis or Tay Sachs disease figures prominently in any general text on lysosomal disorders. It has such a high incidence amongst Aschkenzic Jewish populations (about 1:30 are heterozygous carriers compared with about one tenth of this incidence in non-Jews) and was one of the first lipidoses to be described and studied as a result of Tay's description of the macular cherry red spot which is almost pathognomonic for this and a few very closely related conditions of abnormal sphingolipid metabolism. As in the case of many lysosomal disorders, GM_2 gangliosidosis has infantile, juvenile and adult forms with considerable phenotypic variability. Clinical presentation is usually that of a hypotonic infant with an exaggerated startle response to noise. The muscle weakness is slowly progressive. Although crawling may be achieved, these infants never walk and pursue a rapid downhill path of motor and mental deterioration from the end of their first year, usually associated with marked feeding problems, blindness, deafness and convulsions, and finally ending in a state of decerebrate cortical rigidity by the age of 2–3 years.

Sandhoff disease is virtually clinically identical. A later onset juvenile form of GM_2 gangliosidosis is often mistakenly diagnosed as Batten's disease or Spielmeyer-Vogt disease in which retinitis pigmentosa is an important differentiating feature. A late onset slowly progressive adult form also exists.

All of these conditions are due to deficient activity of β-D-N acetyl hexosaminidase, essential for degradation of GM_2 gangliosides. Two lysosomal forms of this enzyme exist, hexosaminidase A which is heat labile and heat stable hexosaminidase B. Deficiency of A is complete in Tay Sachs disease, at least when pure GM_2 ganglioside is used as substrate, and partial in the juvenile and adult forms while both enzymes are affected in Sandhoff disease. The B enzyme is not involved in GM_2 ganglioside catabolism but is important in degradation of oligosaccharides so that Sandhoff disease is sometimes classified as an oligosaccharidosis. Infantile, juvenile and adult forms of that condition also exist. The situation has been complicated by the discovery of an activating polypeptide for hexosaminidase activity, synthesis of which is also genetically determined and absence of which may cause a similar disorder.

The mean hexosaminidase A activity (measured as a ratio of heat labile activity to heat stable activity) in serum of heterozygous carriers is about half that found in homozygous normal individuals and follows a Gaussian distribution curve which overlaps the lower end of the reference range for non-carriers. Where the results in the overlap area are inconclusive, designation of genetic status can be confirmed using leucocytes. These tests are now widely used in mass population screening in communities at risk for Tay Sachs disease thus enabling sound genetic advice and prenatal diagnosis to be offered to couples who are both carriers. Such programmes have reduced the incidence of Tay Sachs disease in North America to about one third of what it used to be and the programmes have provided a prototype for the detection of other genetic diseases in high risk populations. Such programmes have proven value in medical audit, having cost less than one fifth of the care for affected individuals born if the screening programme had not been initiated.

Sulphatidoses

Metachromatic leukodystrophy

Metachromatic leukodystrophy (MLD) encompasses a group of at least six disorders with similar clinical presentation associated with increased urinary galactosyl sulphate (cerebroside sulphate) excretion and tissue accumulation of cerebroside sulphates due to defective action of cerebroside sulphatase (arylsulphatase A).[16] The most common variant, a late infantile form, presents at about 18 months to 2 years of age with delayed neuromuscular development, hypotonia, a progressive loss of speech and onset of ataxia ultimately ending with spastic quadriparesis within about 5 years. This is rapidly followed by a downhill course leading to death at about the age of

7 years. Optic atrophy is also a prominent feature also seen in a later onset juvenile form which shows slower progression. An adult form may be difficult to diagnose clinically and presents with dementia and psychosis associated with ataxia which may also progress very slowly to spastic quadriparesis. This diagnosis is probably quite often missed.

A congenital form of the disease is thought to exist but this is based on limited information on two infants presenting with apnoea and cyanosis, seizures with muscular weakness and death in the first few weeks of life. The biochemical lesion in this condition has not been confirmed but in the other types described above there is deficient activity of arylsulphatase A with accumulation of metachromatic material in neuronal tissues which has been identified as cerebroside sulphates and is associated with progressive demyelination. There is also a markedly raised protein concentration in cerebrospinal fluid.

Arylsulphatase A is a heat labile component of cerebroside sulphatase which is associated with a heat stable activator of the enzyme, deficiency of which can also lead to a rare form of metachromatic leukodystrophy. These patients show arylsulphatase A activity in the heterozygous range in cultured fibroblasts but the activity can be enhanced to normal levels by the addition of the heat stable protein activator. These patients present clinically with the features of juvenile MLD.

Another condition presents with all the features of late infantile MLD plus abnormal coarse facies, hepatosplenomegaly, dysostosis multiplex, ichthyosis and deafness. Not only do these patients excrete metachromatic cerebroside sulphate but they also have excess glycosaminoglycan excretion of a similar pattern to I-cell disease with heparan sulphate, dermatan sulphate and possibly keratan sulphate present. Metachromatic granules are seen in leucocytes which also distinguishes it from other forms of MLD. This fascinating condition results from a single gene mutation which affects several sulphatases and is thus usually designated multiple sulphatase deficiency. The disorder thus represents a complex presentation of the features of MLD (aryl sulphatase A deficiency), Maroteaux-Lamy disease (MPS IV, arylsulphatase B deficiency), X-linked ichthyosis (aryl sulphatase deficiency), Hunter disease (MPS II, iduronate-2-sulphate sulphatase deficiency), Sanfilippo A disease (MPS III A, heparan-N-sulphamidase deficiency), Morquio disease (MPS IV, N-acetyl-galactosamine-6-sulphate sulphatase deficiency) and DiFerrante disease (MPS VIII, N-acetyl-glucosamine-6-sulphate sulphatase deficiency).

Diagnosis of MLD no longer requires histological confirmation or identification of urinary metachromatic granular deposits since arylsulphate A activity is easily measured with p-nitrocatechol sulphate as substrate. The enzyme is less stable in urine and plasma than in leucocytes. The enzyme assay can be made more specific by separating the various arylsulphatases before assay or by using the natural cerebroside substrate. Heterozygote detection is possible but the presence of a low activity allele for arylsulphatase activity among some otherwise normal members of the population may produce low results suggestive of MLD if the artificial substrate is used. Prenatal diagnosis is feasible and potential treatment now exists in the form of bone marrow transplantation if only one could be assured that the enzyme could be targeted to the oligodendroglial cells across the 'blood-brain barrier'.

Other lipid storage disorders

Acid lipase deficiency

Hydrolysis of the cholesteryl esters derived from low density lipoprotein requires active lipase which is deficient in the two related disorders, Wolmans disease and cholesteryl ester storage disease. Wolmans disease is usually fatal in the first year of life with progressive failure to thrive, hepatosplenomegaly and adrenal calcification. The condition is untreatable but prenatal diagnosis has been achieved and heterozygotes can be detected. Cholesteryl ester storage disease which has a slower, more benign course, may be confused clinically with Type I glycogenosis. (see also p. 379)

Ceramidase deficiency (Farbers lipogranulomatosis)

Farbers lipogranulomatosis is a very rare lipid disorder resulting from a deficiency of lysosomal acid ceramidase thus leading to the accumulation of ceramide. The latter leads to painful deformity of the joints, multiple subcutaneous nodules especially in pressure bearing areas and a hoarse voice due to laryngeal and lung involvement. This clinical triad is unique to Farbers disease. Death is usually early and there is no treatment.

Mucopolysaccharidoses

Mucopolysaccharidosis IH (Hurler syndrome)

This condition is the classic mucopolysaccharide storage disorder described by Hurler in which there is a distinctive bone dysplasia (dysostosis multiplex) associated with severe mental retardation.[13]

Patients with this condition usually present in infancy and early childhood with progressive deterioration of mental and physical ability associated with distinctive facial features. The head is large and bulging with a marked increase in the antero-posterior diameter due to premature closure of the sagittal sutures, thus producing a scaphocephalic skull. These patients have coarse features and thick hair with marked hypertelorism, flattening of the bridge of the nose making it saddle shaped, wide nostrils, thick patulous lips, an enlarged protruding tongue and open mouth which, with their coarse facial skin and hair, gives them a distinctly ugly appearance. Narrowing of the nasopharynx and the enlarged tongue lead to a snuffling respiration associated with chronic rhinitis.

There is progressive clouding of the cornea during the early months of life associated with retinal degeneration. The neck is short so that the head appears to rest directly on the thorax. The abdomen is protuberant and inguinal and umbilical herniae are common. The liver and spleen are both grossly enlarged from about 6 months of age. Progressive kyphosis and gibbus formation of the lumbar region of the spine give these patients a cat-like position. The hands are broad and stubby, flexion contractures of the elbows and hands develop progressively (claw-hand deformity), and the fifth finger is usually bent radially. Bilateral dislocation of the hip is common.

Growth is rapid during the first year of life but falls below the third percentile later. Neurological development may appear normal at first but eventually there is a delay in sitting and walking, and toilet training is rarely achieved. The progressive thickening of the skull due to hyperostosis is ultimately associated with a conductive deafness. These children reach a learning plateau before the age of 2 years, and death from respiratory or cardiac failure usually occurs before the age of 10 years. Respiratory infections are frequent.

The radiological features are distinctive with thickening of the calvarium, microcephaly and a J shaped sella turcica. The ribs are spatulate and the chest is wide. The vertebrae are immature and there is usually anterior beaking of T12 and L1. The ilia are flared and the femoral epiphyses are dysplastic and there is marked shortening of the shafts of the long bones with irregular diaphyses. Short bones show metaphyseal widening and dysplastic epiphyses. The terminal phalanges are particularly hypoplastic, and the metacarpals broad and tapering proximally.

The biochemical defect is due to deficient activity of α-L-iduronidase, a lysosomal enzyme which is required for the degradation of heparan sulphate and dermatan sulphate. Those two glycosaminoglycans accumulate in the tissues within the lysosomes and can be seen as metachromatic granules in peripheral blood lymphocytes. Heparan and dermatan sulphate are excreted in the urine with dermatan sulphate in excess. There also appears to be a partial deficiency of β-galactosidase activity which may be due to the inhibition of the enzyme by accumulated glycosaminoglycans.

Mucopolysaccharidosis IS (Scheie syndrome)

This condition was first described as a variant of Hurler syndrome with which it has many features in common. Patients have coarse facial features with a large tongue and broad mouth associated with a square mandible. Very marked clouding of the cornea occurs, maximal at the periphery, and associated with retinitis pigmentosa and glaucoma later in life. Inguinal herniae are common and the liver may be enlarged. There are marked joint contractures which are usually more severe than seen in Hurler syndrome with a particularly severe claw-hand deformity.

In common with other mucopolysaccharidoses these patients have excessive body hair. Their stature is usually normal although their bone age is retarded. Their neurological development is normal except that they may develop carpal tunnel syndrome. Scheie syndrome shows a later progression than that seen in Type IH, and intellect is normal. Spinal changes are minimal and there are only mild changes in the femur and long bones.

The condition is allelic with Hurler syndrome, and the biochemical abnormality is identical in that α-L-iduronidase activity is defective, and the patients excrete excessive amounts of dermatan sulphate and heparan sulphate.

An intermediate condition between Type IH and Type IS has also been described which has all the features of Hurler syndrome but milder radiological features associated with severe joint contractures and later progression of the disease.

Mucopolysaccharidosis II (Hunter syndrome)

This condition is less severe than Hurler syndrome and there appear to be two allelic types based on the severity and survival, a juvenile and a late form. These patients have plethoric facies with many of the features of Hurler syndrome. There is no corneal clouding except in older patients, and this is usually only revealed by slit lamp examination. A form of retinitis pigmentosa may occur in older patients as well as papilloedema secondary to hydrocephaly both of which may lead to blindness. These patients also have a protuberant abdomen with hepatosplenomegaly. Although they develop kyphoscoliosis they do not develop the lumbar gibbus seen in Hurler syndrome. Stiffness of the joints occurs with the typical claw-hand deformity.

There is marked hypertrichosis, the hairs showing nodular or ridged thickening. Growth is retarded so that these patients become severely dwarfed. Mental retardation is slowly progressive and commonly associated with deafness. Patients with late onset type Hunter syndrome appear to preserve mathematical ability longer than they do verbal ability and some patients are known to retain a fair intelligence into adult life. They also have longer survival, usually up to the fourth decade, and occasionally up to the seventh. Patients with the juvenile type tend to die before they reach their teens. Most patients develop osteoarthritis of the hips in later life, and death is usually due to cardiac failure associated with pulmonary hypertension.

The condition is seen in Caucasians, but is rare in other ethnic groups. Inheritance is X-linked recessive and occurs only in boys, although a similar condition has been described in patients, including girls, who appear to be homozygous for an autosomal recessive gene. The biochemical deficiency is in the activity of iduronate sulphatase, and results in excessive excretion of dermatan sulphate and heparan sulphate, although the relative proportions of the two glycosaminoglycans is somewhat variable.

Mucopolysaccharidosis III (Sanfilippo syndrome)

The clinical features in this mucopolysaccharidosis are usually less marked than they are in Hurler syndrome. The skull is usually normal although the circumference may be increased early in life but tends towards normal circumference later. The nasal bridge is only slightly flattened, and the facies often appear normal. The eyes are usually normal although corneal stippling may be seen on slit lamp examination, but this does not usually interfere with vision. The neck is short as in Type IH. The abdomen is only moderately enlarged, and the spine is usually normal externally. The spleen is enlarged in about 20% of patients, and inguinal herniae occur in about one third of males. Four different genotypes are now recognised, designated IIIA, IIIB, IIIC and IIID. Liver enlargement occurs in all patients with Type IIIA but does not appear to be as common in patients with the other varieties. All patients may show moderate contractures of various joints and genu valgum is often present. The hair is dry and coarse as seen in the other mucopolysaccharidoses.

Growth tends to be accelerated in infancy, and patients maintain good height up until puberty, although bone age is retarded. Early neurological development is normal, but is followed by regression between the age of 1 to 4 years, during which speech loss associated with deafness are common features. These patients seem to find speech control most difficult and develop stuttering. Dementia is not a cardinal feature of the disease early on, and the neurological findings are not consistent. The deafness is of a conductive type in two thirds of the patients, and approximately one third learn to speak late. Mental retardation seems to be a more prominent feature of Type IIIB, whereas behaviour disturbances, sometimes associated with violence and hyperactivity, especially if the patient is restrained, are more common in Type IIIA. About half of the patients show abnormalities before the age of 3 years, although patients with Type IIIB may present later during their school years, and disturbances of sleep may be the first sign of the disorder.

The course of the disease is extremely variable, and the mean life expectancy is usually beyond adolescence, although patients with Type IIIA tend to die earlier. Cardiovascular problems are rare, and death is usually due to respiratory difficulties, recurrent respiratory infection being a common feature. Other clinical features commonly seen are episodes of diarrhoea, polyphagy and pica.

Radiological features are less marked than they are in Hurler syndrome, tend to revert to normal in later childhood, and are not detectable before 18 months of age. Biconvex vertebral bodies are common in the thoracic region. The disease is mainly seen in Caucasians and it is the commonest mucopolysaccharidosis in the United Kingdom and in Holland where Type A exceeds Type B by fourfold, and Type A exceeds C by twofold. The incidence at birth has been calculated as 1:24 000.

The enzyme deficient in Type A is heparan sulpha amidase, in Type B N-acetyl-D-glucosaminidase, in Type C acetyl CoA-glucosaminide-N-acetyl-transferase and in Type D N-acetylglucosamine-6-sulphate sulphatase. All patients excrete excessive amounts of heparan sulphate.

Mucopolysaccharidosis IV (Morquio syndrome)

Neurological abnormalities are not a prominent feature of this rare muco-polysaccharidosis in which skeletal abnormalities are more obvious. It is basically a spondyloepiphyseal dysplasia with extra-skeletal features which may include corneal opacities, aortic valve disease, and rarely mental retardation. These patients have the broad mouth seen in Hurler syndrome with prominent maxillae, a short nose and widely spaced teeth. The neck is short and the abdomen may be protuberant. There is beaking of the lumbar vertebrae as seen in other mucopolysaccharidoses. The joints are hyperextensible, the wrists are enlarged and the shape of the hands is distinctly odd. Growth is markedly retarded so that these patients are strikingly dwarfed.

Development appears to be normal in the first year of life but between the ages of 2 and 3 growth slows, and the patients usually present with abnormal gait. On examination flared ribs, large joints, knock-knees and a dorsal kyphosis are usually evident, and all of these become worse with age. The radiology is quite distinctive, particularly the marked platyspondyly in the lumbar spine. Patients excrete excessive amounts of keratan sulphate early in childhood although this excretion pattern may revert to normal in adulthood, and a similar pattern may be seen in other bone dysplasias.

Two types are now recognised, a severe condition with distinctive bone changes, cloudy corneae and aortic regurgitation (Type A) and a milder type (Type B). Both types of patients excrete excessive amounts of keratan sulphate, but the enzyme defect is different being galactosamine-6-sulphatase in Type A and β-galactosidase in Type B.

Mucopolysaccharidosis VI (Maroteaux-Lamy syndrome)

Patients with this extremely rare disorder show similar skeletal changes to patients with Type IH mucopolysaccharidosis, but are usually of normal intellect, and bone changes are more severe. They have a very poor survival. Dwarfism is extremely marked and noticeable at the age of 2–3 years with growth ultimately ceasing at the age of 7 years.

The most striking radiological features occur in the pelvis. The acetabula are small with a sloping roof and the ilia are flared. Ossification of the femoral heads is irregular, and this condition is often confused with Legg-Perthes disease. A distinctive feature is constriction of the metaphyses which is not seen in that condition or other mucopolysaccharidoses.

Patients excrete excessive amounts of dermatan sulphate, and cytoplasmic inclusions are more common than they are in the other mucopolysaccharidoses, usually being seen in over 75% of peripheral blood leucocytes. The enzyme defect is in the activity of aryl sulphatase B (N-acetylgalactosamine 4-sulphatesulphatase) which is thought to result from a mutation on chromosome 5.

Mucopolysaccharidosis VII (Sly syndrome)

This rare mucopolysaccharidosis was described by Sly and colleagues in 1973. Their patient, a black infant, had odd facies with hypertelorism, small epicanthic folds, depressed nasal bridge, and an increased head circumference later in infancy. The cornea were clear, the abdomen was protuberant with enlargement of spleen and liver associated with diastasis recti and umbilical hernia. There was a marked lumbar gibbus, and radiological examination revealed a J shaped sella turcica, flared ribs and hypoplastic odontoid. The enzyme which was defective was β-glucuronidase. Both parents and several other relations had intermediate activity of this enzyme, indicating autosomal recessive inheritance. The locus for this enzyme has been identified on the long arm of chromosome 7. Urinary mucopolysaccharide excretion was only increased in the early weeks of life, and consisted of chondroitin sulphate excretion in excess, therefore difficult to distinguish from some normal infants.

Mucopolysaccharidosis VIII (Di Ferrante syndrome)

This disorder combines clinical and biochemical features of the Morquio and Sanfilippo syndromes.

The first patient described in detail was a 5-year-old boy with growth and mental retardation, mild osteochondrodystrophy, hypoplasia of the odontoid process, hepatomegaly, and excessive, coarse hair. He excreted excessive amounts of both heparan sulphate and keratan sulphate in the urine. Study of cultured fibroblasts from this patient revealed virtual absence of N-acetyl-glucosamine sulphate sulphatase.

The principal enzyme defects in the mucopolysacharidoses are summarised in Figure 3.3.

Oligosaccharidoses

The common feature of this group of disorders is the excretion of oligosaccharides in the urine. They are difficult to classify at present since some of them result from faulty degradation of the oligosaccharide fragment of glycoproteins and others result from faulty degradation of the oligosaccharide fraction of gangliosides.[12] They include some conditions which have previously been classified as glycoproteinoses and others which have been

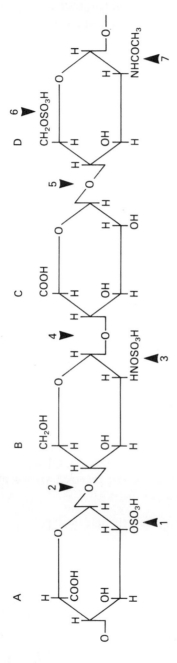

Fig. 3.3 Catabolism of heparan sulphate and associated lysosomal disease
1. iduronate sulphatase (MPS II Hunter)
2. iduronidase (MPS I Hurler or Scheie)
3. heparan-N-sulphamidase (MPS III Sanfilippo A)
4. N-acetyl-glucosaminidase (MPS IIIB Sanfilippo B)
5. glucuronidase (MPS VII Sly)
6. N-acetyl-glucosaminide-6-sulphate sulphatase (MPS IIID Sanfilippo D)
7. acetyl CoA glucosaminide transferase (MPS IIIC Sanfilippo C)
1, 3 and 6 (Multiple sulphatase deficiency)
1–7 (I-cell disease/Pseudo Hurler)
A = Iduronic acid-2-sulphate B = N-sulphated glucosamine C = Glucuronic acid D = N- acetyl-glucosamine-6-sulphate

classified as mucolipidoses. Since there is no evidence to suggest that the protein part of the glycoprotein is involved and since mucolipids as chemicals in the strict sense of the term do not exist, it seems preferable to use the term oligosaccharidoses which more directly reflects the abnormality of catabolism although that too is deficient in the sense that it creates overlap between other classifications such as the ganglioside storage disorders. In the following paragraphs only those conditions affecting the oligosaccharide portion of glycopeptides or glycoproteins are discussed and the ganglioside storage disorders have been described under the heading of lipidoses.

Sialidosis

This disorder, or group of disorders, is due to failure to remove sialic acid residues from the oligosaccharide side chains of both glycoproteins and gangliosides.[17] Two major types of this very rare condition are now recognised—a normosomatic type seen in infantile form in Japanese, with a later onset juvenile presentation seen in Italians and a dysmorphic type of variable clinical presentation usually seen in Caucasians. The normosomatic types present with diminishing visual acuity associated with development of a red spot in the macular region of the fundus. The condition has previously been called cherry red spot myoclonus syndrome since a progressive action type myoclonus is a distinctive feature which is uncontrollable with a wide range of therapeutic agents and is seen in the majority of patients. Intelligence in this condition does not seem to be grossly impaired although it is difficult to measure because of the myoclonic spasms.

Only a small number of patients with dysmorphic sialidosis has been described and they show the same clinical signs as the normosomatic patients but associated with coarse facial features of the Hurler type and a similar bone dysplasia, hepatomegaly and corneal opacities. Another condition, largely affecting the kidney, called nephrosialidosis and a further disorder with a combined defect of sialidase and beta galactosidase have also been described.

Accumulation of a wide range of sialyloligosaccharides probably occurs in most tissues and many are found in the urine with a preponderance of those with sialyl linkages of the α-2-6 configuration, some of which have not yet been found in glycoproteins. The defect is due to a deficiency of a neuraminidase (sialidase) isoenzyme required for degration of sialyloligosaccharides with α-2-6 sialyl linkages. (The other isoenzyme digests α-2-3 linkages found in gangliosides.) Laboratory diagnosis may be achieved by thin layer chromatography of sialyloligosaccharides and verified by enzyme assay on peripheral blood leucocytes. Patients with I-cell disease may show similar results and it is important to assay other lysosomal enzymes in dysmorphic patients. Enzyme activity is greater in fibroblasts and these may be used for confirmation. However, the enzyme is difficult to assay without experience because it is unstable on sonication and freezing.

Mannosidosis

This disorder is clinically reminiscent of the mucopolysaccharidoses but mucopolysacchariduria is not a prominent feature, although it has been recorded. Less than 100 patients have been described so far and there does not seem to be any ethnic predilection. Pyschomotor retardation, coarse facies, ataxia and hearing loss appear as principal features associated with dysostosis multiplex. Marked clinical heterogeneity exists even within a family and it has been suggested that two forms of the disease exist with a mild form surviving into adulthood.

Mannose-rich oligosaccharides accumulate in the tissues and are excreted in the urine. The condition is due to deficiency of α-mannosidase and has been described in cattle and cats. Isoenzymes with acidic and neutral pH optima exist and it is the acidic component which is defective. Enzyme assay on serum is unreliable because of the relatively low content of the acidic lysosomal fraction even in normal individuals whereas in leucocytes that is the major component. Even so, activity varies with different leucocyte populations and may be influenced by infections. Definitive diagnosis relies on the combination of clinical features, demonstration of abnormal urinary oligosaccharides as well as enzyme assays under carefully controlled conditions. Heterozygote detection is not easy but prenatal diagnosis is feasible.

About 10% of the New Zealand stock of Aberdeen Angus cattle are heterozygous carriers of an abnormal α-mannosidase gene. Homozygous cattle show a similar progressive ataxic disease to that seen in humans and experimental enzyme replacement therapy has been tried but failed to normalise the neurological deficit. In spite of problems with isoenzymes, screening for heterozygotes has been successful using serum or plasma, followed by confirmatory studies on lymphocytes in borderline cases, provided that results are compared with age and sex matched controls. A similar neurodegenerative disorder due to deficiency of β-mannosidase has been described in goats and has recently been found in man.

Fucosidosis

Less than 20 patients, mainly of Italian descent, have been described with this condition which presents in either an infantile or a chronic form of similar presentation but slower progression. Early hypotonia progresses to hypertonia and spasticity. Some infants have Hurler-like facies and most of them have hepatomegaly and cardiomegaly associated with progressive neurological deterioration and failure to thrive.

The disorder is due to the accumulation of fucoglycoconjugates such as fucose-containing glycopeptides, oligosaccharides, H isoantigen and keratan sulphate. Laboratory diagnosis is based on demonstration of vacuolated lymphocytes, raised sweat sodium chloride content, identification of abnormal urine oligosaccharide excretion and demonstration of α-L-fucosidase deficiency in leucocytes and fibroblasts. Serum assay is not reliable as about 6–10% of phenotypically normal individuals show diminished activity due to inheritance of a variant enzyme. Heterozygote detection is not easy in either leucocytes or fibroblasts because the enzyme activity appears to change with the growth cycle of the cells but prenatal diagnosis is feasible nevertheless.

Aspartlyglucosaminuria

This disorder of glycoprotein metabolism is almost unknown in all races other than Finns where the incidence is about 1:26 000, rising to 1:2000 in a population of Finnish extraction now living in Northern Norway. Aspartylglycosamine residues form the linkage of the carbohydrate moeity to the polypeptide in many glycoproteins including red cell membrane sialoglycoprotein, thyroglobulin, IgM and IgE, transferrin, ceruloplasmin, α_2-macroglobulin and chorionic gonadotrophin. The disorder is due to deficiency of the specific amidohydrolase required to hydrolyse the linkage, which results in accumulation and excretion of aspartylglucosamine (2-acetamido-1-(β-2-aspartamido)-1, 2-dideoxy-β-D-glucose) and some higher asparagines.[18]

Clinical presentation may be confused with that of the mucopolysaccharidoses. Normal early development and facial appearance is complicated by episodes of unusual diarrhoea in about one third of patients and recurrent infections in all of them during the first year of life. Gradual and progressive hypotonia and mental deterioration, heralded by loss of speech, occur with development of skeletal abnormalities similar to those seen in the mucopolysaccharidoses and almost indistinguishable from those seen in mannosidosis. The facial characteristics are also indistinguishable from those seen in Hurler syndrome but occur much later and eventually become quite grotesque as the mental handicap worsens. Over half of the patients have a systolic murmur possibly due to infiltration of the mitral valve which has been described in the few postmortem examinations recorded.

Deficiency of 1-aspartamido-β-N-acetylglucosamine amidohydrolase (AADG ase) is demonstrable in leucocytes, serum and cultured fibroblasts; but the enzyme assay is not easy to do and requires long incubation times because the Morgan-Elsen reaction, used to measure the release of N-acetylglucosamine, is relatively insensitive and tissue enzyme activity, even in normal tissues, is very low. Aspartylglucosamine excretion can be detected in amino acid chromatograms stained with ninhydrin and heated to 120°C for 5 minutes to give a characteristic deep blue spot. One dimensional chromatography of urinary oligosaccharides stained with resorcinol yields a purple brown spot with associated minor components in the area of the chromatogram usually occupied by tetrasaccharides (i.e. low Rf).

There is no successful treatment currently available but heterozygotes may be detected by enzyme assay on lymphocytes. Prenatal diagnosis is feasible but rarely requested as most parents have completed their family by the time the index patient has been diagnosed.

Disorders of lysosomal enzyme transport

I-cell disease and pseudo Hurler polydystrophy

I-cell disease and pseudo Hurler polydystrophy (sometimes referred to as mucolipidosis II and III but for which multiple hydrolase deficiency seems a preferable term) are closely related diseases but clinically very different. Several acid hydrolases are absent from the lysosomes because the mannose-6-phosphate recognition marker has not been added to the pro-enzyme so that it can be pinocytozed into the lysosome.[19] The enzymes thus appear in the intracellular fluids and blood plasma since they cannot be taken up by lysosomes. The macromolecules which they should have digested accumulate in the lysosomes, hence the name I-cell or inclusion cell disease. The enzymes so affected may also exhibit slightly different physicochemical properties since they have not undergone partial proteolytic digestion within the lysosome to convert them into their most active form.

Clinical presentation of I-cell disease may be difficult to distinguish from that of Hurler syndrome. I-cell disease is also difficult to differentiate biochemically from pseudo Hurler polydystrophy but the latter exhibits a milder course, and is presumed to be due to a partial phosphorylation defect. The presentation of I-cell disease is usually neonatal with gargoyle facies and development of severe dysostosis multiplex with progressive neurological degeneration culminating in death in early infancy. Corneal opacities are usually present but difficult to demonstrate and the only distinguishing features from MPS I are the very early presentation and the development of very marked gingival hyperplasia.

Since many different lysosomal hydrolases may be involved the urine may contain abnormal oligosaccharides or mucopolysaccharides (particularly heparan sulphate) and either of these macromolecules as well as sphingolipids may accumulate in tissues. Diagnosis may be confirmed by demonstrating increased activity of β-hexosaminidase and arylsulphatase A in plasma or serum, associated with diminished activity of these, and other enzymes, in leucocytes and fibroblasts.

β-galactosidase, although deficient in cells, is not usually raised in plasma, whereas fucosidase and mannosidase which may be raised in plasma, may still exhibit normal activity within cells. These findings may be due to partial phosphorylation defects and may prove useful in differentiating the two conditions which currently appear to be inseparable on chemical grounds. The primary enzyme defect is in UDP-N-acetylglucosamine glycoprotein-N-acetylglucosaminyl phosphotransferase responsible for phosphorylating mannose in the carbohydrate side chain of the lysosomal hydrolases. The reaction catalysed by this enzyme still proceeds, but at a very low rate, in pseudo Hurler polydystrophy fibroblasts so that partial phosphorylation, and hence enzyme uptake, probably occurs in that condition and accounts for its milder clinical presentation.

Cystinosis

It is far from clear whether this disorder should be classified with defects of amino acid metabolism or with the lysosomal storage diseases. It is quite unlike the other conditions described in this chapter since complex carbohydrates or lipids do not accumulate. With the exception of thiolprotein disulphide oxidoreductase, no lysosomal enzymes are involved in cystine/cysteine metabolism and yet in cystinosis we see excessive accumulation of free cystine, largely confined to lysosomes, and for which extensive research has failed to find a satisfactory explanation. It is therefore only considered here tentatively as a lysosomal storage disease with a suspicion that it may represent a specific lysosomal membrane transport defect, or that it is not a lysosomal disorder at all but the accumulation is a secondary phenomenon due to a cytoplasmic disorder of cystine metabolism. The former seems the more likely since the lysosomal membrane is impermeable to non-metabolisable amino acids so that there must be a transport mechanism for cystine. Furthermore, penicillamine cysteine (a cystine analogue) accumulates in cystinotic fibroblasts but not in normal fibroblasts. There is a 50–100 times normal accumulation of free cystine in peripheral blood leucocytes, which is diagnostic, while smaller increases may be observed in heterozygotes.

Two clinical presentations are recognised, in a nephropathic form and a benign form, both inherited in an autosomal recessive manner with a few patients showing intermediate expression. Considerable genetic heterogeneity exists with patients in the same family often showing variable expression.

Early development is normal but gradual onset of polyuria and polydypsia precedes the renal tubular damage which is a feature of the nephropathic form. Hyperpyrexia is a common and unusual early feature often associated with severe dehydration. As the renal tubular damage due to cystine accumulation worsens there is a progressive development of a Fanconi type syndrome with a potassium wasting acidosis, aminoaciduria and glycosuria associated with stunted growth and the development of hypophosphataemic rickets. Many children have fair hair, a fair complexion and exhibit photophobia with a poor melanotic response to sunlight. Cystine deposits may be demonstrated by slit-lamp examination of the anterior two thirds of the cornea and with an associated peripheral retinopathy are pathognomonic of cystinosis. The renal disease progresses to renal failure before puberty. In the benign form, cystine deposits seem to be confined to the eyes, bone marrow and leucocytes and appear to lead to no disability.

Treatment is largely symptomatic with adequate fluid intake supplemented by potassium in the form of potassium citrate which helps to correct the acidosis and vitamin D with or without phosphate to correct the rickets, always being mindful that excess phosphate with alkali may precipitate tetany. Prenatal diagnosis may be achieved by following the uptake of ^{35}S cultured cells. The label usually appears in protein, cysteine and glutathione in normal cells but ends up as cystine in cystinotic cell lines.

LABORATORY DIAGNOSIS OF LYSOSOMAL STORAGE DISEASE

It will not have escaped the reader's notice that there is considerable clinical heterogeneity within the presentation of any single lysosomal storage disorder and that there is an impressive degree of overlap in clinical presentation between diseases, even those due to accumulation of different macromolecules.[14]

Gargoyle-like facies, dysostosis multiplex and mental and motor retardation with visual loss are seen in nearly all of the mucopolysaccharidoses, oligosaccharidoses and GM_1 gangliosidosis, although they may be absent from variants of these conditions. Seizures are rare in all but the most severe disorders of glycoprotein catabolism but myoclonus should make one think of sialidase deficiencies. Hypotonia is usually the initial feature of fucosidosis, GM_1 gangliosidosis and Sandhoff disease with rapid progression to spasticity.

The laboratory investigations are very important[20] and a suspected clinical diagnosis of any one of these conditions should alert the biochemist to search more widely and carefully if the initial clinical diagnosis proves to be wrong. In the author's laboratory all of the patients diagnosed as having a mucopolysaccharidosis Type IV A (Morquio) had all been thought to have Hurler syndrome at initial presentation below the age of 5 years, the diagnosis only being modified as the clinical picture and radiological changes unfolded and biochemical identification of abnormal keratan sulphate was made. Careful note should be made of specific clinical features such as a cherry red macula, corneal clouding or gingival hypertrophy which often helps as much to exclude a disorder as to confirm it.

Demonstration of vacuolated lymphocytes or foam cells in marrow are highly suggestive of a lysosomal disorder. Enzyme assays can be done on serum, plasma, tears, saliva, leucocytes, hair follicles and cultured fibroblasts.[21,22] Assay on cultured individual hair follicles may be useful in detection of carriers of X-linked disease based on the principle that some follicles will show normal enzyme activity and others will have very low activity depending on which X chromosome is active.

Simple urine screening tests are available for initial help in the diagnosis of the mucopolysaccharidoses but those such as filter paper spot tests which do not take urine concentration into account are likely to give false results.[23] A positive screening test can be confirmed by estimation of alcian blue precipitable material or the hexuronic acid precipitated by a suitable detergent. The excretion pattern may be discerned by two dimensional electrophoresis or sequential thin layer chromatography but considerable experience is required to identify abnormalities with certainty. Patients with Sanfilippo syndrome may only have moderately increased excretion and the abnormal heparan sulphate is sometimes difficult to identify by thin layer chromatography. Patients with I-cell disease excrete mucopolysaccharides and may be difficult to differentiate from MPS disorders, while the diagnosis of Morquio disease by detection of abnormal keratan sulphate excretion (also seen in GM_1 gangliosidosis and fucosidosis) is particularly difficult since it may not persist throughout the life of the patient.

Urinary oligosaccharide excretion may also be evaluated by simple thin layer chromatography[24,25,26] but careful examination of urine from healthy children reveals several oligosaccharides and interpretation of a chromatogram from a patient may require considerable experience. Simple chromatographic techniques can also suggest which enzymes should be studied in blood or tissues.

Looking for the right enzyme first time may be a problem. Because of this some laboratories operate a selective screening approach in which several of the lysosomal enzyme activities are estimated in any patient with progressive neurological handicap but no single feature to indicate a specific diagnosis. Such an approach may be valuable and often helps to diagnose the unexpected, but there are limitations since, unless the list of enzyme assays available is comprehensive, some conditions will inevitably be missed and a partial list of conditions which have been excluded, especially if lengthy, may give the clinician the idea that all possible lysosomal defects have been excluded and the opportunity for prenatal diagnosis in subsequent pregnancies is lost.

The laboratory staff offering a diagnostic service must ensure that they have experience of all the enzymes referred to in this text, as well as new ones which may be identified in the future, and have adequate information culled from their own experiments to identify optimal conditions for enzyme assay and provide adequate information on reference ranges. Special care may be required with those enzyme assays where isoenzymes are likely to interfere, or the enzyme is labile or affected by the stage of cell development or cultural growth conditions. It is becoming increasingly clear that, although many lysosomal enzymes appear to be as easy to perform as a serum alkaline or acid phosphatase assay, there are many pitfalls for the unwary and these tests should probably be done in specialised laboratories providing specific services for the investigation of inherited metabolic disease. This is an absolute requirement when prenatal diagnosis is being considered and adequate lists of suitable laboratories are available throughout the countries of Europe and the United States.

TREATMENT OF LYSOSOMAL STORAGE DISEASE

Treatment of these conditions has been largely palliative and supportive, often requiring institutional care for the severely and progressively handicapped. Orthopaedic surgery plays an important part in some of the conditions where skeletal abnormalities predominate. Fusion of the atlanto-occipital axis in Morquio disease is essential to prevent early death or quadriplegia and relief of carpal tunnel syndrome may be required in all the mucopolysaccharidoses. Corneal grafting may be temporarily helpful but the graft usually becomes opaque quite rapidly.

Recent attempts to replace the missing enzyme by leucocyte or plasma infusion and fibroblast implantation[5] have been unsuccessful while bone marrow transplantation,[6] although resulting in biochemical and clinical improvement, has been bedevilled by graft-versus-host disease.[7] Recent attempts to avoid this problem by using amniotic tissue transplants have produced temporary resolution of corneal clouding but little change in biochemical parameters. Any treatment is unlikely to reverse the neurological damage already sustained unless it can be given in utero. Such an approach would be possible since prenatal diagnosis of most of these conditions is feasible and widely available. However, termination of affected pregnancies is probably the more logical if not always ethically acceptable course. Where the condition has a specific ethnic predilection and heterozygous status can be readily identified, sound genetic advice may be given to help irradicate the disease.

REFERENCES

1 Callahan J W, Lowden J A (eds) 1981 Lysosomes and lysosomal storage disease. Raven Press, New York
2 Haselik A, Neufeld E F 1980 Biosynthesis of lysosomal enzymes in fibroblasts: phosphorylation of mannose residues. Journal of Biological Chemistry 255: 4946–4950
3 Hers H G, Van Hoof F (eds) 1973 Lysosomes and storage disease. Academic Press, New York
4 O'Brien J S 1975 Molecular genetics of GM_1 galactosidase. Clinical Genetics 8: 303–313
5 Gibbs D A, Spellacy E, Tomkins R, Watts R W E, Mowbray J F 1983 A clinical trial of fibroblast transplantation for the treatment of mucopolysaccharidoses. Journal of Inherited Metabolic Disease 6: 62–81
6 Hobbs, J R 1981 Bone marrow transplantation for inborn errors. Lancet ii: 735–740
7 O'Reilly J R, Brochstein J, Dinsmore R, Kirkpatrick D 1985 Marrow transplantation for congenital disorders. Seminars in Hematology 21: 188–222
8 Stoddart R W 1984 The biosynthesis of polysaccharides. Croom Helm, London
9 Varma R, Varma R S 1983 Mucopolysaccharides—Glycosaminoglycans—of body fluids in health and disease. Walter de Gruyter, Berlin
10 McKusick V A 1972 Heritable disorders of connective tissues, 4th edn. C V Mosby Co, St Louis
11 Leroy J G 1982 The oligosaccharidoses: Proposal of a new name and a new classification for the mucolipidoses. Birth Defects: Original Article Series, 18: 3–12
12 Durand P, O'Brien J S O (eds) 1982 Genetic errors of glycoprotein metabolism. Springer-Verlag, Berlin
13 McKusick V A 1978 Mendelian inheritance in man, 5th edn. The Johns Hopkins University Press, Baltimore

14 Whiteman P, Young E 1977 The laboratory diagnosis of Sanfilippo disease. Clinica Chimica Acta 76: 139–147
15 Suzuki K. 1984 Gangliosides and disease: A review. Advances in Experimental Medicine and Biology 74: 407–418
16 Roy A B 1976 Sulphatases, lysosomes and disease. Australian Journal of Experimental Biology and Medical Science 54: 111–135
17 Lowden J A, O'Brien J S 1979 Sialidosis: A review of human neuraminidase deficiency. American Journal of Medical Genetics 31: 1–18
18 Maury C P J 1982 Aspartylglucosaminuria: An inborn error of glycoprotein catabolism. Journal of Inherited Metabolic Disease 5: 192–196
19 Sly W S, Sundaram V 1985 The I-cell model: the molecular basis for abnormal lysosomal enzyme transport in mucolipidosis II and mucolipidosis III. In: Genetics and Metabolic Disease in Pediatrics Lloyd J K and Scriver C R (eds) Butterworth, London, p. 91–110
20 Applegarth D A, Toone J R, Macleod P M 1983 Laboratory diagnosis of inborn errors of metabolism in children. Pediatric Pathology 1: 107–130
21 Hall C W, Liebaers I, DiNatale P, Neufeld E F 1982 Enzymic diagnosis of genetic mucopolysaccharide storage disorders, In: Colowick S P, Kaplan N C (eds) Methods in Enzymology 83: 439–455
22 Suzuki K 1982 Enzymic diagnosis of sphingolipidoses. In: Colowick S P, Kaplan N C (eds) Methods in Enzymology 83: 456–488
23 Pennock C A 1980 Investigation of the mucopolysaccharidoses. Broadsheet 93: Association of Clinical Pathologists British Medical Association, London, p. 1–11
24 Humbel R, Collart M 1975 Oligosaccharides in urine of patients with glycoprotein storage diseases. Clinica Chimica Acta 60: 143–145
25 Sewell A C 1980 Urinary oligosaccharide excretion in disorders of glycolipid, glycoprotein and glycogen metabolism. European Journal of Pediatrics 134: 183–194
26 Sewell A C 1983 The simple detection of neuraminic acid-containing urinary oligosaccharides in patients with glycoprotein storage disease. Journal of Inherited Metabolic Disease 6: 153–157

Amino acid disorders

INTRODUCTION

The amino acids show great chemical diversity, the only common feature being the presence of a primary or secondary amino group and an acidic function, usually a carboxyl group but in some cases an acidic sulphono or phosphono residue. Biochemically too this group is very heterogeneous. Many of the amino acids serve as primary components of proteins but some also act as intermediates in important metabolic cycles, function as neuro-transmitters, and perform a variety of other roles. Many of these functions are essential to life even in utero so that the defects that present as inherited metabolic disease are mainly confined to the catabolic pathways of amino acid metabolism. In keeping with the varied biochemisty of the amino acid disorders the associated clinical features differ markedly. Only the disorders of the urea cycle share a common theme; the other groupings in this chapter reflect an attempt at biochemical order rather than a clinically useful classification.

DETECTION OF AMINO ACID DISORDERS

In contrast to the great biochemical and clinical heterogeneity of disorders of amino acid metabolism, their laboratory investigation follows a relatively simple common pattern. Nearly all the disorders covered in this chapter can be detected by chromatographic examination of the urinary amino acids and in many cases the results of this investigation lead directly to the diagnosis. The ninhydrin reagent provides a sensitive and selective method of detecting and measuring amino acids and related compounds, and their chemical diversity facilitates chromatographic separation. The success of these chromatographic methods led to a rapid growth in knowledge of amino acid disorders during the late 1950s and the 1960s and amino acid chromatography is still the most commonly performed investigation for symptomatic inherited metabolic disease.

For urinary amino acids most laboratories rely on paper or thin-layer chromatographic methods[1,2] which, if critically applied, are highly satisfac-

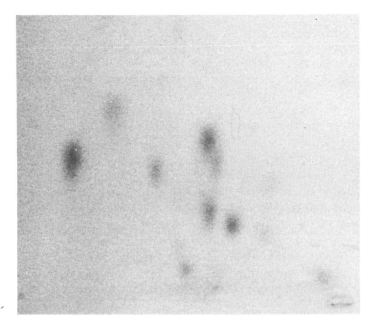

Fig. 4.1 Urinary amino acids from a case of tyrosinaemia Type 2 separated by 2-dimensional thin-layer chromatography on cellulose coated plates. Running solvents: 1, butan-2-one—aqueous ammonia (25% w/v)—water (3:1:2 by vol.); 2, butan-1-ol—acetone—acetic acid—water (7:7:2:4 by vol.). The second dimension has been run twice. The most intense spot, on the far left-hand side, is tyrosine which is not normally visible when this amount of urine is applied.

tory. A good two-dimensional system with normal adult urine will show clear spots of glycine, alanine, serine, threonine, glutamine, histidine and taurine and probably other minor or more variable components (Fig. 4.1). Many disorders of amino acid metabolism will produce clearly unusual patterns, with normal components increased many fold or abnormal components at least as prominent as the normal urinary amino acids, but in a few the abnormality may be quite subtle and easily missed. Critical overlaps in the position of the amino acids vary with the exact system used and may obscure an abnormality, but given the low diagnostic yield from amino acid investigations it is probably impracticable to design a routine procedure that will infallibly detect all known abnormalities.

One-dimensional chromatography is quicker and cheaper than two-dimensional procedures but the more polar amino acids tend to be poorly separated. One-dimensional chromatography is valuable for the emergency investigation of the critically ill neonate for specific disorders such as maple syrup urine disease, argininosuccinic aciduria and citrullinaemia but its use in definitive investigations of patients with suspected metabolic disorders is to be deprecated. High-voltage electrophoresis at pH2 (Fig. 4.2) performed in duplicate with and without hydrogen peroxide oxidation is

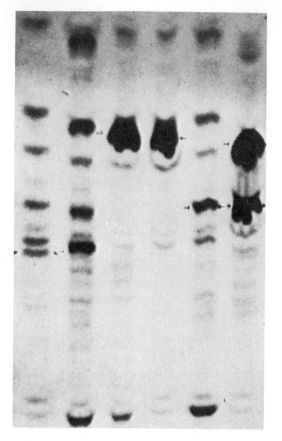

Fig. 4.2 Urinary amino acids separated on paper by high-voltage electrophoresis at pH 2. Samples from left to right: phenylketonuria; normal subject, twice the usual volume applied; non-ketotic hyperglycinaemia with neonatal onset; non-ketotic hyperglycinaemia with late onset; homocystinuria due to cystathionine synthase deficiency; argininosuccinate lyase deficiency. The five most intense bands in the normal sample are, from top to bottom, histidine, glycine, alanine, serine, glutamine, and taurine (close to the point of application).

probably the most useful one-dimensional system available and, particularly if run in parallel with a one-dimensional thin-layer chromatogram to reveal minor increases in the non-polar amino acids, is adequate for preliminary investigations.

Though many disorders are readily detected by examination of urine alone, those affecting amino acids with a high tubular reabsorption, particularly phenylalanine, tyrosine, methionine and the branched-chain amino acids, are more reliably diagnosed by the examination of plasma. In the immediate neonatal period and in mild or intermittent variants the plasma concentration of affected amino acids may be insufficiently high to produce any marked increase in urinary excretion. Moderate increases in the plasma

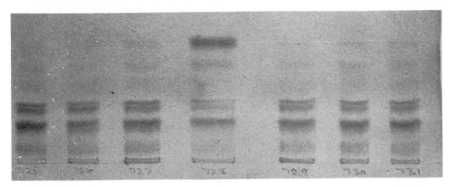

Fig. 4.3 Amino acids eluted from a dried blood spot separated by 1-dimensional thin-layer chromatography on cellulose using butan-1-ol—acetone—acetic acid—water as in Figure 4.1. All the samples are from 6-day-old babies, that in lane 4 showing the characteristic elevation of the branched-chain amino acids seen in maple syrup urine disease.

concentration of these amino acids are, however, readily detectable by one-dimensional chromatography (Fig. 4.3) which is widely used in neonatal screening programmes.

Quantitative amino acid analysis is seldom required for the initial detection of a disorder but may be important in confirming a diagnosis and for monitoring any form of treatment. Semiquantitative methods, such as thin-layer chromatography with visual comparison with standards, are sometimes used for such treatment monitoring but quantitative analysis is much to be preferred. Some amino acids, e.g. phenylalanine, may be estimated by specific methods but for most applications it is simpler and more satisfactory to use an automated amino acid analyser. The traditional form of automatic amino acid analyser separates the amino acids on a column of finely divided ion-exchange resin using an aqueous buffer system. Depending on the application, instrument design, and the resin used, the buffer may be a continuous or a stepped gradient of increasing pH and ionic strength and based on lithium or sodium citrate. The amino acids in the column effluent are detected in a continuous flow system using either ninhydrin with absorptiometry or o-phthalaldehyde with fluorometry. A typical chromatogram is shown in Figure 4.4. Often resolution is deliberately sacrificed for speed of analysis and this may cause problems when the instrument is used for diagnosis rather than for monitoring known conditions. Because the structural features determining mobility on the ion-exchange column differ from those which operate in partition chromatography the amino acid analyser provides useful confirmation of the identity of unusual metabolites.

A detailed account of the methods just described together with a comprehensive review of the chemistry of amino acids found in human body fluids in health and disease is given in the monograph by Bremer et al.[2]

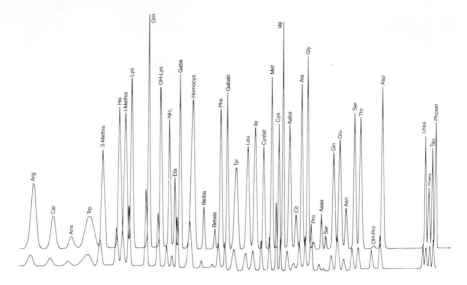

Fig 4.4 Separation of a standard mixture of amino acids likely to be found in physiological fluids using a modern amino acid analyser (Biotronic LC5001). Non-standard abbreviations: Phoser, phosphoserine; Phoeta, phosphoethanolamine; Aaaa, alpha-aminoadipic acid; Aaba, alpha-aminobutyric acid; Cystat, cystathionine; Gabab, gamma-aminobutyric acid; Betala, beta-alanine; Beiba, beta-aminoisobutyric acid; Eta, ethanolamine; Ans, anserine; Car, carnosine. (Reproduced with permission of Biotronic Gmbh).

PHENYLKETONURIA, HYPERPHENYLALANINAEMIA AND RELATED CONDITIONS

Phenylalanine hydroxylase deficiency (McKusick 26160)

Phenylketonuria due to phenylalanine hydroxylase deficiency is the commonest of the amino acid disorders resulting in mental subnormality in most European populations. The disease was discovered by Følling in 1934 following the observation that the urine of two mentally deficient brothers who had a peculiar musty odour gave a green coloration with ferric chloride solution. For an interesting account of the history of phenylketonuria and a review of more recent developments see Bickel[3].

Biochemistry

In man phenylalanine is entirely of dietary origin. The major catabolic pathway is by the action of phenylalanine hydroxylase (phenylalanine monooxygenase, EC 1.14.16.1) to produce tyrosine (Fig. 4.5). This enzyme is present mainly in liver but kidney also shows activity. It cannot be detected in leucocytes, cultured fibroblasts or amniotic fluid cells. Tetrahydrobiopterin is necessary as a co-factor, being oxidised to quinonoid dihydrobiopterin in the course of phenylalanine hydroxylation. The enzyme

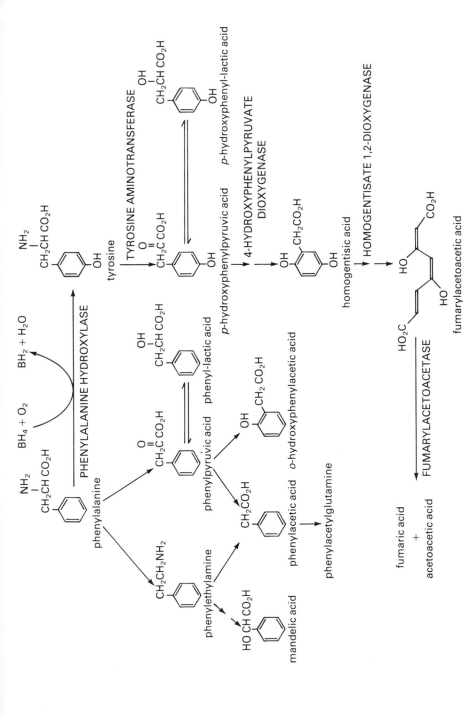

Fig. 4.5 Outline of phenylalanine metabolism showing the origin of major abnormal metabolites found in phenylketonuria.

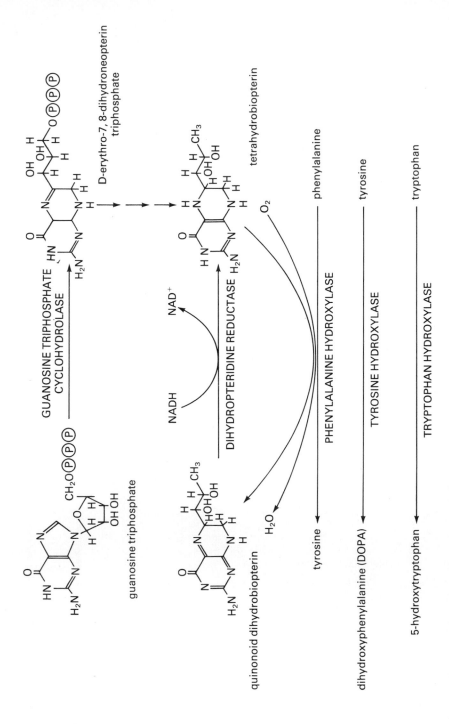

Fig. 4.6 Summary of tetrahydrobiopterin metabolism.

dihydropteridine reductase recycles the quinonoid dihydrobiopterin to tetrahydrobiopterin (Fig. 4.6).

In classical phenylketonuria there is a complete absence of phenylalanine hydroxylase activity, or at most very low residual activity, presumably due to defective enzyme structure or reduced rate of synthesis. In affected individuals phenylalanine concentrations are near normal at birth but rise rapidly once feeding is established and usually reach 1.2–6.0 mmol/l in plasma within 2–3 weeks. Transamination leads to a series of overflow metabolites which appear in the urine: phenylpyruvic acid, phenyllactic acid, o-hydroxyphenylacetic acid, phenylacetic acid and phenylacetylglutamine. The last two metabolites may also arise following phenylalanine decarboxylation as does mandelic acid, also excreted in excess. Phenylacetic acid is responsible for the characteristic smell of patients with untreated phenylketonuria. Phenylpyruvic acid gives a dark apple-green coloration with ferric chloride solution, as first observed by Følling. The increasing capacity for transamination with age is probably responsible for the lower plasma phenylalanine levels seen in older untreated patients compared to infants.

Patients with slight to moderate impairment of phenylalanine hydroxylation are often grouped together under the heading of hyperphenylalaninaemia, also referred to as mild, or atypical, phenylketonuria (McKusick 26158). Strict definition holds that there should be no phenylketonuria (i.e. no urinary excretion of phenylpyruvic acid) but in practice there are borderline patients who will occasionally excrete phenylpyruvic acid in readily detectable amounts depending on dietary phenylalanine intake and other factors. Thus there is a complete gradation between classical phenylketonuria and normal. In some hyperphenylalaninaemic patients the phenylalanine decay curves following intravenous loads show that the residual phenylalanine hydroxylase is susceptible to substrate inhibition, suggesting an abnormal structure. In a few patients hyperphenylalaninaemia has been ascribed to defective phenylalanine transamination but as levels of phenylalanine are regulated by the action of phenylalanine hydroxylase this seems unlikely.

Diagnosis

In many countries with a high incidence, phenylketonuria is detected by neonatal screening for increased blood or plasma phenylalanine concentrations (see p. 108). The diagnosis is usually based entirely on the raised phenylalanine levels in the absence of excess of any other plasma amino acid. Tyrosine is normal or somewhat reduced in concentration. With the prompt initiation of treatment it is unusual for more than trace amounts of the abnormal phenolic acids to be found in urine in the neonatal period but in older patients on an unrestricted diet these metabolites should be present. Enzyme studies (which involve liver biopsy) are unnecessary provided that the possibility of tetrahydrobiopterin deficiency (p. 107) is excluded by other methods.

The classification of patients with partial defects of phenylalanine hydroxylase is an unsolved problem. Not only is there a continuum from classical phenylketonuria to normality but it is difficult to tell in the neonatal period whether a patient will need very strict or only moderate restriction of dietary intake to control plasma phenylalanine levels later in childhood. Assay of hepatic phenylalanine hydroxylase, dietary challenges and phenylalanine load tests, even those involving stable isotopic labelling, yield no reliable prognostic information in the individual patient.

Clinical features

Rapid exchange across the placenta keeps the phenylalanine levels in the fetus with phenylalanine hydroxylase deficiency essentially normal. After birth, however, the accumulation of phenylalanine and its metabolites inhibits mental development and progressively damages the brain. The baby with phenylketonuria usually appears normal for the first few months with no specific neurological signs, but by 6 months of age mental development is often obviously delayed. Untreated phenylketonuria usually leads to severe mental retardation with a high proportion of patients showing microcephaly and having seizures and other neurological abnormalities. Agitated and aggressive behaviour is common, often with autistic features. The hair and eye pigments are diluted, giving a tendency to blond hair and blue eyes. Eczema is found in about a quarter of the patients. A small proportion of untreated patients with the biochemical features of classical phenylketonuria are of normal intelligence. Others may escape with only mild mental retardation and perhaps a sixth of the untreated cases are living within the general community. The reason for this variability is unknown. Retrospective studies have suggested that patients with partial deficiency of phenylalanine hydroxylase whose blood phenylalanine concentrations remain for the most part below 1.2 mmol/l (20 mg/dl) are unlikely to become mentally retarded. Most paediatricians err on the side of safety and choose a lower limit, often 0.9 mmol/l, below which they do not treat.

The pathogenic mechanisms in phenylketonuria are still in dispute. Phenylalanine and its metabolites affect numerous areas of metabolism including the synthesis of indolamine and catecholamine neurotransmitters. Given the individual variations in the threshold at which transamination becomes rapid and the likelihood that phenylalanine itself plays a major role in pathogenesis it is unsound to take the absence of urinary phenylpyruvic acid as a sign that dietary treatment is unnecessary.

Treatment

The aim of treatment is to prevent excessive phenylalanine accumulation by strict control of dietary protein intake coupled with the administration of a phenylalanine-free amino acid supplement to allow for the requirements of normal growth[4]. The original amino acid supplements were derived from acid-hydrolysed natural protein, the phenylalanine being removed by absorption on a charcoal column. Tyrosine is also retained by this column and tryptophan is destroyed during the hydrolysis, so that both must be added to the final product. Such preparations invariably have a most unpleasant taste and some of the earlier ones produced metabolic acidosis and anorexia. For older patients they are being superseded by mixtures of synthetic amino acids which are less distasteful. Such a diet requires careful attention to avoid vitamin and trace element deficiency and, as the patient grows older, to provide a degree of variety and to ensure palatability. Many special dietary products that help in these respects are now commercially available.

The blood phenylalanine concentration should be monitored regularly. Sufficient phenylalanine must be provided for the requirements of growth and tissue repair and it is usual to aim for a slight excess. The lower limit of acceptability for blood phenylalanine is usually set somewhere in the range of 0.1–0.2 mmol/l, normal being 0.06 ± 0.02. The upper limit is less generally agreed and varies with age. A reasonable aim is 0.6 mmol/l to the age of 8 years, relaxing slowly thereafter to achieve a nearly normal diet, apart from some restriction of protein, by the age of 12 years. Patients whose treatment started within the first month of life and who have been moderately well controlled have normal intelligence. Early practice was to completely abandon dietary treatment at around the age of 5 years when, it was argued, brain development would be substantially complete. This led in many cases to slow but very definite developmental regression[5] and it is now realised that the period of vulnerability is much longer. Even with controlled relaxation, allowing plasma phenylalanine to reach no higher than 1.2 mmol/l, some patients show deterioration in the EEG and there is still slight anxiety about possible long-term effects. However for most children with phenylketonuria some degree of relaxation becomes unavoidable as they grow older and seems to be well tolerated.

Genetics

Autosomal recessive inheritance has been demonstrated by showing a 1 in 4 incidence of phenylketonuria in sibs of index cases and an equal sex ratio. The heterozygotes have reduced capacity to hydroxylate phenylalanine and can as a group be distinguished by phenylalanine loading tests or by various measurements of plasma phenylalanine and tyrosine.[6] In individual cases, though, classification may be impossible because of overlap between the normal and heterozygote ranges.[3] The incidence of phenylketonuria varies from country to country and even within regions of the United Kingdom. The overall average in the UK approximates to 10:100 000.

The recently developed technique of DNA restriction fragment length polymorphism analysis (p. 4) can be applied to the prenatal diagnosis of phenylketonuria. A cloned human cDNA probe is used to detect restriction-enzyme generated fragments containing the phenylalanine hydroxylase gene and at present with three restriction enzymes a diagnosis is possible in about 75% of affected families.[7] This method is based on genetic linkage rather than direct detection of the mutation responsible and thus is not universally applicable. There must already be a case of phenylketonuria in the family and the chances of success are increased if DNA samples from unaffected sibs and grandparents are available for analysis. Prenatal diagnosis of phenylketonuria by phenylalanine hydroxylase assay on fetal liver biopsy should also be possible since the enzyme becomes active at 7 weeks gestation. The favourable outcome of early treatment means that in practice there is little justification for either of these procedures which, in any case, would have only a small impact on the total number of cases born. Proponents of prenatal diagnosis point to the somewhat uncertain long-term outcome in treated phenylketonuria after dietary discontinuation and to the difficulties faced by phenylketonuric women who wish to have children (see below). The ability to combine DNA analysis with chorion biopsy may make prenatal diagnosis tempting in individual cases.

Pregnancy in phenylketonuria

The fetus is adversely affected by high phenylalanine concentrations and unless counter measures are taken babies born to phenylketonuric women show a very high incidence of microcephaly and mental retardation and an increased frequency of congenital heart defects and other abnormalities. Such babies are said to suffer from maternal phenylketonuria. In the past this problem has been limited by the relatively small number of women with classical phenylketonuria who were of sufficient intelligence to participate in the general community but it is increasing as more early-treated patients with good intellectual function reach sexual maturity. It seems likely that careful dietary control of maternal phenylalanine levels prior to conception and throughout pregnancy will prevent fetal damage, though as yet there have not been sufficient well-treated pregnancies to allow a reliable estimate of residual risks. A detailed analysis[8] suggests that maternal blood phenylalanine concentration needs to exceed 0.6 mmol/l to produce significant fetal damage. If this figure proves to be correct, patients with partial phenylalanine deficiency who were not considered to need treatment themselves in infancy may need dietary restriction during pregnancy. It has been belatedly recognised that long-term follow-up of female patients with phenylketonuria, with very active counselling as the reproductive years approach, is essential if cases of fetal damage due to maternal phenylketonuria are to be prevented.

Tetrahydrobiopterin deficiencies

For each molecule of tyrosine synthesised by the action of phenylalanine hydroxylase a molecule of tetrahydrobiopterin is oxidised to quinonoid dihydrobiopterin. Normally this quinonoid dihydrobiopterin is rapidly reduced by dihydropteridine reductase (EC 1.6.99.7), back to tetrahydrobiopterin a deficiency of which effectively prevents phenylalanine hydroxylation (Fig. 4.6). Patients with dihydropteridine reductase deficiency (McKusick 26163) may show typical biochemical features of classical phenylketonuria though they often have a fairly high tolerance to dietary phenylalanine. However tetrahydrobiopterin is also a cofactor for tyrosine hydroxylase and tryptophan hydroxylase, enzymes essential for the formation of the catecholamine neurotransmitters (dopamine, noradrenalin and adrenalin) and 5-hydroxytryptamine (serotonin) respectively and in dihydropteridine reductase deficiency depletion of these neurotransmitters often leads to progressive neurological deterioration with feeding difficulties, hypotonia, seizures and death. A similar biochemical and clinical picture can arise from enzyme deficiencies on the pathway of de novo biopterin synthesis from guanosine triphosphate (McKusick 26164 and 26169). Guanosine triphosphate cyclohydrolase (EC 3.5.4.16) deficiency has been demonstrated in some biopterin-deficient patients but the defect in other patients is obscure as the remaining steps from dihydroneopterin triphosphate to tetrahydrobiopterin have not been fully characterised.

These disorders[9] are sometimes referred to collectively as malignant or lethal hyperphenylalaninaemias but in fact some patients may be only moderately affected, presenting late with mental retardation. Patients with dihydropteridine reductase deficiency may have only marginally increased blood phenylalanine concentrations and it is uncertain how many escape detection during neonatal screening for phenylketonuria. In caucasian populations only 1–2% of cases of phenylketonuria and hyperphenylalaninaemia detected by neonatal blood-spot screening have biopterin deficiency defects.

Detailed discussion of diagnosis is beyond the scope of this chapter and some aspects are still controversial.[10] Dihydropteridine reductase is widely distributed in the body and may be assayed in fibroblasts, leucocytes or dried blood spots.[11] The *Crithidia fasiculata* assay for total blood biopterin, also applicable to dried blood spots,[11] may be a useful screen for disorders of biopterin synthesis. High performance liquid chromatography of urinary biopterins is recommended in doubtful cases. In most cases of tetrahydrobiopterin deficiency an oral dose of tetrahydrobiopterin produces a temporary reduction in blood phenylalanine concentrations. This could be a useful preliminary test but has given misleading results on occasions.

Treatment is by dietary phenylalanine restriction together with neurotransmitter replacement using carefully controlled doses of L-DOPA and L-5-hydroxytryptophan together with a peripheral decarboxylase inhibitor.

Though the short term effects are dramatic it remains to be seen whether such a regime can be supported on a long-term basis.

Dihydropteridine reductase deficiency can be diagnosed prenatally by enzyme assay on cultured amniotic fluid cells.

Screening for phenylketonuria and other amino acid disorders

The demonstration in 1954 of the feasibility of dietary control of phenylketonuria created the need for a routine method for detecting babies with this condition before irreversible brain damage occurred. The first large-scale screening programmes[12] were based on the colour reaction of phenylpyruvic acid with ferric chloride. Initially this was performed by applying ferric chloride solution from a dropping bottle to the urine-soaked nappy, this solution being replaced later by a dry test-stick (Phenistix[R]) containing buffered ferric salts. Because of the time taken for blood phenylalanine concentrations to increase after birth and for transamination to become established this test had to be performed at about 6 weeks of age and even so gave a false negative rate of about 10%. A more significant problem was the general inconvenience of nappy-testing in the baby's home in this way, with the frequent need for return visits if a wet nappy was not available, which, together with the lack of central control, led to many babies not being tested at all. With the development of the Guthrie bacterial inhibition assay (1960) it became possible to estimate the phenylalanine content of dried blood spots on a large scale and this became the method of choice for screening for phenylketonuria. In the Guthrie method discs from the blood spot are applied to a nutrient agar gel containing spores of *Bacillus subtilis*. The medium also contains β-thienylalanine which inhibits the growth of the organism, this inhibition being overcome by phenylalanine. Thus after an overnight incubation each blood disc is surrounded by a zone of bacterial growth, the higher the phenyalanine content of the disc, the larger the growth zone. Use of a blood-based assay for the metabolite immediately before the metabolic block increased the sensitivity of detection of impaired phenylalanine hydroxylation and enabled screening to be carried out at an earlier age. In the UK it is recommended that the test be performed on, or soon after, the sixth day of life, providing that full protein feeding has been established for at least 48 hours. Centralising testing in the laboratory allows for proper quality control and also for checking that all babies are being screened.

The introduction of blood testing for phenylketonuria produced almost universally about twice the number of patients anticipated, a common problem with screening programmes. A proportion of the excess could be ascribed to cases of classical phenylketonuria that would have been missed by the urine test but most was due to the detection for the first time of patients with mild to moderate impairments of phenylalanine hydroxylase activity. These variants raised difficult problems in drawing the dividing line for non-treatment.

Whilst many areas still use the original Guthrie method or an alternative specific fluorometric assay to screen for phenylketonuria alone, others have taken advantage of the availability of blood samples to screen for additional amino acid disorders.[13] One-dimensional chromatography has proved popular, over a quarter of the babies born in the UK being screened by chromatographic methods. The Efron technique uses dried blood spots. The Scriver method uses plasma and gives better chromatograms. Maple syrup urine disease, tyrosinaemia, some cases of homocystinuria, some of the urea cycle defects, and other rarer disorders may be detected in addition to phenylketonuria but except in special areas the yield of treatable disorders other than phenylketonuria is rather low.

TYROSINAEMIAS

Three well-recognised inherited disorders of tyrosine metabolism produce tyrosinaemia. The best known, *tyrosinaemia Type I* or tyrosinosis (McKusick 27670), affects predominantly the liver and kidneys and has clinical features which may be confused with those of hereditary fructose intolerance and transferase-deficiency galactosaemia. It has recently been shown that the majority of cases are due to fumarylacetoacetase (EC 3.7.1.2) deficiency. This enzyme is on the tyrosine degradation pathway but follows homogentisate dioxygenase (Fig. 4.5). As a deficiency of the latter enzyme causes homogentisic aciduria but not tyrosinaemia it follows that the amino acid abnormalities in tyrosinaemia Type I are secondary to liver damage. Indeed similar amino acid abnormalities are seen in advanced cases of galactosaemia and hereditary fructose intolerance. Tyrosinaemia Type I is therefore primarily a disorder of organic acid metabolism (see Ch. 5).

A rare condition, *hawkinsinuria*, so far reported only from Australia, is due to a blockage in one of the steps in *p*-hydroxyphenylpyruvic acid oxidation and results in transient tyrosinaemia in infancy. Hawkinsin, 2-cystein-*S*-yl-1,4-dihydroxycyclohex-5-enylacetic acid, is detectable on amino acid chromatography and is a conjugate of a reactive intermediate in the oxidation sequence. This is a dominant condition suggesting that successive steps in the overall reaction occur with the substrate closely associated with a multienzyme complex.

Tyrosinaemia Type II (McKusick 27660) is associated with hyperkeratotic erosions of the palms and soles, corneal erosion and ulceration and variably with mild to moderate mental retardation. The dermatological features were described as the Richner-Hanhart syndrome before the biochemical nature of the disease became apparent. The biochemical features are a marked tyrosinaemia of 0.7–3.4 mmol/l together with urinary excretion of excess tyrosine and *p*-hydroxyphenyllactic and *p*-hydroxyphenylpyruvic acids. The primary defect is in hepatic tyrosine aminotransferase (EC 2.6.1.5) which is responsible for the first step in tyrosine catabolism. This is a cytosolic enzyme. Mitochondrial aspartate aminotransferase will accept tyrosine as a substrate and this reaction occurring in tissues which lack p-hydroxy-phenylpyruvate dioxygenase accounts for the paradoxical high urinary output of p-hydroxy acids. A diet low in phenylalanine and tyrosine leads to rapid resolution of the dermatological problems and presumably if started early will remove the risk of mental retardation. Inheritance is autosomal recessive and the disease is particularly prevalent in populations of Italian origin.

Transient neonatal tyrosinaemia is particularly associated with prematurity and is ascribed to a temporary deficiency of p-hydroxyphenylpyruvate dioxygenase (EC 1.13.11.27) though there is no direct biochemical evidence for this. It is not usually treated, and probably has little ill-effect. It cannot be easily distinguished from Type II tyrosinaemia except for the generally lower tyrosine levels. The incidence has declined over recent years with the reduction in the protein level of artificial infant feeds and the trend to breast-feeding.

Other less well-defined disorders of tyrosine metabolism have been reported, some apparently due to defective p-hydroxyphenylpyruvate dioxygenase.

DISORDERS OF BRANCHED-CHAIN AMINO ACID CATABOLISM

The first two steps in catabolism are similar for the three branched-chain amino acids, leucine, isoleucine and valine (Fig. 4.7). In each case trans-amination yields the corresponding 2-oxo acid which then undergoes oxidative decarboxylation to yield a branched-chain carboxylic acid. This second step is mediated by the same enzyme for all three substrates.

Maple syrup urine disease (McKusick 24860)

In this disease there is deficient activity of the branched-chain oxo-acid dehydrogenase (2-oxoisovalerate dehydrogenase (lipoamide), EC 1.2.4.4). Many of the clinical and biochemical features of maple syrup urine disease are due to accumulation of the branched-chain 2-oxo acids but the striking accumulation of branched-chain amino acids often leads to the condition being diagnosed by amino acid chromatography. This accumulation reflects the reversibility of branched-chain amino acid transamination under physiological conditions. Leucine is usually the most markedly elevated amino acid, in plasma sometimes reaching 5 mmol/l, with isoleucine and valine around 1 mmol/l, giving rise to the alternative name of leucinosis. That valine accumulates to a smaller extent than might be expected is probably due to the very ready reduction of 2-oxoisovaleric acid to 2-hydroxyisovaleric acid. The 2-oxo acid arising from isoleucine retains a chiral centre at the 3-position and in maple syrup urine disease chemical racemisation followed by transamination gives rise to alloisoleucine, found in plasma at up to 0.4 mmol/l.

The classical form of maple syrup urine disease is associated with a

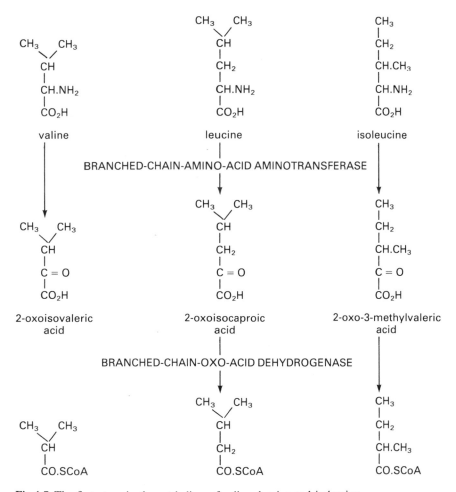

Fig 4.7 The first steps in the catabolism of valine, leucine and isoleucine.

virtual absence of branched-chain oxo-acid dehydrogenase activity whilst milder and intermittent forms show significant residual activity. A thiamine responsive variant is known. Dihydrolipoyl-CoA dehydrogenase deficiency will also produce biochemical features of maple syrup urine disease and branched chain amino acids are occasionally increased in some other organic acid disorders. For further details of maple syrup urine disease and these other conditions see Chapter 5.

Disorders of branched-chain amino acid transamination

The branched-chain amino acid transaminases so far isolated and studied in vitro have shown activity with all three natural substrates but two rare diseases in man are most easily explicable in terms of functionally separate transaminases. Hyperleucine-isoleucinaemia has been reported in two sibs who showed other unexplained biochemical abnormalities. Hypervalinaemia (McKusick 27710) has been found in three families and appears to be associated with mental retardation or neurological problems. Plasma valine concentrations were in the range 0.8–1.7 mmol/l.

DISORDERS AFFECTING SULPHUR-CONTAINING AMINO ACIDS

The pathway from methionine through cysteine to inorganic sulphate (Fig. 4.8) has long been assumed to be the major catabolic route. However transamination of methionine to 2-oxo-4-methylthiolbutyrate undoubtedly occurs in man, at least at high plasma methionine concentrations, and this may form the first step in an alternative catabolic pathway. The methionine to homocysteine sequence serves also to provide methyl groups for a variety of important metabolic reactions including catecholamine neurotransmitter inactivation and creatine synthesis. The demand for methyl groups usually exceeds the methionine supply and a remethylation cycle, converting homocysteine back to methionine, makes up the deficiency. Two remethylation reactions occur, one using betaine as the methyl donor, the other 5-methyltetrahydrofolate. Catabolism of homocysteine is by conversion to cystathionine as the first step in the transfer of the -SH group to cysteine. Cystathionine β-synthase requires pyridoxal phosphate as cofactor, as also does cystathionine-γ-lyase.

Hypermethioninaemia

Plasma levels of methionine exceeding 1 mmol/l have been reported in patients with a variety of clinical conditions and in apparently healthy individuals too. This cannot always be explained as a simple deficiency of methionine S-adenosyl transferase (EC 2.5.1.6) activity. The condition is probably harmless though in the absence of adequate biochemical characterisation of the underlying metabolic defect(s) and correlation of these with clinical disorders the possibility remains that this is a heterogeneous condition and that some forms are pathogenic. A mild degree of hypermethioninaemia is seen in cystathionine synthase deficiency (see below). More severe hypermethioninaemia associated with other amino acid abnormalities is found as a secondary feature of severe liver damage in, for example, advanced cases of tyrosinaemia Type I and uridyl transferase deficiency galactosaemia.

Homocystinuria: cystathionine synthase deficiency (McKusick 23620)

Biochemistry

Cystathionine-β-synthase (EC 4.2.1.22) deficiency leads to the accumulation and excretion of homocysteine, homocystine, cysteine-homocysteine

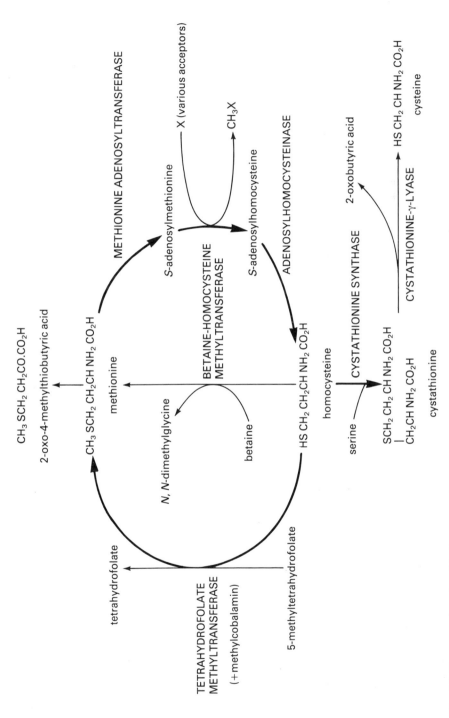

Fig. 4.8 The conversion of methionine to cysteine.

mixed disulphide and a number of other sulphur-containing amino acids. The homocystine levels in plasma range from 0.02–0.25 mmol/l and the 24 hour urine excretion may reach 2 mmol. Plasma methionine is usually increased (up to 2 mmol/l but usually much less) and plasma cystine tends to be low. These biochemical abnormalities are much less pronounced in some patients with pyridoxine-responsive homocystinuria (see below) and also vary with protein intake.

Diagnosis

Chromatographic examination of the urine is the most satisfactory method of detecting homocystinuria. Care is needed as in some patients, particularly in the neonatal period, homocystine is excreted in quite small quantities and unless it runs to a unique position in the system used it can easily be obscured by other amino acids. High-voltage electrophoresis at pH2 after hydrogen peroxide oxidation is very satisfactory. Normally at most only the faintest trace of homocystine should be seen, though small amounts may be excreted in cystinuria, during penicillin treatment and in deficiencies of pyridoxine or vitamin B_{12}. The cyanide-nitroprusside test is sometimes used as a preliminary screening test when homocystinuria is suspected but it may give false negative results, is less sensitive than chromatography, and gives positive results with other conditions such as cystinuria. Screening for cystathionine synthase deficiency in the neonatal period using chromatography or a bacterial inhibition test to detect hypermethioninaemia has proved unreliable as methionine is not always significantly increased at this time.

Whilst the increased plasma methionine concentrations usually found in cystathionine synthase deficiency distinguish this condition from the homocystinurias due to remethylation defects (see below) some older patients with untreated cystathionine synthase deficiency develop a partial defect in remethylation due to folate deficiency and may show normal methionine levels. In these cases the diagnosis may be confirmed by the increase in plasma methionine concentrations following correction of the folate deficiency or by assay of cystathionine synthase. This enzyme is widely distributed amongst the tissues and can be assayed in cultured fibroblasts and in phytohaemagglutinin-stimulated lymphocytes as well as in liver biopsy. Occasionally unexpectedly high residual activity is found in a patient with an otherwise typical biochemical and clinical picture.

Clinical features

Subjects with homocystinuria due to cystathionine synthase deficiency appear normal at birth but progressively develop a wide range of clinical abnormalities. Dislocation of the lens is the most universal finding. In mild cases this may be the first clear sign of the disease though it may be

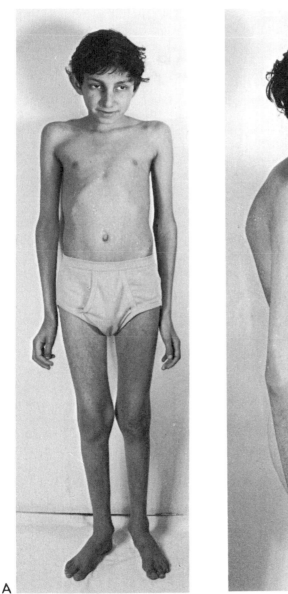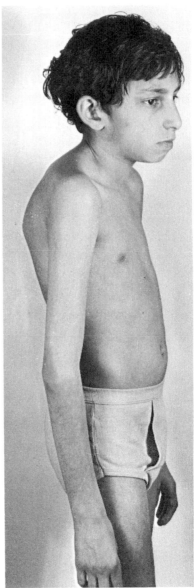

A   B

Fig. 4.9 A patient with untreated cystathionine synthase deficiency.

preceded by myopia. In severe cases mental retardation is usually the first sign and there may be convulsions. Osteoporosis is common, often leading to spinal deformity. In later childhood excessive lengthening of the arms, legs and often fingers occurs giving a physical appearance similar to that of Marfan's syndrome (Fig. 4.9). Knock knee often develops and the patient may walk like Charlie Chaplain. The clinical picture is further complicated by a marked tendency to arterial and venous thrombosis which may lead to a marked malar flush and livido reticularis. Thrombosis is a major cause of death.

Treatment

A marked biochemical response to high doses of pyridoxine (vitamin B_6) is seen in about half the patients. Responders presumably have a structural variant of cystathionine synthase apoprotein that leads to defective binding of the pyridoxal phosphate cofactor. The dose required varies, some patients responding to as little as 2 mg of pyridoxine per day, others requiring 500 mg/24 h. Some authorities hold that such high doses should be continued for several weeks before a patient is definitely classified as non-responsive but caution is required as very high doses of pyridoxine may produce sensory neuropathy in the adult. In general, patients who are found to respond to low doses of pyridoxine will have shown a mild clinical course prior to diagnosis. It may be necessary to correct any co-existing folate deficiency if the full response to pyridoxine is to be achieved.

Patients who do not respond adequately to pyridoxine should be treated with a low-methionine high-cystine diet, following the same general principles as those used in the treatment of phenylketonuria, maple syrup urine disease, etc, and monitoring plasma methionine and homocystine levels. Plasma cystine tends to remain low despite dietary supplementation. As an adjunct to this treatment supplementary betaine or choline may be administered to promote the remethylation of homocysteine. The long-term effects of treatment have not been evaluated in sufficient early-diagnosed patients to draw firm conclusions but it appears that in patients with the more complete deficiencies of cystathionine synthase activity the degree of dietary control achieved has not always been sufficient to completely halt the progression of the disease.

Genetics

Cystathionine synthase deficiency is inherited as an autosomal recessive disorder. The disease has a world-wide distribution. The estimated incidence in Northern Ireland is 4:100 000 but elsewhere it appears to be much less common. Obligate heterozygotes have on average less than half the normal cystathionine synthase activity in liver, cultured fibroblasts and phytohaemagglutinin-stimulated lymphocytes but individual results may be within the normal range. Carefully standardised methionine load tests with analysis of homocystine and other metabolites will also distinguish the majority of heterozygotes.[14] Overlap of the normal and heterozygote ranges is to be expected in view of the heterogeneity of the biochemical disorder in clinically affected patients, many of whom presumably carry different mutations on the homologous chromosomes. Prenatal diagnosis using cultured amniotic fluid cells should be possible.

Homocystinuria: remethylation defects

These conditions are less common than cystathionine synthase deficiency and are associated with impaired remethylation of homocysteine by 5-methyl-tetrahydrofolate. Two are well characterised, both showing moderate homocystinaemia, homocystinuria and sometimes cystathioninuria with normal or slightly low plasma methionine levels. Vascular changes similar to those in cystathionine synthase deficiency are seen.

Methylenetetrahydrofolate reductase deficiency (McKusick 23625)

In this disorder there is a reduced supply of 5-methyltetrahydrofolate for homocysteine remethylation. The clinical severity correlates with the decrease in methylenetetrahydrofolate reductase (EC 1.1.99.15) activity in cultured fibroblasts. The most severely affected cases die in early infancy with convulsions and other neurological symptoms. Less severe cases show mental retardation and spasticity and tend to die of thrombosis, presumably related to the homocystinuria. The late-onset form of the disease may present with a schizophrenia-like psychosis. There is no effective treatment.

Combined homocystinuria and methylmalonic aciduria (McKusick 27740 and 27741)

Methylmalonyl-CoA mutase (see Ch. 5) requires adenosylcobalamin as a cofactor. 5-Methyltetrahydrofolate-homocysteine methyltransferase requires methylcobalamin. Two closely-related defects in cytosolic cobalamin metabolism, so far only distinguished by fibroblast complementation studies, result in a deficiency of both cofactors and hence in combined methylmalonic aciduria and homocystinuria. The clinical course is usually severe with failure to thrive, developmental delay, seizures and early death. The exact sites of the defects have not been determined. Biochemical improvement has followed the administration of very large doses of hydroxycobalamin but it is not known if this treatment is clinically effective.

A combined methylmalonic aciduria and homocystinuria may develop in severe nutritional B_{12} deficiency and with defective B_{12} absorption.

Cystathionuria (McKusick 21950)

This is probably a harmless biochemical abnormality and is due to a deficiency of cystathionine-γ-lyase, the enzyme that converts cystathionine to cystine and 2-oxobutyrate. Cystathionine excretion varies with dietary methionine intake and may be as high as 12 mmol/24 h. In the majority of cases the cystathioninuria is reduced or abolished by large doses of pyridoxine. Diagnostic confusion may arise from bacterial contamination of cystathioninuric urine leading to the formation of homocystine. Cystathionine and homocystine may be excreted in modest quantities in pyridoxine deficiency.

Sulphite oxidase deficiency

Isolated deficiency of sulphite oxidase (EC 1.8.3.1) is extremely rare, having been reported in only two patients (McKusick 27230). Combined deficiency of sulphite oxidase and xanthine oxidase is slightly more common and is caused by deficiency of a specific pterin (molybdenum cofactor) necessary for the action of these molybdenum-requiring enzymes (McKusick 25215). Though not strictly amino acid disorders, both forms may be detected by the urinary excretion of S-sulphocysteine (1–7 mmol/g creatinine) formed by the reaction of sulphite with cyst(e)ine. Plasma cystine is very low and urinary taurine is increased. Both forms lead to severe neurological problems and early death. Dislocation of the occular lens often occurs. Patients with the molybdenum cofactor defect may show characteristic slight abnormalities in the shape of the head. No treatment is available but sulphite oxidase can be measured in cultured amniotic fluid cells and this should enable prenatal diagnosis.

DISORDERS OF UREA SYNTHESIS

Any impediment in the synthesis of urea, the main nitrogenous excretion product in man, leads to accumulation of the ammonium ion which is toxic. Thus most of the urea cycle disorders[15] share a similar spectrum of clinical presentations and many of the treatment strategies are common to the entire group. In addition to disorders directly or indirectly affecting the activity of urea-synthesising enzymes, pathological impairment of the urea cycle occurs in two other disorders which seem to be primarily amino acid transport defects.

Deficiencies of urea cycle enzymes

Biochemistry

The synthesis of urea (Fig. 4.10) starts with the formation of carbamoyl phosphate from inorganic ammonia. A second nitrogen atom is introduced in the form of aspartate, derived from oxaloacetate by transamination. The complete reaction is essentially confined to liver but the three enzymes catalysing the sequence from citrulline to ornithine are present in a variety of tissues. There is normally a slow net outflow of citrulline from the liver and uptake of arginine and ornithine so that this part of the cycle is physio-

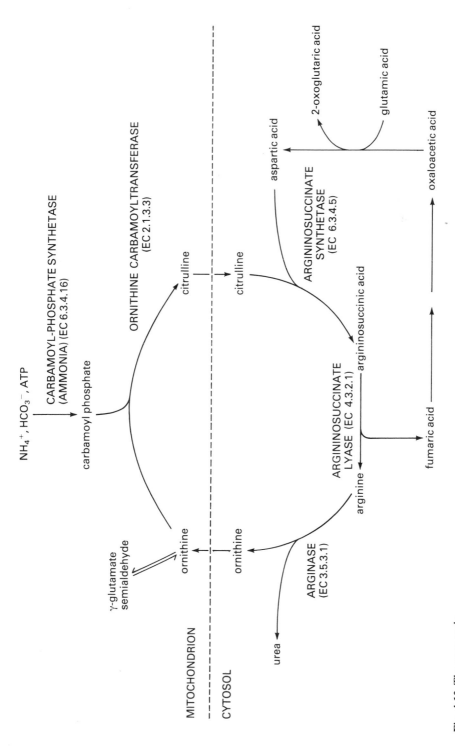

Fig. 4.10 The urea cycle.

logically active in peripheral tissues. Metabolic defects occur in the synthesis of carbamoyl phosphate and at each of the enzymatic steps of the cycle proper. *Ornithine carbamoyltransferase (transcarbamylase), deficiency* (McKusick 31125) is sometimes called hyperammonaemia Type I with *carbamoyl phosphate synthetase* deficiency as Type II (McKusick 23730). This terminology is confusing and has no advantages. Deficiencies of *argininosuccinate synthetase*, (McKusick 21570), *argininosuccinate lyase*, (McKusick 20790) and *arginase* (McKusick 20780) result in *citrullinaemia, argininosuccinic aciduria* and *argininaemia*, respectively and are often referred to under these names though again there is sometimes scope for ambiguity.

The simplest biochemical picture is seen in carbamoyl phosphate synthetase deficiency. Blood ammonia levels are much increased and glutamine, used to transport ammonia from the periphery to liver, is usually increased in plasma. Plasma glutamate is also increased and 2-oxoglutarate decreased because of the effect of the excess ammonia on the glutamate dehydrogenase reaction. Plasma alanine is raised and there may be other non-specific changes in plasma amino acids. Blood urea is often low. Carbamoyl phosphate synthetase requires N-acetylglutamate as an activator and in the single patient reported to have a deficiency of N-acetylglutamate synthetase the biochemical picture was similar to that of carbamoyl phosphate synthetase deficiency.

In ornithine carbamoyltransferase deficiency additional biochemical features stem from the accumulation of carbamoyl phosphate some of which passes into the cytosol and stimulates the synthesis of carbamoyl aspartate and thence pyrimidines. (Carbamoyl phosphate for pyrimidine biosynthesis is normally supplied by a cytosolic carbamoyl phosphate synthetase that uses glutamine as a substrate.) Orotic acid, uracil, and uridine are excreted in excess in urine.

All these biochemical features—hyperammonaemia, increased glutamine, and pyrimidinuria—are seen, though often to a lesser degree, in the remaining three urea cycle enzyme defects in addition to the specific amino acid accumulations. Urinary pyrimidines are excreted in unexpectedly large amounts in arginase deficiency, possibly due to the combination of low mitochondrial ornithine levels with a stimulation of N-acetylglutamate synthetase by arginine.

Clinical features

Hyperammonaemia is thought to be the main damaging factor in all the urea cycle defects other than arginase deficiency which is discussed separately below. The severity is very variable, each disorder having a form which proves rapidly fatal and milder forms usually with chronic presentations. Most patients who survive the first few days of life probably have residual enzyme activity.

The acute neonatal presentation is that of poor feeding, vomiting, lethargy, hypotonia or spasticity, irritability and twitching leading to convulsions, apnoea and death. Pulmonary and gastric haemorrhages occur particularly in deficiencies of carbamoyl phosphate synthetase or ornithine carbamoyl transferase. In the chronic presentation with non-specific mental retardation there is often some history of episodic vomiting, lethargy, irritability or headache, often associated with high-protein meals, to indicate occasional ammonia intoxication and there may have been seizures or even periods of coma. Some late onset cases remain healthy until presenting in infancy or later childhood as an acute illness, often associated with an infection. An adult-onset form of citrullinaemia is found particularly in Japan.

Brittle hair with trichorrhexis nodosa is often seen in argininosuccinate lyase deficiency but improves with age.

In arginase deficiency there are usually only minor symptoms of irritability and mild developmental delay in infancy but over the next few years progressive spasticity of the lower limbs, tremor, ataxia, choreoathetosis, seizures and severe mental retardation develop. These symptoms are presumed to be due mainly to direct toxic effects of arginine rather than to hyperammonaemia.

Diagnosis

Though all urea cycle disorders have hyperammonaemia as a common feature this is often intermittent in cases with sub-acute or late onset presentation. Deficiencies of argininosuccinate synthetase, argininosuccinate lyase and arginase are more easily detected by amino acid chromatography. In argininosuccinate synthetase deficiency plasma citrulline levels vary from 0.23 to over 4 mmol/l (normal 0.012–0.030 mmol/l) depending on protein intake and urinary citrulline is grossly increased (3–15 mmol/24 h). Care is needed in patients with plasma citrulline at the lower end of the quoted range to distinguish between argininosuccinate synthetase deficiency and the acute neonatal variant of pyruvate carboxylase deficiency (plasma citrulline approximately 0.2 mmol/l) described in Chapter 5. A modest increase in plasma citrulline is also seen in argininosuccinate lyase deficiency but here the outstanding feature is the gross excretion of argininosuccinic acid and its anhydrides (combined output 5–30 mmol/24 h), with lower levels (0.12–0.5 mmol/l) in plasma. Arginase deficiency leads to a 5–15 fold increase in plasma arginine. The urinary excretion is very variable and may be normal at times. When arginine is excreted in large amounts it is accompanied by lysine, cystine and traces of other amino acids giving a pattern rather like that seen in cystine-lysinuria due to defective renal tubular reabsorption. In all three disorders the specific amino acid abnormalities are accompanied by increased plasma and urinary glutamine levels and, particularly in the neonatal forms, by a number of less specific changes. Urinary pyrimidine excretion is increased.

The presumptive diagnoses of carbamoyl phosphate synthetase deficiency and ornithine carbamoyl transferase deficiency are usually made on the basis of hyperammonaemia (and increased plasma glutamine) in the absence of specific amino acid abnormalities. The increased urinary pyrimidine excretion secondary to accumulation of carbamoyl phosphate serves to distinguish ornithine carbamoyl transferase deficiency from carbamoyl phosphate synthetase deficiency and from N-acetylglutamate synthetase deficiency. Care is needed, however, not only with the technical aspects of blood ammonia estimation but also in interpretation. Asymptomatic hyperammonaemia occurs in a large proportion of neonates with birth weights under 2500 g, is also common following perinatal asphyxia, and accompanies certain types of infection. Valproate therapy is a common cause of mild hyperammonaemia and other drugs have from time to time been implicated. Hyperammonaemia also occurs in liver disease and is a particular feature of Reye's syndrome. Many of the organic acidaemias (Ch. 5) produce hyperammonaemia, probably by depleting hepatic intra-mitochondrial acetyl-CoA and thus preventing N-acetylglutamate synthesis, so that a careful examination for such disorders, particularly propionic acidaemia which is easy to miss, should be made in any child with hyperammonaemia and normal urinary orotic acid levels.

The urea cycle enzymes can all be assayed in a single needle biopsy specimen of liver.[16] Such direct enzyme assays are needed for the firm diagnosis of carbamoyl phosphate synthetase and ornithine carbamoyl transferase deficiencies but as liver biopsy is particularly hazardous in such patients the alternative source of the enzymes in rectal mucosa may be prefered. Other tissues, particularly cultured fibroblasts and lymphocytes, can be used to confirm argininosuccinate synthetase and argininosuccinate lyase deficiency if required, though for argininosuccinate lyase deficiency several studies have shown discordant results between liver and other tissues. Erythrocytes are a ready source of arginase and show the defect in argininaemia.

Treatment

The hyperammonaemia of the severe neonatal forms must be corrected promptly if irreversible neurological damage is to be avoided. Haemodialysis is the best method currently available for rapid removal of ammonia, though peritoneal dialysis is also effective.[17] Protein intake must be reduced to a minimum and essential amino acids may be supplied as their 2-oxo-analogues. Amino nitrogen may also be trapped and removed as hippuric acid by giving sodium benzoate orally or intravenously.[18] Phenylacetic acid, excreted as phenylacetylglutamine, may be used analogously but doubts persist as to its possible toxicity.

Restriction of dietary protein intake is the mainstay of long term treatment, particularly for the milder or late-onset forms of urea cycle disorder. If natural protein intake is to be kept very low supplementary essential amino acids may be needed and in all disorders except arginase deficiency supplementary arginine is beneficial. Chronic oral sodium benzoate is a very useful additional treatment. In argininosuccinate synthetase and argininosuccinate lyase deficiencies substantial amounts of nitrogen are eliminated in the urine as citrulline and argininosuccinate respectively. The excretion of these metabolites may be yet further increased by supplementing the supply of the ornithine skeleton, either as ornithine itself or as arginine. Intravenous arginine may be given acutely to forestall hyperammonaemic coma in the neonatal period and is undoubtedly beneficial but anxieties arise over possible long-term effects of the accumulating metabolites themselves.

In spite of very vigorous application of these and other treatment strategies, the neonatal onset forms of urea cycle disorders carry a very high immediate mortality rate. If hyperammonaemia is prolonged the survivors show considerable handicap. Life-threatening hyperammonaemic crises are apt to recur unpredictably. Patients with the milder varieties may show normal development if promptly recognised and effectively treated but they too are susceptible to hyperammonaemic crises, particularly during infectious illness. Though arginase deficiency is seldom associated with severe illness in the neonatal period, the long-term outlook is problematical as it is probably necessary to control the arginine accumulation as well as the hyperammonaemia.

Genetics

With the exception of ornithine carbamoyl transferase deficiency which is discussed in more detail below, the urea cycle disorders are inherited as autosomal recessive characters. Reduced levels of the appropriate enzyme have been demonstrated in various tissues of heterozygotes but the dependence of hepatic urea cycle enzyme activity on dietary protein intake must be remembered if this tissue is to be used for carrier detection. In practice carrier detection is of little importance as these urea cycle defects are sufficiently rare for the risk of a carrier marrying (non-consanguineously) another carrier to be very low.

The main preventive measure is prenatal diagnosis but this is not always straightforward. Carbamoyl phosphate synthetase deficiency can only be diagnosed by fetal liver biopsy. Cultured amniotic fluid cells have detectable levels of argininosuccinate synthetase, as measured directly or by the incorporation of ^{14}C from [carbamoyl-^{14}C] citrulline into protein as arginine, but activity varies with the cell type. The slower-growing epithelial cells have low activity whereas the fibroblastoid amniotic fluid cells show high activity. This leads to a very broad normal range and may cause difficulties if the index case showed significant residual activity. The citrulline concentration in the amniotic fluid may provide a better guide or fetal liver biopsy may be performed. Argininosuccinate lyase may be determined in cultured amniotic fluid cells, directly or by protein incorporation assay, or argininosuccinic acid may be determined in the amniotic fluid. Arginase deficiency can presumably be detected in the fetal erythrocytes obtained by fetoscopy. Though the use of all these techniques is growing rapidly the experience so far accumulated is limited. Therefore caution is required in performing and interpreting this type of investigation.

The gene for ornithine carbamoyl transferase is carried on the X-chromosome. Transmission from generation to generation is to be expected and in any one family the males will be more severely affected than the females. Where the male cases are mild or of late onset the female hemizygotes are usually clinically normal. Severe forms of ornithine carbamoyl transferase deficiency, usually lethal in the neonatal period in affected males, may also produce symptoms in the female hemizygotes. The severity of these symptoms is variable within a single family and reflects the degree to which Lyonisation, the random inactivation of one X-chromosome in each somatic cell, has been unfavourable to the normal allele. A mosaic of normal and ornithine carbamoyl transferase deficient cells can be demonstrated by enzyme histochemistry in the liver of affected females. As in other X-linked metabolic diseases it may be difficult to assess carrier status in apparently healthy females as the proportion of cells carrying the mutant gene may be very low. Needle biopsy may show an essentially normal activity of ornithine carbamoyl transferase activity. The urinary excretion of orotic acid following a protein load may be a better guide but a clear result in all cases cannot be expected.

Prenatal diagnosis by enzyme assay on fetal liver biopsy should be possible in the male but will be unreliable if the fetus is female. Probes for regions of the X-chromosome adjacent to the ornithine carbomoyl transferase gene are now available so that in favourable families early prenatal diagnosis by analysis of restriction fragment length polymorphism is possible. Markedly impaired ammonia metabolism in the mother may conceivably damage the fetus irrespective of its genetic composition, further complicating family studies. Ornithine carbamoyl transferase deficiency is probably the most common urea cycle defect and its X-linked mode of inheritance gives considerably greater scope for prevention by genetic counselling and prenatal diagnosis than the sporadically occurring disorders of enzymes coded on autosomal chromosomes.

Hyperammonaemic hyperornithinaemia with homocitrullinuria
(McKusick 23897)

The operation of the urea cycle within the hepatocyte requires the transport of ornithine into the mitochondria and citrulline out (Fig. 4.10). The mitochondrial ornithine transporter is thought to be defective in a syndrome characterized by hyperammonaemia, hyperornithinaemia and homocitrullinuria (HHH). The hyperammonaemia arises through the impairment of the urea cycle by mitochondrial ornithine deficiency and is accompanied by

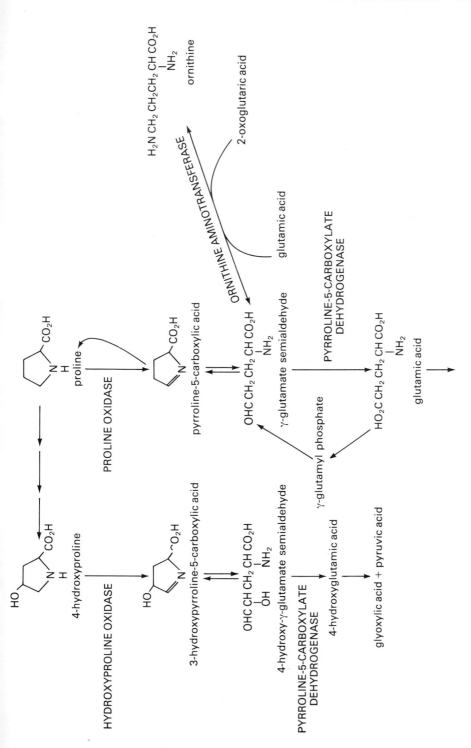

Fig. 4.11 The catabolism of ornithine, proline and hydroxyproline.

a modest orotic aciduria. Ornithine catabolism also occurs within the mitochondria so that extramitochondrial ornithine concentration is increased. The homocitrulline seems to be synthesised directly from lysine and its output increases with the plasma lysine concentration and the load on the urea cycle. Clinically HHH presents as a relatively mild urea cycle disorder with typical symptoms of intermittent hyperammonaemia, though spasticity is a marked feature in some of the older patients (cf. argininaemia).

Diagnosis is based on the finding of all three cardinal biochemical features (HHH) but the first clues may be difficult to spot. The hyperammonaemia is intermittent, though it can exceed 1 mmol/l. The hyperornithinaemia is relatively modest, 0.4–0.9 mmol/l compared to a normal of below 0.12 mmol/l, and could be missed in the many chromatographic systems where lysine and ornithine run together. In some patients the ornithinaemia gives rise to an overflow amino aciduria but in others the urinary amino acids appear normal except for the presence of homocitrulline. This may occur at levels of up 0.13 mol/ mol creatinine but may be barely noticeable during clinical remission. The widespread use of sterilised cows' milk formulae in infant feeding militates against a chance finding of homocitrullinuria being taken seriously. Urea is present in high concentration in cows' milk and during the heat treatment this carbamylates the *epsilon*-amino groups of protein lysyl residues, the homocitrulline thus produced being liberated during digestion and excreted in the urine. In an acutely ill infant an unequivocal diagnosis of HHH may be difficult to establish rapidly and confirmation may be obtained by demonstrating a reduced rate of incorporation of [14C] ornithine (as proline and glutamate, see Fig. 4.11) into cell protein by phytohaemagglutinin-stimulated lymphocytes or cultured fibroblasts. This will not distinguish HHH from ornithine aminotransferase deficiency (see below) but this latter disorder is unlikely to be under consideration in the ill infant.

Treatment is primarily by protein restriction. Some patients respond to ornithine supplementation (oral ornithine or arginine hydrochlorides) with a reduction in hyperammonaemia. A parallel increase in the rate of ornithine-14C incorporation into protein in response to increased ornithine concentration in the medium has been shown by fibroblasts from an ornithine-responsive patient and this may provide a convenient way of assessing ornithine-responsiveness in vivo. The association of hyperornithinaemia with gyrate atrophy of the choroid and retina (p. 127) should prompt caution in the long-term use of ornithine supplements. So far no patient with HHH has shown any indication of these occular lesions.

Lysinuric protein intolerance (McKusick 22270)

Defective urea cycle operation in this disorder is evident from post-prandial hyperammonaemia and increased orotic acid excretion. The disorder is ascribed to a functional deficiency of ornithine in the hepatic mitochondria but the exact mechanism is problematical [19]. Defective transport of dibasic amino acids at the baso-lateral membrane of the jejunal epithelium has been clearly demonstrated and is also present in the renal tubule. Plasma concentrations of ornithine, arginine and lysine are subnormal but the citrulline concentration is elevated. Paradoxically the overall concentrations of these amino acids in liver are normal or increased. Diagnosis is based on the finding of a dibasic amino aciduria (usually without cystinuria) together with low plasma dibasic amino acid concentrations and hyperammonaemia.

The disease is particularly common in Finland (approximately 1.3:100 000 births) but is also found elsewhere. The symptoms include those of intermittent hyperammonaemia but lens opacities, hyperelastic skin, hyperextensible joints, and sparse, brittle hair are also commonly found. Treatment consists of a protein-restricted diet and supplementary citrulline.

ORNITHINE AMINOTRANSFERASE DEFICIENCY (McKusick 25887)

Ornithine synthesis and degradation (Fig. 4.11) are mediated by the same enzyme, ornithine-oxoacid aminotransferase (EC 2.6.1.13) which is present in the mitochondria of many cell types. Deficiency of this enzyme leads to hyperornithinaemia (0.4–1.4 mmol/l) with normal or low blood ammonia levels and no homocitrullinuria. A cystine-lysine-ornithinuria may be present.

The main clinical feature of ornithine aminotransferase deficiency is progressive loss of vision due to a characteristic degeneration (gyrate atrophy) of the choroid and retina. Symptoms usually become apparent in the first decade of life and progress to produce complete blindness at ages varying between 20 and 50 years. Histological changes are seen in liver mitochondria and in muscle but are asymptomatic.

Ornithine aminotransferase is a pyridoxal phosphate requiring enzyme and a minority of patients respond biochemically (and presumably clinically) to large doses of pyridoxine. In the absence of any clear idea of the direct cause of the gyrate atrophy, no generally agreed treatment strategy for pyridoxine unresponsive ornithine aminotransferase deficiency has emerged. The slow and irregular progression of the untreated disease makes it impossible to evaluate treatments except over a very long period. Plasma ornithine levels may be reduced to near normal by restricting dietary arginine intake but as ornithine cannot be synthesised in the absence of ornithine aminotransferase care is needed to avoid ornithine deficiency which rapidly leads to hyperammonaemia. Based on the finding of low creatinine excretion, the administration of creatine (1.5 g/24 h orally) has also been tried and improves the histological appearance of muscle. Proline supplementation has been used to correct a hypothetical deficiency of proline in the retina, where both ornithine aminotransferase and pyrrolidone-5-

carboxylate reductase are normally particularly active. None of these approaches can yet be confidently recommended.

Ornithine aminotransferase deficiency is inherited as an autosomal recessive condition, can readily be detected in fibroblasts and presumably would be susceptible to prenatal diagnosis using cultured amniotic fluid cells.

NON-KETOTIC HYPERGLYCINAEMIA (McKusick 23830)

Hyperglycinaemia is a non-specific feature of several organic acidurias and in these cases is usually associated with intermittent ketosis (Ch. 5). Non-ketotic hyperglycinaemia[20] is a specific disorder of glycine catabolism due to a defect in the glycine cleavage system (Fig. 4.12). This system is present in liver, brain, and probably other organs but not in cultured fibroblasts. Four proteins are involved in the overall reaction: a pyridoxal phosphate dependent glycine decarboxylase (P-protein), a lipoic acid containing aminomethyl carrier protein (H-protein), a lipoamide dehydrogenase (L-protein) and a tetrahydrofolate-requiring methylene-group acceptor (T-

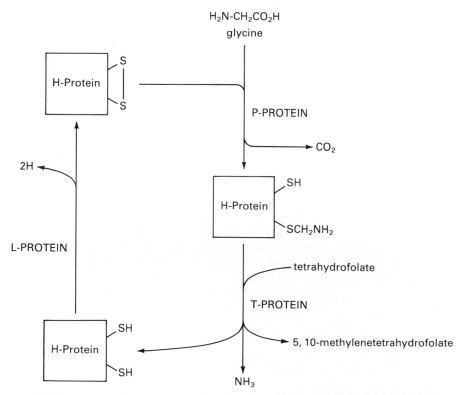

Fig. 4.12 The glycine cleavage system. H-protein is the aminomethyl-carrier protein and contains lipoic acid. P-protein is a pyridoxal phosphate dependent glycine decarboxylase. L-protein is a lipoamide dehydrogenase.

protein). In the majority of cases of non-ketotic hyperglycinaemia the site of the defect has not been determined but of three studied in detail, two had a deficiency of the decarboxylase and one had a deficiency of the methylene group acceptor.

In the most common form of non-ketotic hyperglycinaemia acute neurological problems may begin only a few hours after birth and generally in the first week of life. Somnolence, lethargy and lack of spontaneous movement progress to deep coma with apnoeic spells. Exaggerated reflexes may be present and there may be myoclonic seizures. The EEG shows a pattern of very low activity interspersed with occasional high-amplitude synchronous bursts. This abnormal pattern may be shown 30 min after birth in spite of apparent clinical normality at this stage. Milder forms of non-ketotic hyperglycinaemia may show rather non-specific mental retardation though some later-onset patients show rapid neurological deterioration. As yet we cannot correlate the clinical variability with the biochemical heterogeneity.

Diagnosis is based on the finding of hyperglycinaemia and hyperglycinuria in the absence of an organic acid disorder. These abnormalities may be obvious but in a minority of cases the diagnosis must be actively sought as the plasma glycine levels may be only marginally increased and the glycinuria modest. If a diagnosis of non-ketotic hyperglycinaemia is suspected on clinical grounds a quantitative amino acid analysis of plasma is mandatory. Spurious hyperglycinaemia can develop in infants fed on very low protein diets. Determination of CSF glycine will provide supporting evidence of non-ketotic hyperglycinaemia since, at least in the more severe forms of the disease, the CSF/plasma ratio (0.2–0.33 compared with normal 0.02–0.03) as well as the absolute CSF glycine concentration (0.09–0.36 mmol/l, normal 0.004–0.010) are abnormally high. Glycine is an important inhibitory neurotransmitter in the central nervous system where the glycine cleavage system may well play a role in terminating its action. In patients with ketotic hyperglycinaemias (secondary to defects in organic acid metabolism) the CSF/plasma glycine ratio is similar to that in normal children, suggesting that in these disorders the liver is the main site of inhibition. This would explain how patients with propionic acidaemia and similar diseases can tolerate high plasma glycine concentrations without severe neurological symptoms.

Treatments aimed at reducing the overall glycine levels in the body by restricting supply or removal as conjugates have met with varied success as measured by the plasma glycine concentration but have been uniformly unsuccessful in allowing normal intellectual development. Supplementing the supply of various cofactors has been equally unsuccessful where it has been tried but there is no reason to suppose that cofactor responsive variants might not occur. Improvement in neurological function can be rapidly achieved by blocking glycine receptors with high doses of strychnine but in most cases the long-term results have been disappointing. A similar approach uses diazepam in high dosage[21] but has not yet been fully evaluated. Prenatal diagnosis using cultured amniotic fluid cells or by amino acid analysis of amniotic fluid has so far proved impracticable, though diagnosis by fetal liver biopsy is a theoretical possibility.

DEFECTS IN LYSINE DEGRADATION

The pathways for lysine catabolism are summarised in Figure 4.13. The major route is through saccharopine, 2-oxoadipic acid and glutaryl-CoA. Three inborn errors of metabolism are known to affect the early part of this pathway—hyperlysinaemia, saccharopinuria, and α-aminoadipic aciduria. In addition, pipecolic acid, apparently an intermediate on a minor metabolic pathway of lysine, is excreted in excess in Zellweger's disease which is possibly due to a defect in peroxisome assembly (see Ch. 5). Pipecolic acid gives a rather unstable ninhydrin coloration, more red-violet than the normal amino acid colour and with an intense red fluorescence in ultraviolet light. Zellweger's disease is untreatable but amenable to antenatal diagnosis.

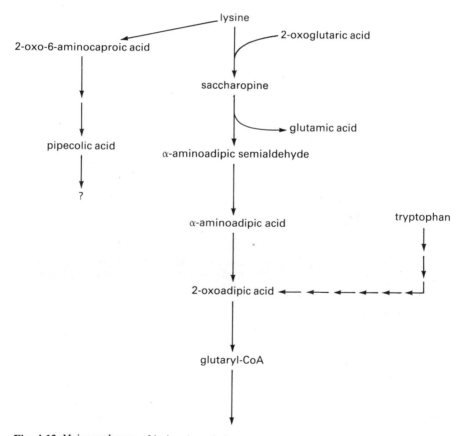

Fig. 4.13 Major pathways of lysine degradation.

Hyperlysinaemia (McKusick 23870)

In this moderately rare condition plasma lysine concentrations range up to 1.5 mmol/l and large amounts of lysine but not of other dibasic amino acids or cystine are excreted in the urine. The lysine metabolites α-N-acetyl-lysine, ϵ-N-acetyl-lysine, homocitrulline and homoarginine are also excreted in excess. The basic defect is in lysine-2-oxoglutarate reductase. This enzyme and saccharopine dehydrogenase are probably combined in a single protein, 'α-aminoadipic semialdehyde synthetase', and at least some patients with hyperlysinaemia have a combined deficiency of both enzymes. A variety of clinical symptoms have been described in association with hyperlysinaemia, mental retardation being prominent. However a limited prospective study[22] based on sibs of index cases and cases detected by neonatal screening suggests that the association of disease and hyperlysinaemia is in most cases fortuitous.

'Congenital lysine intolerance with periodic ammonia intoxication' (McKusick 23875) has been reported as a single case which is not easily explained in terms of current biochemical knowledge. Whilst there are theoretical reasons to predict that accumulation of lysine might interfere with the urea cycle, most cases of hyperlysinaemia show at most only marginally increased blood ammonia levels. Plasma lysine is sometimes increased in infants with ornithine carbamoyl transferase deficiency.

Saccharopinuria (McKusick 26870)

A deficiency of saccharopine dehydrogenase has been reported in only three patients. Saccharopine is excreted in large amounts (2 mmol/24 h) together with lysine, α-aminoadipic acid and, in one patient, citrulline. The clinical significance of this metabolic anomaly is unknown.

α-Aminoadipic aciduria (McKusick 20475)

Excessive excretion of 2-hydroxyadipic and 2-oxoadipic acids accompanies the α-aminoadipic aciduria in most, and possibly all, cases of this disorder. The output of these metabolites is very variable, all in the range 0.05–1.5 mmol/24 h. Plasma α-aminoadipic acid, below 5 μmol/l normally, is from 30–120 μmol/l. A deficiency of 2-oxoadipate dehydrogenase has been demonstrated in some cases but in another a defect in mitochondrial α-aminoadipate aminotransferase (EC 2.6.1.39) seemed more likely. The clinical presentations of the 11 cases so far reported have been very varied and could well be unrelated to the biochemical defect.

HISTIDINE METABOLISM

Histidinaemia (McKusick 23580)

The first step in the metabolism of histidine is the elimination of ammonia

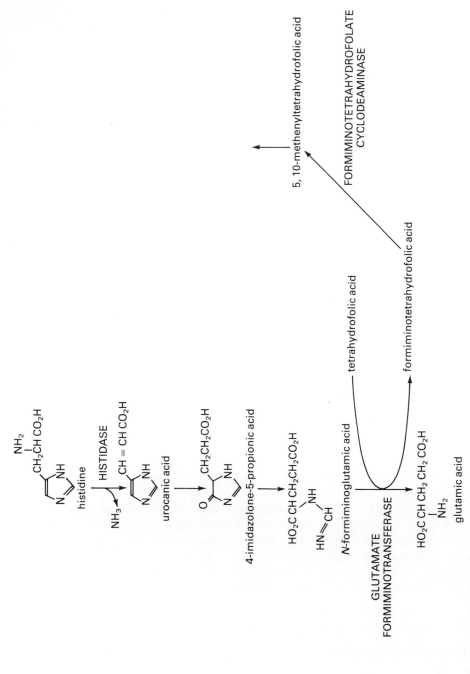

Fig. 4.14 Histidine catabolism.

to form urocanic acid (Fig. 4.14). The enzyme histidine ammonia lyase (histidase, EC 4.3.1.3) is absent in histidinaemia. Histidine accumulates, plasma concentration 0.3–1.6 mmol/l (normal 0.05–0.2 mmol/l), and is excreted in excess in urine. Transamination leads to Imidazolepyruvic acid, Imidazolelactic acid and Imidazoleacetic acid. With ferric chloride solution Imidazolepyruvic acid gives a green coloration, similar to that given by phenylpyruvic acid only more transient, so that there is a danger of confusion with phenylketonuria. Histidine ammonia lyase can be measured in liver biopsy or in fresh skin, but not in cultured fibroblasts.

In Caucasian populations histidinaemia occurs with a frequency approaching that of phenylketonuria and it is also common in Japan. For some years it was believed that histidinaemia caused mental retardation, generally less severe than that seen in phenylketonuria and with a high proportion of patients with speech difficulties. However it has slowly become apparent that for the vast majority histidinaemia is a harmless biochemical anomaly, though the possibility remains that for a small number of individuals, at most 1%, histidinaemia has been a contributing factor in the development of some form of central nervous system dysfunction. This subject, and the difficulty of reconciling data from retrospective study of selected (diseased) populations with that derived from whole population screening has been well reviewed by Scriver and colleagues.[23,24,25] Similar problems have arisen for other amino acid disorders and are particularly difficult to resolve for rare conditions.

Formiminoglutamic aciduria (McKusick 22910)

Further catabolism of urocanic acid produces formiminoglutamic acid (FIGLU, Fig. 4.14). The formyl group is then passed to tetrahydrofolate to form in turn 5-formiminotetrahydrofolate and 5, 10-methyltetrahydrofolate. Patients described as having formiminotransferase deficiency are suspected to fall into two groups[26]. A deficiency of glutamate formininotransferase (EC 2.1.2.5) itself results in excretion of FIGLU (up to 3.9 mmol/l) and a relatively mild clinical presentation, mainly of psychomotor retardation and hypotonia. A second type, reported from Japan, results in severe mental and physical retardation with cortical atrophy. This type has a partial deficiency of glutamate formiminotransferase, coupled (it is hypothesised) with a severe deficiency of formiminotetrahydrofolate cyclodeaminase (EG 4.3.1.4). The excretion of FIGLU is less marked than in isolated formiminotransferase deficiency. In both types urinary FIGLU may at times be normal and a histidine load test should be performed if the diagnosis is doubtful.

FIGLU does not normally react with ninhydrin though it may give a weak colour with some formulations and if the chromatogram is overheated. However it decomposes to glutamic acid in alkaline chromatographic solvents or may be revealed by ninhydrin after in situ conversion to glutamate by exposure of the chromatogram to ammonia vapour. FIGLU also gives a peak on some automatic amino acid analysers.

DISORDERS OF PROLINE AND HYDROXYPROLINE METABOLISM

Proline is oxidised to pyrroline-5-carboxylic acid (which is in equilibrium with γ-glutamate semialdehyde) by proline oxidase, an enzyme that is tightly bound to the inner mitochondrial membrane (Fig. 4.11). γ-Glutamate semialdehyde can then be oxidised to glutamic acid by pyrroline-5-carboxylate dehydrogenase (EC 1.5.1.12) or can be converted to ornithine by ornithine aminotransferase. In *hyperprolinaemia Type 1* (McKusick 23950) proline oxidase activity is absent and proline accumulates in tissues (concentration in plasma 0.7–2.6 mmol/l) and is excreted in excess in the urine. In *hydroxyprolinaemia* (McKusick 23700) there is a deficiency of the specific hydroxyproline oxidase, leading to increased tissue levels of hydroxyproline and to increased urinary excretion. In *hyperprolinaemia Type 2* (McKusick 23951) pyrroline-5-carboxylate dehydrogenase activity is deficient. This enzyme participates in the degradation of proline, hydroxyproline and ornithine but only proline accumulates, again giving hyperprolinaemia (up to 2.8 mmol/l in plasma) and prolinuria. The urine does however also contain pyrroline-5-carboxylic acid (0.10–0.24 mmol/g creatinine) and 3-hydroxypyrroline-5-carboxylic acid. Both types of hyperprolinaemia show increased urinary excretion of hydroxyproline and glycine due to partial saturation by proline of common renal transport sites. All three conditions are believed to be harmless.

Prolidase (proline dipeptidase, EC 3.4.13.9) cleaves proline or hydroxyproline from the C-terminus of peptides. *Prolidase deficiency* (McKusick 26413) results in the accumulation and excretion of proline- and hydroxyproline-containing peptides derived from the turnover of collagen and other proteins. These peptides form an elongated streak in many one-dimensional chromatographic systems, darker areas marking the positions of the major peptides such as glycylproline and leucylproline. Urinary bound proline and hydroxyproline are much increased. The diagnosis may be confirmed by assay of prolidase in erythrocytes, leucocytes or cultured fibroblasts, affected subjects generally showing less than 7% of normal activity.

Patients with this disorder show a wide range of symptoms, dermatitis and leg ulceration being the most common. Splenomegaly, mental retardation and bony deformities, particularly affecting the shape of the skull, are also frequently seen. A preliminary report[27] suggests that treatment with oral manganese salts and supplementary ascorbic acid (vitamin C) is beneficial.

SPECIFIC DEFECTS OF RENAL TRANSPORT

There are many amino acid transport systems in the body. Of those concerned with transport within the cell, the systems of the mitochondrial inner membrane have been particularly well studied. They are in general highly specific, mediating the transport of a single metabolite or the counter-transport of a metabolically-related pair. Some information is available on transport across the lysosomal membrane (see cystinosis p. 91). Transport systems across the outer cell membrane vary with cell type and function, and in epithelial cells from one face of the cell to another. Most of the systems studied in vitro will transport a range of amino acid substrates and most amino acids seem to be transported by more than one system. In vivo such transport systems are most conspicuous by their absence and the clearest examples are seen when the deficiency is expressed in the renal tubules.

Cystine-lysinuria (McKusick 22010)

The formation of cystine stones in bladder or kidney has been a recognised phenomenon for over 150 years, the name cystine being derived from the greek *kystis* (bladder). Cystinuria was one of Garrod's original four inborn errors of metabolism. It is now recognised that the defect in cystinuria lies not in the metabolism of cystine but in its transport by the renal tubule since plasma cystine levels are normal or even low. In the most common form (cystine-lysinuria) the cystinuria is accompanied by excessive excretion of lysine, ornithine, and arginine which share with cystine a high affinity (low Km) renal tubular transport system. This transport system is not expressed in cultured fibroblasts but many cystinuric patients show intestinal malabsorption of cystine and the dibasic amino acids indicating that the affected transport system is normally active at the brush border membrane. The unabsorbed dibasic amino acids are converted by bacterial action to putrescine, cadaverine and related products that may then appear in the urine. In those patients with a severe defect in the intestinal transport system some uptake of the affected amino acids still occurs in the form of dipeptides which are hydrolysed intracellularly by the mucosal cell. By contrast, in lysinuric protein intolerance (p. 126) the intestinal defect in dibasic amino acid transport is at the basolateral membrane of the mucosal cell so that intestinal absorption as free amino acids or as dipeptides is equally affected, the lysinuria in this condition showing that a transport system of this type also exists in the kidney.

Isolated cystinuria (no excessive excretion of dibasic amino acids) is rarer than combined cystine-lysinuria and is thought to reflect a defect in a low-affinity transport system that is not shared with the dibasic amino acids. Hyper-dibasic aminoaciduria without cystinuria, which is very rare, is presumably due to a defect in the low-affinity transport system specific for the dibasic amino acids. Thus it appears that in the kidney and probably many other organs there is a multiplicity of transport systems, the malfunction of any one of which can significantly affect the overall efficiency of amino acid transport in the organ concerned.

Diagnosis and classification

Diagnosis is based on the demonstration of grossly excessive urinary excretion of the appropriate amino acid(s) in the absence of any increase in their plasma concentration and, in the case of hyper-dibasic aminoaciduria, the absence of hyperammonaemia after a protein load. Amino acid excretion patterns superficially similar to those in cystine-lysinuria may be seen at times in hyperargininaemia and in hyperlysinaemia, the excessive load of the amino acid primarily affected hindering renal reabsorption of others sharing the same transporter.

The grossly excessive excretion of cystine in cystine-lysinuria and in isolated cystinuria may be detected by the cyanide-nitroprusside test. Though this is a convenient side-room test for the renal clinic the use of solid sodium cyanide under these conditions is hazardous, and doubtful or false-positive results are common. In the laboratory context this test is not worth performing if the specimen is to be examined for amino acids in any case. The other classical procedure, microscopy of urine sediment, has more to recommend it, in that the demonstration of the characteristic hexagonal crystals of cystine at least confirms that cystine is present in potentially stone-forming concentrations, but should not be relied on to definitely exclude the possibility of significant cystinuria.

The excretion of amino acids in homozygous cystine-lysinuria is rather variable, ranging from 2–3, 4–13, 2–8, and 1–6 mmol/g creatinine for cystine, lysine, arginine and ornithine respectively. The disorder is clearly heterogeneous. Some heterozygotes for cystine-lysinuria excrete cystine and lysine at about one tenth the levels seen in the homozygous condition whilst others show no excessive excretion and this is used as a basis for classification. In Type 1 cystine-lysinuria the heterozygotes show no abnormality in urinary amino acid excretion and the homozygotes have a complete deficiency in intestinal absorption of cystine and dibasic amino acids. In Type 2 the heterozygotes show the amino aciduria but the homozygotes have some residual activity for the intestinal transport of cystine (but not lysine). Some authorities recognise a third type, similar to Type 2 but with a less severe intestinal transport defect.

Clinical expression and treatment

The only medical problems clearly associated with defects in the renal transport of cystine are those due to stone formation. Symptoms may first occur at any time from infancy to old age but onset is most common in the second and third decades of life. Renal colic, urinary obstruction, recurrent infection, and progressive loss of renal function develop as in urolithiasis from other causes.

Biochemical treatments aim at preventing saturation of the urine with cystine. Restriction of methionine intake, unless very drastic, probably has little effect on plasma cystine concentrations and hence on the filtered load. The simplest therapeutic measure is to maintain a high water intake so that the urine is always dilute. This requires particular attention at night, when the most concentrated urine is usually produced, and is not without its inconveniences. Alkalinisation of the urine by oral intake of sodium bicarbonate or citrate should help to decrease the possibility of the urine becoming saturated as the solubility of cystine increases rapidly at pH >7.5. Small stones may even redissolve. If these simple measures fail, treatment with D-penicillamine, N-acetylpenicillamine or mercaptopropionylglycine, all of which form soluble mixed disulphides with cystine, may be effective but these drugs, particularly penicillamine, have severe side-effects in some patients. Without adequate treatment chronic renal failure can result and renal transplantation may be necessary. The transplanted kidney will not be affected by the transport defect elsewhere in the body and should remain disease-free (see cystinosis, p. 91, and hyperoxaluria, p. 208).

Cystine-lysinuria can easily be detected in neonatal urine screening programmes. The incidence detected by such programmes has ranged from 6–50:100 000 which is much higher than that expected from the prevalence of cystine stones. Presumably many biochemically affected individuals never develop clinically significant stones so that the institution of alkalinisation and hydration therapy on a lifelong basis following such neonatal detection does not seem justified.

There have been several reports of an increased frequency of cystine-lysinuria in mentally retarded or psychiatrically disturbed populations but the reason for this association is unclear[28]. It is also unclear whether isolated hyper-dibasic aminoaciduria (very rare) has any clinical significance.

Iminoglycinuria (McKusick 24260)

The iminoacids proline and hydroxyproline share a renal tubular transport site with glycine. Deficient carrier activity at this site results in an hereditary iminoglycinuria. As in cystine-lysinuria different types occur, some of which also express the transport defect in the intestine. Heterozygotes may show isolated glycinuria. For a full discussion see Scriver[29]. These abnormalities appear in general to have no clinical significance. Though the earliest cases were discovered in the course of investigation of patients with mental retardation or convulsions subsequently the disorder has been found in healthy individuals. Babies discovered to have iminoglycinuria by newborn screening have remained healthy without treatment. The temptation to dismiss all the reported associations of iminoglycinuria with disease as coincidental is very strong. However, there is a multiplicity of transport systems within the body and, at present, methods of characterising them are much less developed than methods for the investigation of enzyme defects. Given this heterogeneity the possibility that in some cases the particular transport defect expressed in the kidney may have more serious effects elsewhere cannot be discounted, lysinuric protein intolerance being an example where this effect has been easy to demonstrate.

Transient iminoglycinuria due to immaturity of renal transport systems occurs frequently in the neonatal period. Iminoglycinuria also occurs through competition at the shared renal site(s) in hyperprolinaemia and hyperhydroxyprolinaemia, but not in hyperglycinaemia.

Hartnup disease (McKusick 23450)

This is a combined renal and intestinal transport defect affecting predominantly the neutral amino acids, especially alanine, asparagine, glutamine, threonine, serine, the branched-chain amino acids, tryptophan, tyrosine, phenylalanine and histidine. These are present in the faeces and are excreted in excess in urine. Bacterial action on unabsorbed tryptophan in the gut gives rise to the rich variety of indoles that are excreted in urine in this condition. Plasma concentrations of the affected amino acids tend to be low.

The affected members of the Hartnup family, in whom the disease was originally discovered, showed symptoms only intermittently. The most striking problem was a pellagra-like rash, but there was also a cerebellar ataxia and psychological changes. These symptoms are relieved by oral nicotinamide and, though only a small proportion of tryptophan is converted to nicotinamide, are most likely to be due to nicotinamide deficiency secondary to the tryptophan malabsorption. The skin rash has been the most commonly reported symptom in subsequently diagnosed cases of Hartnup disease but expression seems to require some marginal degree of nutritional inadequacy. In newborn screening programmes in USA and in Australia Hartnup 'disease' has been detected with a frequency of 5.6 and 4.3 per 100 000 births respectively. However, the clinical presentation is virtually unknown in these areas, which traditionally have a high meat consumption, and the condition is regarded as harmless. In this context it is interesting to note that tryptophanaemia (probably due to tryptophan pyrrolase deficiency) also appears to be asymptomatic.

OTHER DISORDERS

It has not been possible to cover all the known abnormalities of amino acid metabolism in man in this chapter. Of the better defined conditions, sarcosinaemia[30] (McKusick 26890), carnosinaemia, (McKusick 21220), hydroxylysinuria (McKusick 23690) and β-alaninaemia (McKusick

$23740)^4$ are the most obvious omissions and the reader is referred to the larger monographs[2,31,32] for information. Except for β-alaninaemia there is a strong possibility that these disorders are benign. In addition there are many individual reports in the literature which cannot be interpreted satisfactorily from the clinical or biochemical points of view and their elucidation must await the discovery of further similar cases. Certain disorders discussed here in other chapters may also be detected through abnormalities of amino acid excretion. In addition to those examples already mentioned in passing, aspartylglycosaminuria may be detected by the excretion of asparaginyl-N-acetylglucosamine (p. 89), hypophosphatasia by increased phosphoethanolamine excretion, some instances of generalised deficiency of acyl-CoA dehydrogenation by the associated sarcosinaemia and sarcosinuria (p. 189) and some disorders of pyruvate metabolism by the associated hyperalaninaemia. Generalised amino aciduria may provide a clue to cystinosis (p. 91) and other causes of Fanconi syndrome, Wilson's disease (p. 392) and galactosaemia (p. 36).

ACKNOWLEDGEMENTS

We would like to thank Mrs A Green and Dr B L Priestley for Figures 4.1 & 4.9 respectively.

REFERENCES

1 Smith I, Seakins J W T (eds) 1976 Chromatographic and electrophoretic techniques. Vol 1: Paper and thin layer chromatography. Vol 2: Zone electrophoresis. Heinemann, London

2 Bremer H J, Duran M, Kamerling J P, Przyrembel H, Wadman S K 1981 Disturbances of amino acid metabolism: clinical chemistry and diagnosis. Urban and Schwarzenburg, Baltimore

3 Bickel H 1980 Phenylketonuria: past, present and future. Journal of Inherited Metabolic Disease 3: 123–132

4 Francis D E M 1987 Diets for sick children, 3rd edn. Blackwell Scientific Publications, Oxford

5 Smith I, Lobascher M E, Stevenson J E et al 1978 Effects of stopping low-phenylalanine diet on intellectual progress of children with phenylketonuria. British Medical Journal 2: 723–726

6 Guttler F, Hansen G 1977 Heterozygote detection in phenylketonuria. Clinical Genetics 11: 137–146

7 Woo S L C 1984 Prenatal diagnosis and carrier detection of classical phenylketonuria by gene analysis. Pediatrics 74: 412–423

8 Levy H L, Waisbren S E 1983 Effects of untreated maternal phenylketonuria and hyperphenylalaninemia on the fetus. New England Journal of Medicine 309: 1269–1274

9 Dhondt J L 1983 Tetrahydrobiopterin deficiencies: preliminary analysis from an international survey. Journal of Pediatrics 104: 501–508

10 Matalon R 1983 Current status of biopterin screening. Journal of Pediatrics 104: 579–581

11 Leeming R J, Barford P A, Blair J A, Smith I 1984 Blood spots on Guthrie cards can be used for inherited tetrahydrobiopterin deficiency screening in hyperphenylalaninaemic infants. Archives of Disease in Childhood 59: 59–61

12 Medical Council Steering Committee for the MRC/DHSS Phenylketonuria Register 1981 Routine neonatal screening for phenylketonuria in the United Kingdom 1964–1978. British Medical Journal 282: 1680–1684

13 Bickel H, Guthrie R, Hammersen G (eds) 1980 Neonatal screening for inborn errors of metabolism. Springer, Berlin

14 Sardharwalla I B, Fowler B, Robins A J, Komrower G W 1974 Detection of heterozygotes for homocystinuria: study of sulphur-containing amino acids in plasma and urine after L-methionine loading. Archives of Disease in Childhood 49: 553–559

15 Urea cycle symposium 1981 Pediatrics 68: 271–297, 446–462

16 Nuzum C T, Snodgrass P J 1976 Multiple assays of the five urea-cycle enzymes in human liver homogenates. In: Grisolia S, Baguena R, Mayor F (eds) The urea cycle, Wiley, New York, ch 21, p 325–349

17 Wiegand C, Thompson T, Bock G H, Mathis R K, Kjellstrand C M, Mauer S M 1980 Management of life-threatening hyperammonemia—a comparison of several therapeutic modalities. Journal of Pediatrics 96: 142–144

18 Batshaw M L, Brusilow S, Waber L, et al 1982 Treatment of inborn errors of urea synthesis: activation of alternative pathways of waste nitrogen synthesis and excretion. New England Journal of Medicine 306: 1387–1392

19 Rajantie J, Simell O, Perheentupa J 1983 'Basolateral' and mitochondrial membrane transport defect in the hepatocytes in lysinuric protein intolerance. Acta Paediatrica Scandinavica 72: 65–70

20 Carson N A J (ed) 1982 Selected reviews from the workshop on non-ketotic hyperglycinaemia. Journal of Inherited Metabolic Disease 5 suppl 2: 105–128

21 Matalon R, Naidu S, Hughes J R, Michals K 1983 Nonketotic hyperglycinemia—treatment with diazepam, a competitor for glycine receptors. Pediatrics 71: 581–584

22 Dancis J, Hutzler J, Ampola M G et al 1983 The prognosis of hyperlysinemia: an interim report. American Journal of Human Genetics 35 438–442

23 Scriver C R, Levy H L 1983 Histidinaemia. Part I: Reconciling retrospective and prospective findings. Journal of Inherited Metabolic Disease 6: 51–53

24 Rosenmann A, Scriver C R, Clow C L, Levy H L 1983 Histidinaemia. Part II: Impact: a retrospective study. Journal of Inherited Metabolic Disease 6: 54–57

25 Coulombe J T, Kammerer B L, Levy H L, Hirsch B Z, Scriver C R 1983 Histidinaemia. Part III: Impact: a prospective study. Journal of Inherited Metabolic Disease 6: 58–61

26 Rowe P B 1983 Inherited disorders of folate metabolism. In: Stanbury J B, Wyngaarden J B, Fredrickson D S, Goldstein J L, Brown M S (eds) The metabolic basis of inherited disease, 5th edn. McGraw-Hill, New York, p 498–521

27 Charpentier C, Dagbovie K, Lemonier A, Larregue M, Johnstone R A W 1981 Prolidase deficiency with iminodipeptiduria: biochemical investigations and first results of attempted therapy. Journal of Inherited Metabolic Disease 4: 77–78

28 Scriver C R, Whelan D T, Clow C L, Dallaire L 1970 Cystinuria: increased prevalence in patients with mental disease. New England Journal of Medicine 283: 783–786

29 Scriver C R 1983 Familial iminoglycinuria. In: Stanbury J B, Wyngaarden J B, Fredrickson D S, Goldstein J L, Brown M S (eds) The metabolic basis of inherited disease, 5th edn. McGraw-Hill, New York, p 1792–1803

30 Levy H L, Coulombe J T, Benjamin R 1984 Massachusetts Metabolic Disease Screening Program: 3: Sarcosinemia. Pediatrics 74: 509–513

31 Nyhan W L 1984 Abnormalities of amino acid metabolism in clinical medicine. Appleton-Century-Crofts, Norwalk

32 Stanbury J B, Wyngaarden J B, Fredrickson D S, Goldstein J L, Brown M S (eds) 1983 The metabolic basis of inherited disease, 5th edn. McGraw-Hill, New York

Disorders of organic acid metabolism

INTRODUCTION

General concepts and definitions

Disorders of organic acid metabolism, more commonly refered to as organic acidurias or organic acidaemias, comprise a diverse group of diseases whose biochemistry encompasses several areas of intermediary metabolism. These include metabolic pathways associated with amino acid metabolism, particularly of L-leucine and other branched-chain amino acids, of L-lysine and of aromatic amino acids, pathways associated with fatty acid metabolism and ketogenesis and also of pyruvate and carbohydrate metabolism including the tricarboxylic acid (TCA) cycle. These disorders share the common feature that they are characterised by the accumulation in body tissues and fluids, particularly urine, of organic acids and their esters and conjugates. Organic acids in this context are carboxylic acids that may contain a variety of other functional groups, for example hydroxyl, oxo (keto) and imino, and include conjugated organic acids, for example acyl-glycines and conjugates with other amino acids, including glutamate and aspartate, and glucuronides, but excludes the amino acids themselves. The characteristic features of such organic acids are high water solubility, acidity and ninhydrin-negativity and the range of biochemical and chemical properties are wide and not limited to relatively few compounds as in the case of physiological amino acids.

In addition to the common features of chemistry and biochemistry these disorders of intermediary metabolism also share some common clinical characteristics, the patients frequently presenting with acute symptoms in early life with acidosis, ketosis, vomiting, convulsions and coma. The disorders are often lethal in the newborn and young child and survivors may be physically or mentally handicapped. Although the incidence of individual diseases may be low, collectively their overall incidence may be as high as 1:3000 liveborn infants, thus presenting a significant clinical and clinical biochemical challenge. Early and precise diagnosis is thus essential since this, coupled with adequate early therapy, may result in greatly improved prognosis with normal subsequent physical and mental development. Other patients may present later in childhood with established failure to thrive or with sudden acute and profound attacks associated with infections and trauma, and careful investigation of such patients for metabolic disease is important.

As a result of their common clinical features, the organic acidurias cannot be diagnosed on purely clinical grounds and organic acid analysis, particularly with use of gas chromatography and mass spectrometry, and other biochemical investigations, are essential for their specific and unambiguous characterisation. Most of these disorders are of proven autosomal recessive inheritance and good genetic counselling and prenatal diagnosis form an essential part of the overall care of the families in which an index case has been identified. This is discussed generally in more detail below in addition to specific examples related to individual diseases.

Diagnosis and screening for the organic acidurias

The primary population at risk for the organic acidurias are acutely ill newborns and infants, since most organic acidurias, including those that may be associated with neurological and physical handicap in later years, present with acute life-threatening illness in the newborn and infant and it is these patients who need to be investigated in detail using the most comprehensive screening methods available. A suitable screening protocol is shown in Figure 5.1 which is also applicable to those presenting in later childhood with failure to thrive and with acute symptoms indicative of a possible underlying metabolic disease. The latter patients include those presenting acutely with Reye's syndrome-like attacks after a previous uneventful history but who may have an underlying metabolic disorder, for example in fatty acid metabolism. The initial clinical presentation giving suspicion of a metabolic disorder prompts the initiation of routine first-line tests and biochemistry designed to rapidly exclude traumatic, infective and acquired disorders (Fig. 5.1), while also providing further indicators for possible metabolic disorders. Second-line tests provide further indicators prior to introduction of more specific and diagnostic tests including quantitative organic acid and amino acid analysis of blood and urine. These latter tests should not be considered as part of the screening tests for metabolic diseases since they are in themselves specific diagnostic procedures. More than one sample should ideally be analysed in order to exclude transient metabolic disorders and careful interpretation of the results is necessary with due attention being made to effects of diet and drugs employed at the time of sampling. Samples obtained during the initial acute phases of an illness are essential to detect those diseases associated with an intermittent abnormal organic aciduria, for example dicarboxylic acidurias due to medium-chain acyl CoA dehydrogenase deficiency. The use of such a screening protocol outlined in Figure 5.1, combined with good analytical methods for organic acids and other metabolites, would be expected to result in the detection

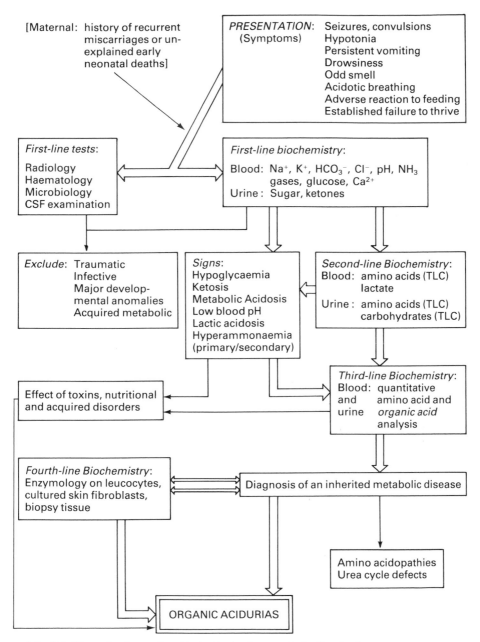

Fig. 5.1 Diagnosis of organic acidurias (and other metabolic disorders).

and diagnosis of the organic acidurias, the amino acidopathies and the hyperammonaemias, comprising in total some two-thirds of the known inherited metabolic diseases, while also providing valuable information and aids towards the diagnosis of other diseases.

Following the diagnosis made from organic acid analysis, further investigations may be introduced ('fourth-line biochemistry') including enzymology on cultured skin fibroblasts, leucocytes or other biopsy material.

Analytical methods for organic acids

The wide variety of organic acids present in human physiological fluids, particularly urine, and especially from patients with disorders of organic acid metabolism and during acute episodes, necessitates the use of a chromatographic procedure to separate the individual components and to identify and quantify them. While simpler procedures, including paper and thin-layer chromatography, have been used successfully in preliminary analyses, and liquid chromatography has been favoured for limited applications,[1] in practical terms the use of gas chromatography is essential for the analysis of organic acids. Most of the known organic acidurias were identified with the use of gas chromatography and gas chromatography-mass-spectrometry (GC-MS) but with the development of capillary gas chromatography, particularly with fused silica columns and chemically-bonded stationary phases, most quantitative and much qualitative diagnostic analysis of organic acids can be achieved with use of gas chromatography alone, although GC-MS is still essential for more detailed studies, quantitation at low concentrations and unambiguous identifications and diagnoses. The current availability of small dedicated and easily-operated GC-MS instruments has placed GC-MS within the capabilities of most large clinical biochemistry departments and has permitted the further development of laboratories capable of diagnosing the organic acidurias. The use of other analytical techniques, particularly proton nuclear magnetic resonance spectroscopy (^{1}H-nmr), for the rapid diagnosis of both organic acidurias and amino acidopathies in unextracted biological fluids, may offer new advances for the future[2] but the very costly instrumentation required precludes extension of this approach outside all but the most specialised laboratories.

Urine is the most readily-available physiological fluid for diagnostic and study purposes, particularly from an acutely-ill baby or young infant, and is obtainable by essentially non-invasive methods. For these reasons urine has been the most extensively studied fluid and has further advantages in that any organic acids that accumulate in blood plasma are also excreted into the urine. In addition many acids are found in measureable quantities only in urine and hence these disorders of organic acid metabolism are characterised more generally by an abnormal organic aciduria than by an organic acidaemia. Random clean urine samples are sufficient for diagnostic purposes while for detailed patient monitoring and therapeutic studies, timed (for example 6-hour) collections are preferred. Because complete 24-hour collections are extremely difficult to obtain and often of less value in detailed studies, and random specimens are frequently employed, an endogenous internal standard to which to relate organic acid concentrations is essential in order to correct for widely differing urine flow rates and volumes. The most widely used standard is creatinine, the excretion of which is related to mean muscle mass and, while not the perfect standard, particularly in young metabolically-unwell infants, it is the generally accepted standard, with results being expressed in terms of mg/g creatinine or mmol/mol creatinine, for example. Heparinised blood plasma is also analysed, with methods scaled to deal with the small volumes available (100–200 μl) and results are expressed in volume terms, for example μmol/l.

Extraction of organic acids from physiological fluids

The organic acids present in urine and other fluids must be extracted as a group prior to gas liquid chromatographic analysis, in order to separate them from neutral and basic components present in the fluid. Organic acids may be extracted from protein-free fluids by solvents, anion-exchange methods or with use of silicic acid columns (Fig. 5.2). The most widely employed methods are those involving solvent extraction with diethylether and ethylacetate and anion-exchange extraction with DEAE-Sephadex. For solvent extraction, acidified urine or other fluid is saturated with salt and extracted successively with diethylether and ethylacetate, the extracts are combined and reduced to dryness with a stream of dry nitrogen gas. Prior stabilisation of keto acids is necessary, usually by alkyloxime formation. Solvent extraction is at best only semi-quantitative, with many polyfunctional acids remaining unextracted, and the analysis may be complicated by the co-extraction of neutral metabolites and by enhanced artefact formation from drugs and dietary metabolites. DEAE-Sephadex extraction is used to quantitatively extract acids as a group, with prior or subsequent alkyloxime stabilisation of keto acids. The acids are usually eluted from the column with aqueous pyridinium acetate buffer and the eluate freeze-dried (lyophilised) prior to derivative preparation and chromatography. Anion exchange analysis may be complicated by the co-extraction of inorganic anions, for example sulphate and phosphate, but these potential problems are generally overcome with the use of capillary gas chromatographic columns. Fuller details of these procedures are given in more specialised texts.[1,3]

Derivative preparation and gas-liquid chromatography

The high polarity, low volatility and thermal instability of the majority of organic acids necessitates their conversion into suitable derivatives prior to gas-liquid chromatography. Many derivatives have been employed but those most favoured are the trimethylsilyl (TMS) esters. Trimethylsilylating reagents, for example BSTFA (N,O-bistrimethylsilyl-trifluoroacetamide), react with all active hydrogens present in the molecule and thus, in addition to esterification of the carboxylic acid group, replace hydrogens on hydroxyl

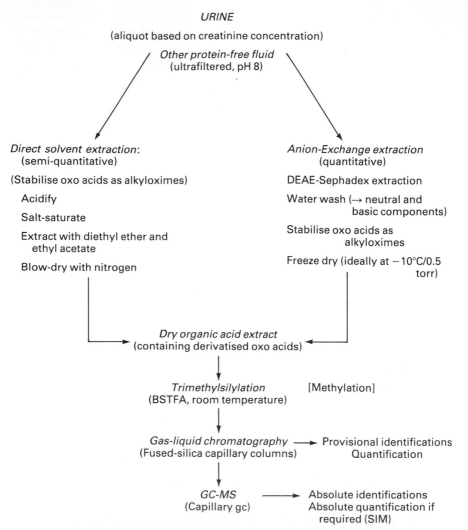

URINE
(aliquot based on creatinine concentration)

Other protein-free fluid
(ultrafiltered, pH 8)

Direct solvent extraction:
(semi-quantitative)

(Stabilise oxo acids as alkyloximes)

Acidify

Salt-saturate

Extract with diethyl ether and
ethyl acetate

Blow-dry with nitrogen

Anion-Exchange extraction
(quantitative)

DEAE-Sephadex extraction

Water wash (→ neutral and
basic components)

Stabilise oxo acids as
alkyloximes

Freeze dry (ideally at −10°C/0.5
torr)

Dry organic acid extract
(containing derivatised oxo acids)

Trimethylsilylation   [Methylation]
(BSTFA, room temperature)

Gas-liquid chromatography ⟶ Provisional identifications
(Fused-silica capillary columns)   Quantification

GC-MS ⟶ Absolute identifications
(Capillary gc)   Absolute quantification if
required (SIM)

Fig. 5.2 Analysis of physiological fluids for organic acids. (For abbreviations see pp. 144, 145, 149)

groups to give TMS ethers, hydrogens on imino groups to give N-TMS derivatives and react similarly with amino groups if present. The reagents and the derivatives are highly moisture-sensitive and dry conditions are required for their use: the products are however very non-polar and volatile and ideally suited for gas-liquid chromatography. In addition to TMS derivatives, methyl esters are also employed in some laboratories, with diazomethane generated as required by alkali action on N-methyl-N-nitroso-p-toluene-sulphonamide. The diazomethane is distilled into diethyl-ether and the solution in ether is used for derivative preparation.

Diazo-methane forms methyl esters with carboxylic acid groups but may form partial methyl ethers with hydroxyacids and generally these derivatives are of less utility than the TMS derivatives, although favoured for some purposes. Keto (oxo) acids present special problems because keto-enol tautomerism will result in two derivatives being formed on esterification (keto ester and enol ether-ester). Such acids are stabilised, either prior to extraction or prior to derivative preparation, by formation of oxime derivatives, with O-ethyloximes (ethoximes) being most favoured.[1,3] In addition to these alkyloximes, quinoxalinols of α-keto (2-oxo) acids have also been usefully employed.

The derivatised organic acids are separated and quantified using temperature-programmed gas-liquid chromatography, in earlier work using glass columns packed with non-polar (for example SE30, OV1, OV101 methylsilicone oils) or polar (for example SE52, OV17, OV22 phenylmethylsilicones) stationary phases on inert deactivated diatomaceous earth supports[3], and more recently on fused silica capillary columns coated with chemically-bonded non-polar or polar phases.[4] Quantification is by reference to internal standards added to the biological fluid prior to extraction or more usually to hydrocarbon standards added during derivative preparation, and the use of response factors for individual acid derivatives, calculated from analyses with authentic standards taken through the same procedure.[5] Compounds are identified by reference to retention data, usually expressed in terms of methylene units[6] but absolute identifications necessitate the use of GC-MS. Extensive compilations of retention index data are available[3,4,7] and modern microprocessor-based instruments with programming facilities enable production of data tabulated with retention time, retention index in methylene units, peak areas and final quantification. Capillary gas-liquid chromatography also has application to specific problems, for example the separation and characterisation of enantiomers of hydroxyacids such as lactic acids and glyceric acids.

Gas chromatography-mass spectrometry

The introduction of capillary gas liquid chromatography on fused silica columns, with the associated improvements in peak separation and reproducibility of retention data of individual components, has greatly improved the quality and reliability of identifications made by gas chromatography alone. Despite these advances, the complexity and variety of organic acids present in physiological fluids, particularly urine, and especially during crises in patients with metabolic disorders, still necessitates the use of gas chromatography-mass spectrometry for their absolute and unambiguous identification. Indeed, the use of fused silica capillary GC-MS has provided the most powerful analytical tool for the study of the organic acidurias.

The processes involved in the GC-MS of organic acids have been reviewed elsewhere[3] but essentially the derivatised organic acids, as they

are separated and elute from the gas chromatographic column, are introduced into the source of the mass spectrometer where they are subjected
to an ionisation process, generally by bombardment with an energised electron beam, electron impact ionisation (EI) or, less usually, by secondary
ionisation induced by collision with an ionised reagent gas such as
ammonia, chemical ionisation (CI). In EI, the electron beam is generated
from a heated filament and the electrons so produced are accelerated,
producing positive ions of separated components presented as neutral
molecules from the gas chromatograph, by transfer of the electron energy.
The excess energy transferred can only be dissipated by resonance stabilisation or by fragmentation of the molecule:

eg:

$$\begin{array}{l} [XZ]^{+}_{\bullet} + Y \\ [XZ]^{+}_{\bullet} + Y\bullet \end{array} \Big\} \quad \text{rearrangements}$$

$$XYZ + e \longrightarrow [XYZ]^{+} + 2\,e \quad \text{molecular ionisation}$$

$$[XYZ]^{+}_{\bullet} \; \Big\} \begin{array}{l} \longrightarrow [XY]^{+} + Z\bullet) \\ \longrightarrow [YZ]^{+} + X\bullet) \end{array} \quad \text{primary cleavages}$$

$$\longrightarrow \text{secondary decompositions}$$

The pattern and intensities of the ions produced in EI are characteristic
of the parent molecule from which it may be identified either by reference
to a mass spectral library or, with previously-unidentified compounds, by
study of the fragmentation pattern and processes, coupled with accurate
mass measurements to aid deduction of the elemental composition of both
parent molecule and ions where possible. In addition, CI will give precise
measurement of the molecular mass of the parent molecule, with little or
no fragmentation of the molecule concerned. In this process, the reagent
gas (ammonia, methane, isobutane etc) is introduced into the ion source at
a relatively high pressure (1 torr) and is ionised preferentially to produce
positively-charged species that then interact with the sample components,
with the latter becoming ionised by proton transfer to produce M^+ and $(M
+ 1)^+$ species in a low energy ionisation reaction.

In the GC-MS process, repetitive scanning with the mass spectrometer
throughout the GC analysis produces a series of spectra from which the
individual component peaks may be identified. The quantity of data
produced (for example, more than 1500 spectra from a 30 minute capillary
GC analysis, using a relatively slow scan speed of one scan over the full
mass range per second), coupled with the need for subsequent data
processing and library searching, makes the use of an on-line data system
(DS) essential and most instruments used are in the form of combined GC-
MS-DS instruments. The detail of such processes and the interpretation of
the spectra produced have been reviewed elsewhere,[3] together with
compilations of mass spectral data of derivatised organic acids. In addition,

in both EI and CI, individual characteristic ions may be monitored selectively (SIM) for accurate quantification against appropriate internal standards and this is of particular value where low concentrations and very precise data are to be measured, for example in prenatal diagnosis of the organic acidurias by direct chemical analysis of amniotic fluid (see below).

Treatment and prognosis of the organic acidurias

Treatment

The large majority of patients with organic acidurias present with acute illness often with associated vomiting, (metabolic) acidosis, ketosis, hypoglycaemia and/or hyperammonaemia. Thus the immediate therapeutic measures undertaken, generally before a precise diagnosis has been made, are generally common to all or most organic acidurias, irrespective of the primary defect: they involve management of the acute episodes by supportive therapy, accompanied by detoxification measures to remove any accumulating metabolites and potentially toxic intermediates. Thus, assisted ventilation, control of acidosis with, for example, bicarbonate, restriction or cessation of protein intake accompanied by oral or i.v. glucose to maintain calories and counter hypoglycaemia, and increased fluid (saline) intake to counter the frequently-associated dehydration and electrolyte loss, are supportive measures introduced to any patient in an acute metabolic crisis. Such crises are often precipitated by an intercurrent infection and this must also be sought for and treated actively where possible. Detoxification measures especially in acute and unresponsive ketoacidosis include exchange transfusions, peritoneal dialysis or forced diuresis.[8] It is most important that such treatment is introduced immediately at first presentation (but not delaying the collection of samples for diagnosis) and not after a more specific diagnosis is made. These patients will often present to local and district hospitals and it is here that this immediate therapy must be instituted. Delay means the eventual referral of the patient, often in a coma, to a more central paediatric hospital where adequate treatment may be applied too late to prevent irreversible neurological damage, giving rise to the poor prognosis often ascribed to many of the treatable organic acidurias.[8]

Once a more specific diagnosis has been established, perhaps by referral of the appropriate diagnostic specimens to a regional centre, more specific and individual therapeutic measures suited to particular disorders may be instituted. Such measures, directed towards the long-term management of the patient concerned, may involve environmental manipulation by reduction of the load of substrate presented to the mutant or absent enzyme, including use of dietary restriction, inhibition of substrate synthesis, substrate removal and coenzyme supplementation at pharmacological levels (Table 5.1). Rarely, where the product of the missing or impaired enzyme

Table 5.1   Treatment of Organic Acidurias

1. Dietary and nutritional management	Protein restriction (1–1.5 g/kg 24 h) Amino acid supplementation Hypercaloric diet Low fat if indicated Frequent feeding, nocturnal/nasogastric if necessary Mineral and vitamin supplements.
2. Co-factor therapy (pharmacological doses)	Hydroxocobalamin (B_{12}) (deoxyadenosylcobalamin?) D-biotin Riboflavin Pyridoxine (Thiamine)
3. Substrate removal	Glycine (isovaleric acidaemia) L-carnitine
4. L-carnitine	(Only in acute episodes in some disorders)

reaction is an important intermediate, product replacement may also be attempted.

The most important general approach to the treatment of the organic acidurias is undoubtedly dietary manipulation, not only by protein restriction, perhaps to 1 to 1.5 g/kg body weight/24 h, but also with use of amino acid supplements omitting those amino acid precursors associated with the particular disorder, to give an adequate amino acid and protein intake for normal growth and development and tailored to the specific requirements of the disease and individual patient. Additional supplements of selected amino acids have also been recommended (e.g. alanine, selected branched-chain acids) to promote growth. The use of hypercaloric diets, particularly during acute episodes, may be advantageous to prevent catabolism, and frequent feeding, either orally or via nasogastric tube, including nocturnal feeding, may prove effective. Mineral and vitamin supplements are also required when partially artificial diets are employed in order to avoid specific deficiencies, such as that of zinc, with the associated secondary clinical complications. Close collaboration between paediatrician, dietitian and biochemist is essential in providing the optimum care and management of patients with organic acidurias. In other organic acidurias, for example defects in β-oxidation of fatty acids and ketogenesis, with associated profound hypoglycaemic attacks and dicarboxylic aciduria, the use of low fat, high carbohydrate diets is of value. In such disorders, the use of medium-chain triglycerides in the diet is to be avoided although such supplements may be of value in the treatment of patients with defects in long-chain fatty acid β-oxidation. Patients with other organic acidurias may also show secondary dicarboxylic aciduria and appropriate measures need to be included in their management (see below).

The second most effective approach to treatment of the organic acidurias, based on the primary defect being associated with a mutant enzyme, rather than total absence, is the use of cofactors at pharmacological doses. Some patients with methylmalonic aciduria may respond to high dose vitamin B_{12} treatment, preferably using hydroxycobalamin, given in doses of 1 mg/24 h intramuscularly or 10 mg/24 h orally, with considerable reduction in the excretion of methylmalonate by enhancement of residual enzyme activity. Similarly, D-biotin, in doses of 10 mg/24 h orally, abolishes the abnormal organic aciduria and prevents the clinical symptoms in patients with multicarboxylase deficiency caused by either holocarboxylase synthetase deficiency or secondary to biotinidase deficiency. Some patients with dicarboxylic aciduria caused by medium-chain acyl CoA dehydrogenase deficiency, or with ethylmalonic-adipic aciduria, may respond well to riboflavin therapy, as do some patients with glutaric aciduria.

Cofactor therapy may also be of value in activating alternative metabolic pathways for substrate removal. An example is of the use of pyridoxine at pharmacological doses in the treatment of some patients with primary hyperoxaluria (glycollic aciduria): in this disorder glyoxylate accumulates because of essentially unidentified disorders in its metabolism, resulting in secondary reduction to glycollate and oxidation to oxalate. Oxalate accumulates in tissues and body fluids leading to renal stones, renal failure and heart block with death in early adult life. The transamination of glyoxylate to glycine is pyridoxine (vitamin B_6) dependent and some patients respond effectively to pyridoxine treatment, with reduced excretion of both oxalate and glycollate. Substrate removal is also an effective means of therapy in isovaleric acidaemia where isovaleryl CoA accumulates because of a specific dehydrogenase deficiency: isovaleryl groups are effectively conjugated with glycine via the action of glycine-N-acylase and glycine therapy has proved valuable in the treatment of such patients, especially during acute episodes, although conjugation with L-carnitine may be better for long-term therapy.

Many organic acidurias including isovaleric acidaemia, propionic acidaemia and methylmalonic aciduria are associated with the accumulation in tissues of acyl CoA esters with consequent toxic effects due directly to the acyl CoA esters and to metabolites produced by alternative pathways. Among the secondary effects of acyl CoA accumulation is the sequestration of available free coenzyme A, resulting in severe inhibition of CoA-dependent metabolic processes including pyruvate oxidation, the tricarboxylic acid cycle and β-oxidation, resulting in secondary lactic acidosis and dicarboxylic aciduria. L-carnitine (4-trimethylamino-3-hydroxybutyric acid) is important in the modulation of the availability of free CoA and may exchange readily with acyl CoA esters to form acylcarnitine esters via the action of carnitine acyltransferases and this occurs in many of the organic acidurias, presumably as an attempt to detoxify acyl CoA esters accumulating in the mitochondria and increasing the removal of acyl moieties into the urine. As a consequence, patients with many organic acidurias exhibit increased acylcarnitine excretion with consequent L-carnitine insufficiency or deficiency and L-carnitine has been advocated and used in the treatment of patients with these diseases, both in acute and long-term therapy. L-carnitine has been of particular value in the treatment of patients with propionic acidaemia, methylmalonic aciduria and isovaleric acidaemia[9] and in the acute treatment of patients with medium-chain acyl CoA dehydrogenase deficiency and 3-hydroxy-3-methylglutaric aciduria, although in the latter disorders it is perhaps contra-indicated for long term maintenance therapy because of the enhancement of long-chain fatty acid transport into the mitochondria for β-oxidation. The efficacy of L-carnitine as a therapeutic measure in the organic acidurias requires careful assessment in each disorder concerned and the individual patient's response to treatment also requires careful monitoring.

Prognosis

The increased efficacy of the combinations of early diagnosis, adequate acute treatment and therapeutic advances and improvements (and understanding) in maintenance care of the patients concerned, particularly with dietary, cofactor and L-carnitine therapy, has greatly improved the prognosis of patients with organic acidurias. Formerly, the large majority of patients with these diseases died during the early months or years of life with surviving patients showing severe neurological problems, poor development and greatly reduced life expectancy, with a totally inadequate quality of life. Long-term survivors were almost certainly those with milder 'variants' of the disorders concerned. Effective and early treatment has demonstrated that many patients with these disorders can show relatively normal growth and development, particularly if successful treatment and management is achieved during the early developmental years of life. Medium-chain acyl CoA dehydrogenase deficiency and 3-hydroxy-3-methylglutaric aciduria can be considered to be treatable disorders, despite their associated acute and profound hypoglycaemic and Reye's syndrome-like attacks, and the prognosis for patients with disorders such as isovaleric acidaemia and methylmalonic aciduria is also much improved. However, it is possibly too early to be definitive about the longer term survival of patients with some of these diseases, particularly those with propionic acidaemia, despite the survival now of some patients into their second and even third decades of life, and long-term assessment is still required in this area. Other disorders, for example glutaric aciduria Type II (presumed electron-transfer flavoprotein dehydrogenase deficiency; multiple acyl CoA dehydrogenase deficiency), are associated with severe and acute neonatal problems and intrauterine disorders or, for example glutaric aciduria Type I (glutaryl CoA dehydrogenase deficiency), with severe progressive and crippling neurological problems, and the prognosis of many such disorders remains extremely poor. Thus, in such disorders prenatal diagnosis must remain an important consideration as an essential part of the overall care of the families concerned.

Prenatal diagnosis of the organic acidurias

The enzymic bases for a considerable number of organic acidurias have now been identified and in many of these the enzyme activity and hence its deficiency in affected cases is demonstrable in cultured skin fibroblasts and also in cultured amniotic cells (amniocytes). Such disorders are thus detectable in utero on the basis of enzyme assays on cultured amniocytes obtained by amniocentesis. Amniocentesis (percutaneous withdrawal of amniotic fluid from the amniotic sac) is generally performed at 15–17 weeks' gestation and a cell culture established from the cells in the fluid. It is a prerequisite that the disorder has been previously diagnosed in the index case from the mother concerned and that she is therefore 'at risk' for the disorder concerned. The procedure is dependent upon obtaining a viable cell culture and sufficient cells for enzymology and some four weeks are required from amniocentesis to a final result. Thus repeat assays are generally not possible within the time scale available and relatively late terminations of affected fetuses are necessary.

As an alternative procedure for earlier prenatal diagnosis of the organic acidurias, direct chemical analysis of the cell-free amniotic fluid supernatant may be applicable for some disorders, with analysis using quantitative selected ion monitoring for specific metabolites by GC-MS.[3,10] Results are available within a few days of amniocentesis at 16 weeks' gestation and repeat assays are possible in cases of ambiguity, thus terminations are possible at around 17–18 weeks' gestation in affected cases. The procedure is based upon the knowledge that the fetal bladder fills with urine from about 10 weeks' gestation onwards and this is excreted into the amniotic fluid with the composition of the fluid changing from being primarily an ultrafiltrate

Table 5.2 Prenatal diagnosis of organic acidurias

Disorder	Enzymology on cultured cells	Direct GC-MS analysis of fluid	Direct enzymology on chorionic biopsy tissue
Methylmalonic aciduria	+	+	(+)
Propionic acidaemia	+	+	+
Branched-chain ketoaciduria	+	−	(+)
Isovaleric acidaemia	+	(+)	(+)
3-methylcrotonylglycinuria	+	(+)	(+)
3-hydroxy-3-methylglutaric aciduria	+	+	+
Methylacetoacetyl CoA thiolase deficiency	(+)	(+)	(+)
2-oxoadipic aciduria	(+)	(+)	(+)
Glutaric aciduria Type I	+	+	(+)
Glutaric aciduria Type II	+	+	(+)
Tyrosinaemia Type I	+	+	(+)
Multicarboxylase deficiency*	+	+	(+)
Medium-chain acyl CoA dehydrogenase deficiency*	(+)	(+)	(+)

+ = achieved; (+) = possible; − = not possible or unknown
* not considered to be indicated in these conditions which are easily treatable with good prognosis

of maternal blood plasma to reflecting changes associated with the fetus itself. Where the organic aciduria is expressed biochemically at birth and in utero the fluid will accumulate fetal metabolites until measureable quantities are present at around 15 weeks' gestation. This approach to earlier and more rapid prenatal diagnosis of organic acidurias is being more generally employed and has been applied to propionic acidaemia, methylmalonic aciduria, glutaric aciduria Type I, glutaric aciduria Type II, multicarboxylase deficiency, tyrosinaemia 'Type I' and 3-hydroxy-3-methylglutaric aciduria. (Table 5.2).

More recently, the possibility of using chorionic villus tissue obtained by biopsy at 8–10 weeks' gestation for direct rapid enzymology and hence even earlier prenatal diagnosis, has developed and is currently being investigated for a number of different organic acidurias. However, as methods of treatment and the prognosis for many organic acidurias improve, the necessity and validity of prenatal diagnosis for some of these conditions becomes questionable.

DISORDERS OF BRANCHED-CHAIN AMINO ACID METABOLISM

Introduction

The three neutral branched-chain amino acids are chemically similar and are all initially metabolised via a B_6 (pyridoxine)-dependent transamination with 2-oxoglutarate and secondly by a thiamine pyrophosphate (TPP)-dependent oxidative decarboxylation (Fig. 5.3). The occurrence of individual transaminases, specific to 6-carbon and to the 5-carbon amino acid, is supported by the finding of isolated hypervalinaemia; but it is more likely that isoenzymes or subunit differences occur in a common protein. The oxidative decarboxylation occurs via the action of a multienzyme complex analogous to pyruvate and 2-oxoglutarate dehydrogenases in which at least the E3 enzyme (Fig. 5.4), dihydrolipoyl dehydrogenase (EC 2.3.1.12), is common to all three dehydrogenase complexes, a deficiency of this latter enzyme (E3) producing a syndrome with features of congenital lactic acidosis, branched-chain ketoaciduria and 2-oxoglutaric aciduria. A deficiency of the specific branched-chain keto acid decarboxylase (E1) leads to a severe disorder in which the metabolism of all three branched-chain amino acids is affected, maple syrup urine disease or branched-chain ketoaciduria. Regulation of the enzyme complex may involve acyl CoA compounds and the activity in muscle, in which relatively large amounts of branched-chain amino acids are transaminated and oxidised, is stimulated by L-carnitine which may also thus exert a regulating or modulating effect on enzyme activity. In addition, the complex is subject to phosphorylation (deactivating) and dephosphorylation (activating) in an analogous manner to pyruvate dehydrogenase and is thus probably also under hormonal control.

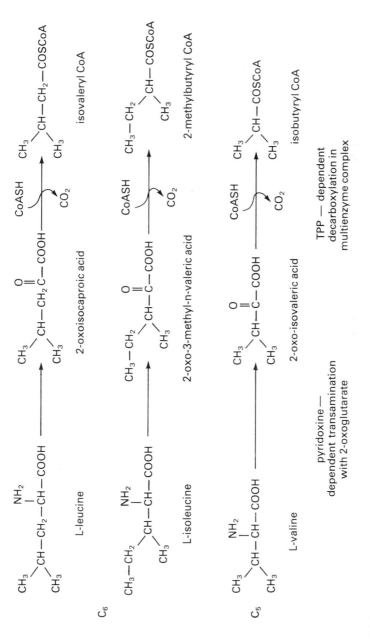

Fig. 5.3 Initial steps in the metabolism of branched-chain amino acids.

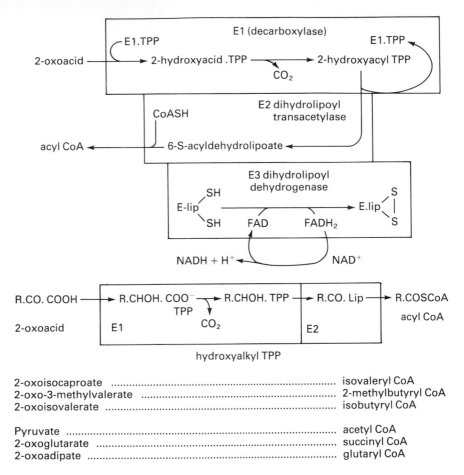

Fig. 5.4 2-oxoacid dehydrogenases and oxidative decarboxylation of 2-oxo acids. A defect in branched-chain keto acid decarboxylase E1 leads to MSUD; in pyruvate decarboxylase E1 to lactic acidosis; in 2-oxoglutarate decarboxylase E1 to 2-oxoglutaric aciduria and in 2-oxoadipate decarboxylase E1 to 2-oxo-adipic aciduria. Deficiency of E3 leads to a combined dehydrogenase deficiency; no cases of E2 deficiencies have been proven. E1 enzymes are $\alpha_2 \beta_2$ tetramers and may share certain subunits. The complexes are deactivated by phosphorylation and activated by phosphatases.

Subsequent to this common 2-oxo acid decarboxylation, the degradative pathways of the three branched-chain amino acids are independent and distinctive. 2-Oxoisocaproic acid (from L-leucine) is metabolised to isovaleryl CoA in the dehydrogenase step and subsequently to 3-methylcrotonyl CoA, 3-methylglutaconyl CoA, 3-hydroxy-3-methylglutaryl CoA and thence to acetyl CoA and acetoacetate, the latter reaction also being an obligate step in 'ketone body' formation. Patients with isolated defects in all stages of this pathway have been identified. The metabolism of 3-methylcrotonyl CoA (and of propionyl CoA and pyruvate) occurs via the action of D-biotin-dependent carboxylases. Defects in the synthesis (holocarboxylase synthetase) and recycling (biotinidase) of the biotin-containing holocarboxylases lead to further disorders related to multicarboxylase deficiency. In contrast to L-leucine metabolism, only one disorder associated with L-isoleucine catabolism, β-ketothiolase deficiency, or methylacetoacetyl CoA thiolase deficiency, has been identified and only one associated with L-valine catabolism, 3-hydroxy-isobutyryl CoA de-acyclase deficiency. These latter two branched-chain amino acids are of particular interest however, since they are both major precursors of propionyl CoA and methylmalonyl CoA, defects in the metabolism of which lead to the relatively common and severe propionic acidaemia and methylmalonic acidurias. These disorders are all described briefly in the following sections.

Branched-chain ketoaciduria (Maple syrup urine disease McKusick 24860)

Branched-chain ketoaciduria is caused by deficient activity of branched-chain keto acid decarboxylase (EC 1.2.4.4., E1 in Fig. 5.4), affecting the metabolism of all three branched-chain oxo and amino acids. In the *classical* form of the disease little or no residual enzyme activity remains and branched-chain amino acids, keto acids and their hydroxy analogues accumulate in body fluids, with the keto acid of isoleucine, 2-oxo-3-methyl-n-valeric acid, apparently being responsible for the maple syrup smell apparent in the urine of some patients. Not all patients exhibit this sweet, caramel-like, odour, best observed in concentrated urine, but it does provide a useful additional indicator of the disease. Allo-isoleucine may also accumulate in the disorder caused by keto-enol tautomerism of 2-oxo-3-methylvalerate.

The disease is inherited by an autosomal recessive mode, with an incidence of 1:120 000 to 1:500 000 dependent upon the geographical area concerned, with high incidence being recorded in Norway and Spain and much lower in southern England and Massachusetts but with all racial types showing cases of the disease. Variant forms of the disease have been recorded including a late-presenting intermittent variant associated with intermittent attacks of acute ataxia that may manifest as the result of an infection or other causes of stress, with affected children being normal between attacks but having the possibility of permanent neurological damage from acute periods. The possibility of 'double heterozygosity' in these patients has been suggested but it would appear most likely that various levels of residual enzyme activity occur (2 to 16%) leading to the spectrum of clinical and biochemical presentations observed. Other so-called variants are even more rare, with a 'mild variant', 'valine toxic' and apparently thiamine-responsive forms being recorded.[11]

Patients are apparently normal at birth with severe symptoms associated with ketoacidosis, poor feeding, vomiting and lethargy occurring within the first week of life. Muscular hypotonicity, abnormal movements and convulsions may occur, death usually intervenes within the first year of life associated with multiple intercurrent infections, with survivors generally suffering severe brain damage. Abnormal branched-chain amino acid and hydroxy and keto acid concentrations in blood and urine are apparent within the first week of life and the disorder may be readily diagnosed from both amino acid and organic acid analysis. CSF concentrations of these metabolites are also increased. Keto acids may be detected using 2,4-dinitrophenylhydrazine (2,4-DNP) or TLC but these and other organic acids are best determined using GC and MS of the TMS oxime, ethoxime or n-butyloxime derivatives and O-TMS quinoxalinols are also of value for 2-oxo acids. The renal clearances of these keto acids are very low (1–2 ml/min/1.73 m^2) and hence there is a tendency to retain the keto acids in the blood, with excess hydroxyacids in the urine, with the retained keto acids probably exacerbating the severe symptoms still further. Lactic acidosis and ketoacidosis with associated organic aciduria may also occur and branched-chain fatty acids are also often elevated in the urine during keto acidotic periods. Acylcarnitines are also elevated in the blood and urine and may be considered consistent with the accumulation of these branched-chain acyl moieties in the disease. The enzyme deficiency is expressed in leucocytes and cultured skin fibroblasts and may be demonstrated by measurement of the rate of oxidation of 1-^{14}C-labelled branched-chain amino acids or keto acids to [14]CO$_2$.

The severity of the disorder requires early diagnosis and vigorous treatment directed at removal of toxic metabolites and prevention of catabolism. Any delay in diagnosis or treatment may result in permanent neurological damage and early death. For effective treatment, diagnosis before about 10 days of age is imperative with initiation of intubation and intensive care for 3–5 days after diagnosis with monitoring of blood amino acids and urinary ketoacids (using 2,4-DNP if required for rapid results). Intensive care may involve peritoneal dialysis for 1–3 days until blood leucine levels plateau (at around 1–1.5 mmol/l) and/or multiple or prolonged exchange transfusions.[8] Coma disappears within six days of treatment and abnormal movements and hypotonia also disappear within 2–3 weeks. Weight gain, associated with near normalisation of blood leucine levels and introduction of an anabolic state, occurs within eight days[8] and is assisted by a high calorie intake via intravenous glucose, with concomitant insulin administration, followed by gradual introduction of a diet low in branched-chain amino acids (40–60 mg/kg body weight/day) supplemented with artificial amino acid mixtures. Most foods have relatively high contents of branched-chain amino acids and treatment with a restricted diet while maintaining normal growth and development is difficult to maintain and requires close laboratory supervision. With adequate therapy, the longer term survival is good but tolerance to dietary leucine and other branched-chain amino acids remains low throughout life except in the variant forms of disease: thus although maintenance of dietary therapy may have been believed to be adequate, ketoacidotic episodes associated with infections are recurrent and the long-term results of evaluation of psychomotor development are disappointing with relatively few patients showing normal development. The severity of the disease and the generally poor prognosis means that prenatal diagnosis is indicated in the management and care of the family concerned.

Disorders of the L-leucine pathway subsequent to isovaleryl CoA

After the transamination of L-leucine and the oxidative decarboxylation of its keto acid, 2-oxo-isocaproic acid, to yield isovaleryl CoA, the further metabolism of the carbon skeleton of L-leucine follows a route that is quite distinct from that of the other branched-chain amino acids. Isovaleryl CoA (Fig. 5.5) is metabolised by the specific FAD and ETF-dependant isovaleryl CoA dehydrogenase to 3-methylcrotonyl CoA, a defect in this dehydrogenase resulting in isovaleric acidaemia. Isovaleryl CoA dehydrogenase activity is also reduced in 'glutaric aciduria Type II' or multiple acyl CoA dehydrogenase deficiency, believed to be caused by a deficiency in the common ETF dehydrogenase responsible for transfer of electrons into the respiratory chain. 3-Methylcrotonyl CoA is carboxylated by the specific D-biotin-dependant 3-methylcrotonyl CoA carboxylase to form 3-methyl-glutaconyl CoA. Deficient activity of the carboxylase apoenzyme causes isolated 3-methyl-crotonylglycinuria with 3-hydroxyisovaleric aciduria. Secondary deficiency may also occur caused by deficient activity of holocarboxylase synthetase, the enzyme responsible for attachment of the D-biotin to the apocarboxylase, and by deficient activity of biotinidase, responsible for recycling of the D-biotin from the lysyl residues (biocytin) arising from holocarboxylase turnover: these disorders also affect other D-biotin dependent carboxylase systems with holocarboxylase synthetase deficiency affecting all three mitochondrial carboxylases, 3-methylcrotonyl CoA carboxylase, propionyl CoA carboxylase and pyruvate carboxylase, and biotinidase deficiency also affecting the cytosolic acetyl CoA carboxylase, to give rise to multi-carboxylase deficiencies. 3-Methylglutaconyl CoA is metabolised by a hydratase to form 3-hydroxy-3-methylglutaryl CoA and possible deficiencies of this hydratase have also been described. Finally, 3-hydroxy-3-methyl-glutaryl CoA is cleaved by a specific lyase to form acetoacetate and acetyl CoA. Deficient activity of the lyase enzyme results in 3-hydroxy-3-methylglutaric aciduria. The lyase deficiency is of interest since 3-hydroxy-3-methylglutaryl CoA is considered as the obligate intermediate in the formation of ketone bodies, i.e. of acetoacetate from acetoacetyl CoA formed from butyryl CoA in the final stage of β-oxidation and lysine metabolism. Patients with the lyase deficiency suffer from episodic acute and profound non-ketotic hypoglycaemia and provide support for this putative pathway of 'ketone body' formation in man.

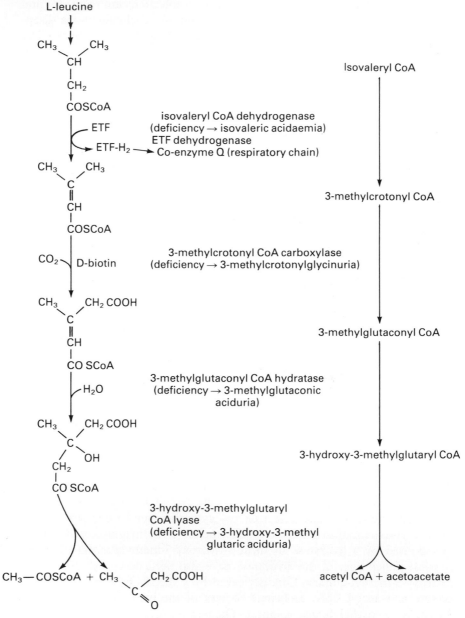

Fig. 5.5 Metabolism of isovaleryl CoA in the L-leucine metabolic pathway.

Isovaleric acidaemia (McKusick 24350)

Isovaleric acidaemia is caused by deficient activity of the specific FAD and ETF-dependent isovaleryl CoA dehydrogenase, leading to intracellular

accumulation of isovaleryl CoA with the appearance of characteristic metabolites in body fluids and of a characteristic odour of *sweaty feet* or *cheese*
during acute episodes. The disorder is characterised clinically by episodes
of acidosis, vomiting, ataxia and tremors that may progress to lethargy and
coma.[3] Many patients present acutely in the newborn period with severe
metabolic acidosis and ketosis, lethargy and severe neurological symptoms
including convulsions and coma. Death has occurred within a few weeks
in about half of such cases with overwhelming sepsis, leucopoenia and
pancytopoenia contributing to the high mortality. Patients who survive this
initial acute period show a subsequent course analogous to those presenting
later in life and the differences of presentation are a reflection of the spectrum of disease associated with residual enzyme activity, environmental
factors and the modifying effects of different enzymatic phenotypes in
different individuals. Mild mental retardation may occur in surviving
patients but prognosis with effective treatment, particularly during the first
1–2 years of life, is good. More than 40 cases are now recorded from 25
sibships with approximately equal numbers of males and females being
affected, consistent with an autosomal recessive mode of inheritance. The
overall incidence of the disease has been estimated at less than 1:200 000.

The accumulating isovaleryl CoA is metabolised to 3-hydroxyisovaleric
acid and, via conjugation through the action of glycine-N-acylase, to isovalerylglycine, the latter being the most characteristic metabolite and always
present in urine specimens. The characteristic odour is due to isovaleric
acid itself which is only present during acute episodes. Some patients
excrete a number of other metabolites during acute ketoacidotic crises,
including methylsuccinic acid, 4-hydroxy-isovaleric acid, methylfumaric
acid, 3-hydroxyisoheptanoic acid and other conjugates including isovaleryl-
glutamate and isovalerylglucuronide.[9] The putative origins of some of
these metabolites is indicated in Figure 5.6. During periods of remission,
only isovalerylglycine is apparent, with concentrations in blood and urine
increasing during crises (to more than 3 g/24 h in urine) and the detection
of this metabolite is essential to the diagnosis. Typical chromatograms of
urinary and blood metabolites have been published elsewhere[3,9] together
with the mass spectra of characteristic metabolites.

The enzyme deficiency is demonstrable in leucocytes and in cultured skin
fibroblasts by reduced oxidation of 1-^{14}C-isovalerate, reduced oxidation of
[2-^{14}C] leucine and reduced incorporation of 1-^{14}C-isovalerate into protein.
Isovaleryl CoA dehydrogenase is a specific mitochondrial dehydrogenase
containing FAD and direct assay of its activity by tritium release assays
using ^{3}H-isovaleryl CoA to measure hydrogen elimination at the 2 and 3
carbons have confirmed the nature of the molecular defect in the disease.
Complementation studies using cultured skin fibroblasts have shown a
single complementation group lending support to the concept of a single
molecular defect (locus) presenting in a variety of manifestations modulated
by environmental and phenotypic differences in individual patients.

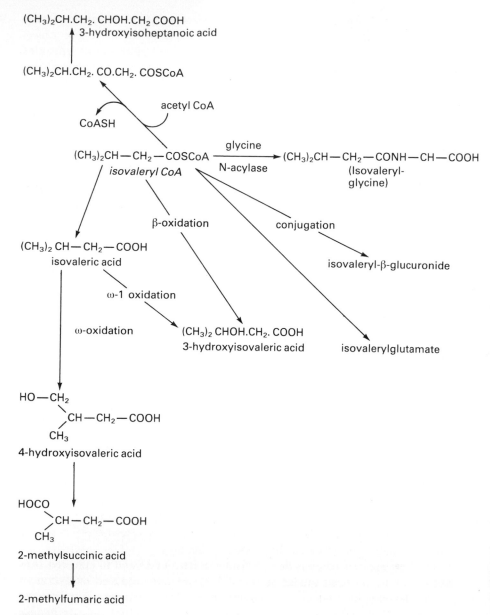

Fig. 5.6 Alternative pathways of isovaleryl CoA metabolism in isovaleric acidaemia.

The free isovaleric acid that accumulates in body fluids including CSF during acute ketoacidotic episodes shows an encephalopathic action in experimental animals and is probably the cause of the coma, in particular, and may be responsible for the mild neurological damage observed in some patients. Treatment of the acute episodes in isovaleric acidaemia may require detoxification by peritoneal dialysis or exchange transfusions and dietary management with a moderately reduced protein intake is also effective for longer term care. The observation that glycine-N-acylase has a relatively high affinity for isovaleryl groups, leading to the increased excretion of isovalerylglycine in isovaleric acidaemia, prompted the use of supplemental glycine therapy in the disease. This was of particular benefit during acute ketoacidotic episodes but of less benefit for long-term management in preventing further attacks.[12] Doses of 250 mg glycine/kg body weight/ 24 h have been used in acute episodes and up to 800 mg/24 h for chronic treatment but some authorities have rejected its use in less severely-affected patients and others have cautioned against the indiscriminate use of glycine therapy after observation of glycine-associated encephalopathy in one patient.[9] Patients with isovaleric acidaemia consistently show reduced free carnitine concentrations in plasma with greatly increased isovalerylcarnitine excretion in urine. Supplemental L-carnitine has been used in the therapy of isovaleric acidaemia both to augment detoxification of isovaleryl groups as isovaleryl-carnitine, and thereby to restore mitochondrial metabolic homoeostasis by release of free CoA and increased ATP synthesis, and through the latter processes also to increase further the formation and excretion of isovalerylglycine.[9] Despite the severity of the acute neonatal ketoacidotic attacks, early diagnosis after presentation and effective treatment provide a relatively good prognosis for patients with isovaleric acidaemia, with survival into adult life. Maternal isovaleric acidaemia, monitored during the pregnancy of one such survivor, also appears to have no adverse effect on mother or baby. However, prenatal diagnosis of isovaleric acidaemia is possible by enzymology on cultured amniocytes and by direct chemical analysis of the cell-free amniotic fluid supernatant for 3-hydroxyisovaleric acid. Direct enzymology on chorionic villus biopsy material at 9 weeks' gestation is also a future possibility.

Isolated 3-methylcrotonylglycinuria with 3-hydroxyisovaleric aciduria (McKusick 21020)

Although many of the earlier reports of 3-methylcrotonyl CoA carboxylase deficiency implied isolated defects of this mitochondrial carboxylase, it has been subsequently shown that the majority of these patients have multi-carboxylase deficiency (see below) and proven cases of isolated 3-methyl-crotonyl CoA carboxylase deficiency are extremely rare. Three cases in two sibships have now been reported. One of two siblings of Vietnamese origin presented with vomiting and coma shortly after arrival in the Netherlands, but the second sibling remained asymptomatic. The third case presented with hypotonia, apnoea and in a collapsed state, with hypoglycaemia, 3-methylcrotonylglycinuria and 3-hydroxyisovaleric aciduria. Isolated 3-methyl-crotonyl CoA carboxylase deficiency was demonstrated in leucocytes and cultured skin fibroblasts.[13] These patients have remained well despite continued abnormal organic aciduria and with a moderate restriction of dietary protein, the prognosis appears good.

3-Methylglutaconic aciduria (McKusick 25095)

Three reports have been made of five patients with isolated 3-methylglutaconic aciduria. Patients have shown normal early development to around 6–12 months of age followed by progressive developmental regression or neurological deterioration, severe in one case, and associated with hypotonia, choreoathetosis with a slowly progressive encephalopathy and moderate dementia, spastic parapareses and optic atrophy. Organic acids in urine showed a marked increase in 3-methylglutaconic acid excretion with increased 3-hydroxyisovaleric aciduria and moderate amounts of 3-methylglutarate. 3-Hydroxy-3-methylglutaric acid excretion was normal. Total combined concentrations of increased metabolites were around 50 mmol/mol creatinine representing only about 2% of daily L-leucine intake and oral loading with L-leucine, while producing some increase in the metabolite levels, did not achieve the expected increase. A preliminary report on 3-methylglutaconyl CoA hydratase activity in sonicates of cultured skin fibroblasts showed this enzyme activity to be greatly reduced in two patients. However, clinical features and other biochemical parameters are inconsistent with a disorder of L-leucine metabolism and further investigation is required.

3-Hydroxy-3-methylglutaric aciduria (McKusick 24645)

3-Hydroxy-3-methylglutaric aciduria (HMG aciduria) is caused by deficient activity of 3-hydroxy-3-methylglutaryl (HMG) CoA lyase, a key enzyme in the degradation of L-leucine and also in the formation of acetoacetate from acetoacetyl CoA and acetyl CoA. A deficiency of this enzyme is characterised by a severe organic acidaemia and aciduria associated with cyanosis, vomiting, apnoea and profound hypoglycaemia with minimal or absent ketosis, leading rapidly to coma and life threatening illness. Indeed, many of the symptoms observed may be ascribed to the inability to form ketone bodies rather than to a disorder of L-leucine metabolism and the disorder could perhaps be better classified as a non-ketotic hypoglycaemia or disorder of ketogenesis. This is of importance when considering the underlying biochemical perturbations in the disease and the necessary therapeutic measures.

More than eleven patients have now been recorded, most patients presenting with acidosis and non-ketotic hypoglycaemia and life-threatening episodes resembling Reye's syndrome (encephalopathy with fatty degeneration of the viscera) and the latter may be the initial diagnosis made. Others have presented initially with mild problems, in particular unusually large head circumference associated with mild hypotonia and poor head control, but have then proceeded at a later date to have acute and profound hypo-glycaemic attacks.[14] The hypoglycaemia is remarkable with glucose levels below 0.1 mmol/l. Blood ammonia is frequently raised (to 500 μmol/l or greater) with associated abnormal liver function tests, again showing marked similarities to Reye's syndrome and emphasising the importance of organic acid analysis in the latter 'condition'. Quantitative analysis is also most important since moderate increases of the same characteristic organic acid metabolites may occur in other Reye's-like syndromes, for example urea cycle defects.

The characteristic and diagnostic organic aciduria (and organic acidaemia) includes greatly increased concentrations of 3-hydroxy-3-methyl-glutaric acid (to above 11 mol/mol creatinine) with associated increases in 3-hydroxy-isovaleric acid (to above 2 mol/mol creatinine), 3-methylglutaconic acid (to above 6 mol/mol creatinine) and 3-methylglutaric acid (to above 1 mol/mol creatinine). During acute episodes, and in the immediate period leading to an acute attack, 3-methylcrotonylglycine is also excreted (Fig. 5.7) in the urine and patients display the very characteristic and distinctive odour of *tom-cats' urine*. Slowing of fatty acid β-oxidation may also occur and a prominent dicarboxylic aciduria with saturated and unsaturated acids and 5-hydroxy-hexanoic aciduria may result.

Acute management must be rapid and positive and is directed at the correction of the profound hypoglycaemia, reduction of the acidosis with concomitant fluid replacement and, in cases of severe hyperammonaemia, with exchange transfusions and peritoneal dialysis. Longer-term management is directed towards reduction of the intake of L-leucine by moderate protein restriction[14] and a reduced fat intake,[15] with careful regulation of blood glucose, especially in early life, by frequent feeding and nocturnal feeding if required to avoid overnight hypoglycaemia. The prognosis of well-treated cases is good although the risk is always present of sudden acute and potentially lethal hypoglycaemic attacks with devastating clinical and residual neurological effects.[15] Careful consideration needs to be given to immunisation in such patients, severe and potentially lethal reactions to such immunisations having occurred in at least two cases.[14] If immunisation is given this should be carried out in hospital with close and appropriate monitoring.

Patients show increased acylcarnitine excretion into urine with evidence for carnitine insufficiency. L-carnitine has been used effectively during acute episodes to assist in the detoxification and removal of accumulating acylmoieties with concomitant restoration of mitochondrial homeostasis evidenced by restoration of normal β-oxidation and aboliton of dicarboxylic aciduria, but may be contra-indicated for chronic therapy because of the unwanted stimulation by L-carnitine of fatty acid β-oxidation and increased attempts to form ketone bodies. Acylcarnitines excreted by these patients have been shown to include 3-methylglutarylcarnitine and 3-hydroxy-iso-valeryl carnitine giving direct evidence for the role of L-carnitine in the

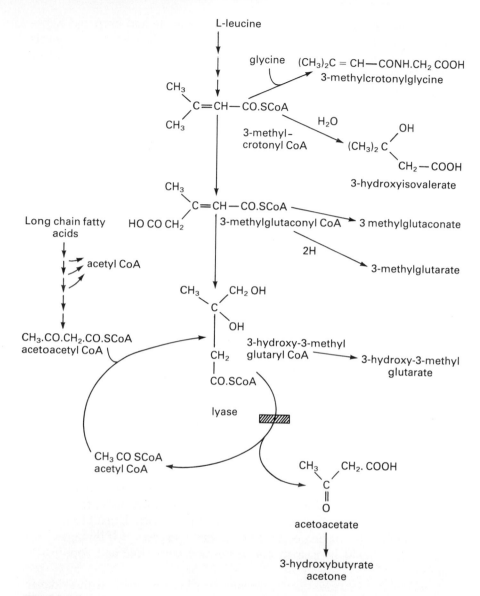

Fig. 5.7 Metabolism of 3-hydroxy-3-methylglutaryl CoA showing its position as the obligate intermediate in the formation of acetoacetate from acetoacetyl CoA and the origins of the metabolites accumulating in 3-hydroxy-3-methylglutaryl CoA lyase deficiency.

transport and metabolism of diacyl and hydroxyacyl moieties. Other acylcarnitines observed included a range from propionylcarnitine to octenoylcarnitine, indicating biochemical abnormalities in the disease that require further investigation for the basis of therapeutic strategies.

The disorder is inherited in an autosomal recessive mode[14] and the HMG lyase deficiency is demonstrable in leucocytes and cultured skin fibroblasts with intermediate levels of activity being recorded in cells of heterozygotes. Prenatal diagnosis may be requested by parents of patients with the disease because of the severity of attacks and uncertain long-term survival and may be carried out on cultured amniocytes, using both direct lyase measurements or measurement of [1-^{14}C] isovalerate incorporation into protein, by direct GC-MS analysis of cell-free amniotic fluid supernatant for metabolites excreted by the fetus into the fluid, and by direct HMG CoA lyase measurements on chorionic villus tissue.

Disorders of L-isoleucine metabolism: 2-methylacetoacetic and 3-hydroxy-2-methylbutyric aciduria (McKusick 20375)

Following the decarboxylation of the 2-oxo-3-methyl-n-valeric acid formed from L-isoleucine, the product, 2-methylbutyryl CoA (Fig. 5.8) undergoes further catabolism to propionyl CoA. 2-Methylbutyryl CoA is dehydrogenated to form tiglyl CoA (2-methylcrotonyl CoA) which is then hydrated across the double bond to give 3-hydroxy-2-methylbutyryl CoA. The latter undergoes dehydrogenation to 2-methylacetoacetyl CoA which is then cleaved (thiolysed) to acetyl CoA and propionyl CoA in an analogous manner to the metabolic steps in mitochondrial β-oxidation of fatty acids. At least three 3-oxoacyl CoA thiolases occur in mammalian tissues, one in the cytosol that is specific for acetoacetyl CoA and two in the mitochondria, one with a broad specificity, perhaps for longer chain acyl groups, and one specific for short-chain acetoacetyl CoA. The acetoacetyl CoA-specific enzymes are activated by K$^+$, whereas the non-specific enzyme is not activated in this way. The cytosolic enzyme may be primarily involved in production of acetyl CoA from ketone bodies for steroid and lipid biosynthesis whereas the specific mitochondrial enzyme is primarily involved in energy production. This is reflected in tissue distribution where the acetoacetyl CoA metabolising enzymes occur in brain while liver shows all three activities including the general catabolic mitochondrial enzyme. The probable occurrence of a more specific methylacetoacetyl CoA thiolase which shares certain subunits with the other thiolases, particularly that with broad specificity, has been supported by studies on cells from patients with the inherited enzyme deficiency and with methylacetoacetic aciduria and 2-methyl-3-hydroxybutyric aciduria.

2-Methylacetoacetyl CoA thiolase deficiency

The disorder is characterised by early presentation with fever, vomiting and diarrhoea, with acidosis and ketosis during acute phases. Moderate hyperammonaemia may occur and frequent recurrent headaches have been an associated phenomenon. The disease is characterised biochemically by

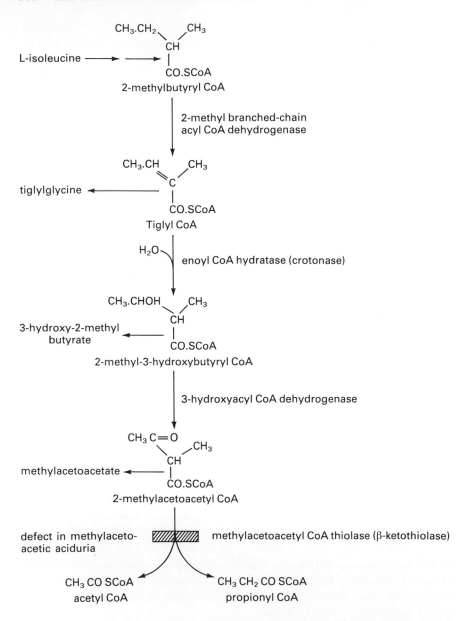

Fig. 5.8 Metabolism of 2-methylbutyryl CoA in the degradation of L-isoleucine showing the defect in β-ketothiolase deficiency and metabolites accumulating in the disorder.

3-hydroxy-2-methylbutyric aciduria and tiglylglycinuria, and 2-methylaceto-acetate and butanone are also excreted during ketoacidosis. Hyperglyci-naemia may also occur. Since all three metabolites may also be excreted in increased amounts by patients with propionic acidaemia it is important to distinguish the two disorders on the basis of the other organic acids excreted by the latter patients. Patients with 2-methylacetoacetyl CoA thiolase deficiency may have intermittent or episodic variants with only moderate excretion of metabolites when clinically well and care must be taken in their diagnosis, isolated tiglylglycinuria with small amounts of 3-hydroxy-2-methyl-butyric aciduria being suggestive of the disorder. More than eight patients have been described with the disorder with wide variation in clinical presentation and with initial onset of symptoms from a few days after birth to 7 years of age. Treatment required has been variable according to the individual needs of the patients concerned but with moderate dietary restriction of isoleucine intake and control of ketoacidotic episodes the prognosis is good with one subject being an asymptomatic 36-year-old.

All the reported patients have partial deficiencies of thiolase activity with the enzyme being expressed in cultured skin fibroblasts as well as other tissues. Various assays have been utilised including oxidation of [U-^{14}C] isoleucine and conversion of tritiated tiglyl CoA into propionic acid. More detailed studies have been carried out into the relationship and specificities of the various 3-oxoacyl CoA thiolases in patients with this disorder and the related acetoacetyl CoA thiolase deficiency associated with congenital ketoacidosis.[16] Using synthesised 2-methylacetoacetyl CoA it has been shown that patients with 2-methyl-3-hydroxybutyric aciduria and tiglylglycinuria show greatly reduced β-ketothiolase activity and no stimulation by K^+ when acetoacetyl CoA was used as substrate, consistent with a deficiency of the mitochondrial (acetoacetyl CoA specific) thiolase with the activity of the broad-specificity enzyme, which is probably involved in fatty acid metabolism, and the cytosolic thiolase being normal. The specificities of the various 3-oxoacyl CoA thiolases (β-ketothiolases) are summarised in Table 5.3.

The disorder is inherited in an autosomal recessive mode and with the deficiency expressed in cultured skin fibroblasts and presumably in amniocytes, prenatal diagnosis is possible. However, in view of the relative ease of treatment once a diagnosis is established, and the good prognosis, prenatal diagnosis may not be indicated.

Table 5.3   Substrate specificities of 3-oxoacyl CoA thiolases in man

Enzyme	cytosolic[1]	mitochondrial branched-chain[2]	mitochondrial straight-chain[3]
Acetoacetyl CoA	+	+	+
Acetoacetyl CoA, K^+ stimulated	−	+	−
2-methylacetoacetyl CoA	−	+	−
3-oxohexanoyl CoA	−	−	+

1. The cytosolic acetoacetyl CoA-specific thiolase is primarily involved in sterol and lipid biosynthesis.
2. The mitochondrial branched-chain, or acetoacetyl-CoA-specific, thiolase is stimulated by K^+ and metabolises both acetoacetyl CoA and 2-methyl-acetoacetyl CoA.
3. The mitochondrial straight-chain thiolase shows broader specificity but is mainly involved in thiolysis of oxoacyl CoA derivatives in fatty acid catabolism.

Other disorders of ketone body metabolism: primary congenital ketoacidosis

Cytosolic acetoacetyl CoA thiolase deficiency

This condition was first described by De Groot et al[17] in a patient who presented from 4 months of age with delayed motor development, ataxia, choreoathetosis, involuntary eye movements and hypotonia associated with greatly and persistently increased 3-hydroxy-butyrate and acetoacetate and raised lactate and pyruvate in blood. Severe neurological symptoms with epileptic fits developed despite treatment. Reduced activity of cytosolic acetoacetyl CoA thiolase was demonstrated in liver biopsy material in the presence of normal activities of several other enzymes studied. Studies on cultured skin fibroblasts confirmed the deficiency which was ascribed to altered kinetic properties of the enzyme. The deficiency has also been described in a severely mentally-retarded boy who presented from 7 months of age and who persistently excreted increased amounts of 3-hydroxy-butyrate and acetoacetate. Other organic acids were normal. Study of cultured skin fibroblasts showed reduced activity of 3-oxoacyl CoA thiolase when acetoacetyl CoA was used as substrate with normal activity with methyl-acetoacetyl CoA and 3-oxohexanoyl CoA, suggesting a deficiency of cyto-solic 3-oxoacyl CoA thiolase. Sterol synthesis rates from acetate were also reduced in the presence of normal fatty acid synthesis, consistent with this deficiency. Succinyl CoA:3-oxoacid CoA transferase activity (see below) was normal.

This disorder is of interest with the association of persistent ketosis and ketonuria with neurological symptoms, and the absence of any other distinguishing biochemical abnormalities, including organic aciduria, clearly distinguishing these patients from those with the mitochondrial thiolase deficiency.

Treatment, with reduced dietary fat intake, has been unsuccessful and, in view of the severe neurological symptoms associated with this condition and with expression of the defect in cultured skin fibroblasts, prenatal diagnosis can be considered in future pregnancies. The condition appears to be inherited by an autosomal recessive mode.

Succinyl CoA:3-oxoacid CoA transferase deficiency (McKusick 24505)

Tildon and Cornblath[18] described a baby who presented from the second day of life with tachypnoea and feeding difficulties associated with severe metabolic acidosis, ketonaemia and ketonuria and hyperuricaemia. Continued severe episodes occurred with intolerance of dietary fat or protein and the infant died at 197 days of life with sepsis, congestive heart failure and respiratory arrest. An apparently slightly milder case presented initially at 7 months and was managed with a high carbohydrate and low fat diet but died at 21 months with acute metabolic acidosis. Thiolase activities were normal but succinyl CoA:3-oxoacid CoA transferase activity was absent in brain, kidney and fibroblasts. This enzyme occurs exclusively in extrahepatic tissues and is responsible for conversion of acetoacetate to acetoacetyl CoA in these tissues for re-utilisation via thiolysis to acetyl CoA. Thus severe neurological symptoms might be expected to occur in both disorders of ketone body metabolism and the two disorders have several features in common. Prognosis appears poor. The relative difficulty in distinguishing and diagnosing such patients with persistent ketoacidosis may mean that several patients have been overlooked in the past.

Disorders of L-valine metabolism

After transamination of L-valine to 2-oxoisovaleric acid and oxidative decarboxylation of the latter to form isobutyryl CoA, the branched-chain acyl CoA ester is dehydrogenated to methacrylyl CoA, followed by hydration to 3-hydroxyisobutyryl CoA in an analogous manner to the metabolism of L-isoleucine (Fig. 5.9). The 3-hydroxyisobutyryl CoA is deacylated to the free acid which is then dehydrogenated to methylmalonyl semialdehyde with further metabolism to propionyl CoA. Only one disorder affecting this pathway has been described, namely 3-hydroxyisobutyryl CoA deacylase deficiency, although in glutaric aciduria Type II (multiple acyl CoA dehydrogenase deficiency) the common deficiency of ETF dehydrogenase affects all ETF requiring dehydrogenase enzymes simultaneously, including isobutyryl CoA (2-methyl branched-chain acyl CoA) dehydrogenase.

3-Hydroxyisobutyryl CoA deacylase deficiency (McKusick 27708)

Only one infant, the first child of healthy first cousin Egyptian parents, who presented with multiple malformations, including dysmorphic facial features, and failure to thrive with poor feeding has been described with this disorder. The infant died at 3 months of age with cardiac malformations and multiple vertebral abnormalities. Routine high voltage amino acid analysis of urine revealed the presence of two unusual sulphur-containing amino acids, subsequently isolated and identified as S-(2-carboxypropyl)-cysteine and S-(2-carboxypropyl)-cysteamine (Fig. 5.9). These compounds were assumed to arise from conjugation of accumulating methacrylyl-CoA with cysteine followed by decarboxylation. Both compounds were found widely distributed in tissues postmortem[19]. The defect was demonstrated in cultured skin fibroblasts by incubation with ^{14}C-valine and ^{35}S-cysteine and isolation of the labelled sulphur-containing acids and by reduced formation of $^{14}CO_2$ from [2-^{14}C] valine. Intermediate levels of enzyme activity were demonstrable in fibroblasts from the parents and a subsequent male child who was clinically normal, consistent with an autosomal recessive mode of inheritance. Prenatal diagnosis is possible as demonstrated by

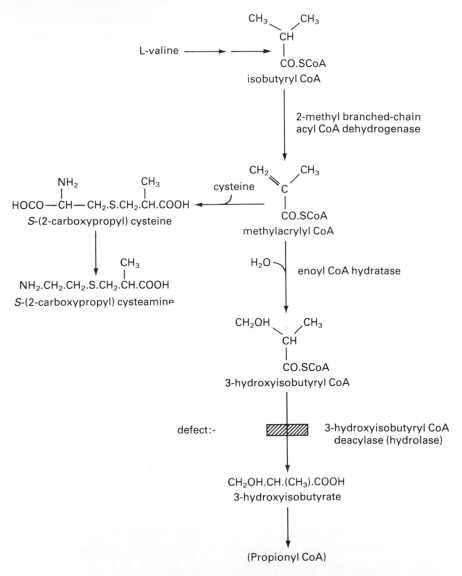

Fig. 5.9 Metabolism of isobutyryl CoA in the degradation of L-valine showing the defect in 3-hydroxyisobutyryl CoA deacylase deficiency and the metabolites that accumulate in this disorder.

the observation of intermediate levels of enzyme activity in the cultured amniocytes from a second pregnancy in this family.

The disorder is of particular interest because the accumulating methacrylyl CoA appears to have teratogenic properties consistent with the known effects of methacrylates in rats. It is also of interest because of the difficulty of detection of the relatively small amounts of abnormal metabolites excreted and the apparent absence of methacrylic acid or other metabolites, indicating potential difficulties in the diagnosis of other disorders of the L-valine (and L-isoleucine) pathway.

Propionic acidaemia (McKusick 23200 & 23205)

L-isoleucine and L-valine are metabolised after the sequences of metabolic pathways described above, to propionyl CoA, with the propionyl CoA being subsequently metabolised via the D-biotin-dependent propionyl CoA carboxylase to S-methylmalonyl CoA. Deficient activity of propionyl CoA carboxylase leads to propionic acidaemia with accumulation of propionyl CoA in tissues and subsequent utilisation of alternative metabolic pathways. Other precursors of propionyl CoA include methionine, threonine, cholesterol and odd-carbon number fatty acids. Propionyl CoA and its alternative metabolites also accumulate when the further metabolism of methylmalonyl CoA is blocked (methylmalonic acidurias) and in multicarboxylase deficiency and they cause many of the symptoms associated with these disorders (described below). Propionate is also produced normally by gut bacteria and thus the intestine is also a potentially important source of propionate in these disorders, this being of relevance to the management of the patients concerned.

Propionyl CoA carboxylase is a mitochondrial enzyme, requiring D-biotin, ATP and magnesium ions for its activity: it is found in most tissues and cells studied including fibroblasts and leucocytes and occurs as a tetrameric protein containing four identical units of 128 000 daltons, made up of two non-identical subunits, α and β, of 72 000 and 56 000 daltons respectively. Four molecules of biotin are bound to each molecule of the apoenzyme, binding to the α subunit under the action of holocarboxylase synthetase, with D-biotinyladenylate being formed initially which is then bound to the ε-lysyl group of the apoenzyme subunits to form the active holocarboxylase. Carboxylation occurs initially by formation of the carboxylated holocarboxylase with the biotin being carboxylated at the 1-N position, and then transfer of the carboxyl group from the biotin to the 2 or α position of the propionyl CoA to form S-methylmalonyl CoA.

Clinical presentation

Propionic acidaemic patients present with severe ketoacidosis, marked hypotonia, areflexia, vomiting, hyperventilation, apnoea, lethargy and coma, usually in early infancy. Hypoglycaemia and hyperammonaemia with neutropoenia, thrombocytopoenia and pancytopoenia may occur and classically the disorder is associated with hyperglycinaemia (ketotic hyperglycinaemia),[20] although this is not observed in all cases. Patients may present acutely in the newborn soon after initial protein feeding, or more chronically with recurrent episodes of ketosis, hyperammonaemia and hyperglycinaemia with periodic thrombocytopoenia and neutropoenia. Others may present with developmental retardation and essentially without ketosis. While some of the acute cases respond to intensive intravenous glucose and bicarbonate therapy, supplemented with peritoneal dialysis and other measures, the disorder is difficult to control and most patients die during such acute episodes. Abnormal EEGs are recorded and CT scans show cerebral atrophy, confirmed on autopsy. These changes are probably secondary to hyperammonaemia, although on autopsy demyelination and spongy degeneration have been observed and lipids containing C_{15} and C_{17} straight chain fatty acids accumulate both in brain and liver.

Early diagnosed and treated cases and the late presenting cases often show no neurological abnormalities. The clinical spectrum observed is illustrative of the heterogeneity of the disease and the modification of the syndrome that can occur, dependent perhaps upon genetically determined molecular variation resulting in differences in the ability of individual patients to metabolise accumulating compounds through alternative pathways and this is underlined by clinical heterogeneity within the same sibships.[20] Similarly, genetic complementation studies using cultured skin fibroblasts have demonstrated at least two major complementation groups in patients with propionic acidaemia.

Biochemistry and diagnosis

Patients with propionic acidaemia consistently show increased excretion of methylcitric acid, generally associated with 3-hydroxypropionate and other metabolites of propionyl CoA including, particularly, propionylglycine and 3-hydroxy-n-valeric acid and its precursor 3-oxo-n-valeric acid, formed by condensation of propionyl CoA with acetyl CoA. Methylmalonate excretion is normal or only very slightly increased. Accumulation of metabolites of isoleucine may also occur and tiglylglycine, 3-hydroxy-2-methylbutyric acid and even 2-methylacetoacetate may be found in urine. 2-methylbutyrylglycine may also be excreted following isoleucine loads. In addition to the characteristic methylcitric acids, 2-methyl-3-oxo-n-valeric acid has also been found consistently, together with the corresponding hydroxy acid, in increased amounts, being formed from the condensation of two molecules of propionyl CoA. Methylcitric acid occurs in two isomeric forms, characterised as the 2R, 3S and 2S, 3S isomers[21] with the two diastereoisomers being excreted in different ratios dependent upon the patient concerned and their metabolic and clinical condition at the time of study. Long-chain ketones may also occur in urine, formed from decarboxylation of 3-oxovaleric acids in an analogous manner to the formation of acetone from acetoacetate (3-oxo-n-butyrate). Similarly, the occurrence of 3-hydroxy-3-ethylglutaric acid in the urine of some patients suggests the substitution of 3-oxo-n-valeryl CoA for acetoacetyl CoA in the hydroxymethylglutaryl CoA synthase reaction and may indicate the free acid is formed via this route in an analogous manner to acetoacetate formation.

Propionyl CoA is the key intermediate in the formation of the majority of the abnormal metabolites observed and is also responsible for the accumulation of odd-carbon number fatty acids and abnormal triglycerides and lipids. Secondary inhibition of other mitochondrial enzyme systems by propionyl CoA also occurs, for example inhibition of N-acetylglutamate synthesis probably underlying the hyperammonaemia observed, and is also the cause of the secondary hypoglycaemia and hyperglycinaemia in patients with the disorder. More direct evidence of the accumulation of propionyl CoA in propionic acidaemia has been presented by the observation of propionylcarnitine as the major acylcarnitine present in increased concentrations in urine, since propionylcarnitine can only be formed by transfer of the acyl moiety from propionyl CoA[22]. Administration of exogenous L-carnitine to patients with the disorder results in increase in the excreted amounts of propionylcarnitine and thus L-carnitine has potential value in the treatment of propionic acidaemia.

Genetics and prenatal diagnosis

Reference has been made above to complementation studies on cultured skin fibroblasts from patients with propionic acidaemia that give evidence for more than one mutation for the defect. Studies of the biochemical properties of enzymes in cells from these patients showed differences in heat lability, potassium affinity and biotin-reactivation following avidin inactivation, suggesting that some patients have a structurally modified enzyme protein in which the ATP and carboxybiotin binding sites are affected.

Propionic acidaemia is inherited in an autosomal recessive mode. The enzyme defect is expressed in cultured skin fibroblasts and amniocytes and reduced enzyme activities have been observed in fibroblasts from obligate heterozygotes of the condition. The difficulty of treatment and relatively poor prognosis make demands for prenatal diagnosis of this condition and this has been carried out on cultured amniocytes using both [1-^{14}C] propionate incorporation into protein and by direct propionyl CoA carboxylase assay. Direct analysis of cell-free amniotic fluid supernatant for methylcitric acid has also been used successfully.[10]

Treatment and prognosis

Treatment of propionic acidaemia, after management of acute ketoacidotic and hyperammonaemic episodes, depends upon dietary manipulation, with minimal natural protein intake (around 1–1.5 g/kg body weight 24 h) supplemented with amino acid mixtures omitting isoleucine and valine, in particular, and with carbohydrate and fat to supply the other calorie requirements. Dietary requirements need to be tailored to suit individual patients and close monitoring of urinary ketones and organic acids is of value particularly during the initial establishment of the diet. Monitoring of growth and development is important and it has been suggested that supplemental L-alanine (100 mg/kg 24 h) may be valuable to promote growth in these patients. Increased fluid intake is also important to avoid the recurrent episodes of dehydration and the use of nasogastric feeding or intravenous treatment may be necessary. Although reports of biotin responsiveness in propionic acidaemia are variable, residual enzyme activity may be enhanced by oral D-biotin (10–50 mg/24 h) and this is always worth investigation. L-carnitine has been shown to increase the urinary excretion of propionyl groups by patients with propionic acidaemia[22] with secondary biochemical effects suggesting increased availability of free coenzyme A and improvements in energy metabolism, although with little direct effect on concentrations of other propionyl metabolites. Administration of L-carnitine (100–400 mg/kg/24 h, orally or up to 50 mg/kg/24 h intravenously) may prove to be of value both for regular therapy and especially in the management of acute episodes. Detoxification and supportive measures, introduced earlier in this chapter, are also essential during acute episodes as are mineral and vitamin supplements during regular therapy.

The prognosis of patients with propionic acidaemia is generally poor by comparison to the majority of other disorders of branched-chain amino acid metabolism, despite advances in therapy, but detailed information on large numbers of patients is relatively limited. Early diagnosis combined with effective acute treatment to prevent irreversible neurological damage and effective regular maintenance therapy with rapid response to acute episodes is improving the prognosis of patients with propionic acidaemia and some patients have now lived into their second and third decades of life.

The methylmalonic acidurias (McKusick 25100, 25110, 25111 & 27741)

Carboxylation of propionyl CoA leads to the formation of S-methylmalonyl CoA which is itself metabolised firstly by racemization to R-methylmalonyl CoA and thence via the action of a specific vitamin B_{12}-dependent mutase to succinyl CoA for entry into the tricarboxylic acid cycle (Fig. 5.10). Methylmalonyl CoA racemase acts by moving the α-hydrogen on S-methylmalonyl CoA and although a single report of a deficiency of this enzyme has appeared, subsequent investigation of cultured fibroblasts from the patient demonstrated a deficiency of methylmalonyl CoA apomutase and thus all patients with methylmalonic aciduria have a deficiency of the apomutase or of the synthesis or attachment of the essential cobalamin cofactor.

The mutase enzyme acts by transfer of the CoA carboxyl group and requires 5′-deoxyadenosylcobalamin as cofactor. The mutase exists as a dimer in which both subunits have a molecular mass of 70 000 daltons and each subunit binds 5′-deoxyadenosylcobalamin (AdoCbl) and both show catalytic activity. The deoxyadenosylcobalamin is itself synthesised from vitamin B_{12}, a molecule composed of a planar corrin nucleus, a 5,6 dimethylbenzimidazole nucleotide and a prosthetic group attached to a central

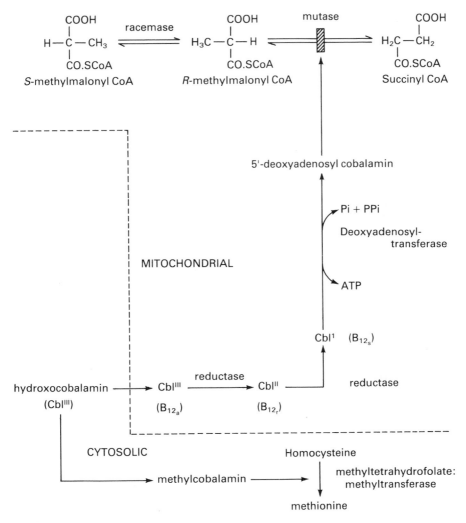

Fig. 5.10 Metabolism of methylmalonyl CoA, hydroxocobalamin (Vitamin B_{12}) and the methylmalonic acidurias. Defects in the mutase apoenzyme (Mut°, Mut⁻), deoxyadenosyltransferase (Cbl B) and mitochondrial Cob III alamin and Cob II alamin reductase (Cbl A) all lead to methylmalonic aciduria with subgroups designated by the complementation groups given. Defects in the cytosolic processing of hydroxocobalamin (Cbl C and Cbl D) lead to combined methylmalonic aciduria and homocystinuria. (See text for further detail.)

cobalt atom in the corrin nucleus. Vitamin B_{12} is an essential vitamin in man, absorbed from the small intestine via the mediation of a glycoprotein intrinsic factor which binds the vitamin and reacts with specific ileal receptor sites in the presence of calcium ions to release the vitamin B_{12} into the portal blood. A deficiency of intrinsic factor leads to pernicious anaemia, secondary to B_{12} malabsorption, associated with mild methylmalonic aciduria (1–2 mmol/24 h) which is responsive to physiological doses of B_{12} given intravenously or intramuscularly. In the blood, the hydroxocobalamin (vitamin B_{12}) is bound to serum β globulin (transcobalamin II) for transport to the tissues. Other transcobalamins (I and III) are also concerned with cobalamin transport in the plasma and with storage of the vitamin. The transcobalamin II-bound hydroxocobalamin is transported in the lysosomes to release the free vitamin. The hydroxocobalamin, in which the cobalt is present as trivalent Co^{III}, undergoes a series of cytosolic and mitochondrial reductions to Co^{I} and is thence metabolised to methylcobalamin and 5′-deoxyadenosylcobalamin in the cytosol and mitochondria respectively. (Fig. 5.10). Deficient activity of the mitochondrial reductases or of the deoxyadenosyltransferase will lead to methylmalonic aciduria, in addition to specific deficiences of the apomutase or of attachment of the AdoCbl to the mutase. Defects in the cytosolic processing of the hydroxocobalamin leads to deficient activities of both methylmalonyl CoA mutase and of the methylcobalamin-dependent methyltetrahydrofolate-homocysteine: methyltransferase, with patients showing both methylmalonic aciduria and homocystinuria. This latter combined defect is also observed in patients with severe vitamin B_{12} deficiency.

Presentation and diagnosis

Patients with methylmalonic aciduria generally present with an acute illness within the first month of life, with low blood pH, failure to thrive, ketoacidosis and frequently with hyperglycinaemia, hyperuricaemia, hypoglycaemia and hyperammonaemia. There is often associated vomiting, dehydration, and lethargy, leading to coma and death if untreated. Neutropoenia; thrombocytopoenia and recurrent acute episodes associated with minor infections are common.

The patients show a greatly increased urinary excretion of methylmalonic acid accompanied by increased excretion of methylcitric acids, 3-hydroxypropionic acid and other metabolites of propionyl CoA. Methylmalonate concentrations in urine are very great, being around 10–30 mol/mol of creatinine or 2–50 mmol/24 h, and increased concentrations are also observed in blood plasma (0.2–3 mmol/l) and in cerebrospinal fluid. Propionic acid may also accumulate during severe acute episodes. A number of reported cases were responsive to pharmacological doses of B_{12} (usually given as cyanocobalamin or hydroxocobalamin, 1 mg/24 h intramuscularly, or 10 mg/24 h orally) with concomitant major reduction of methylmalonate concentrations and of propionyl CoA metabolites. Withdrawal of therapy restored the metabolite concentrations to pretreatment levels, this being the true evaluation of vitamin responsiveness in this and other metabolic disorders.

Patients with combined methylmalonic aciduria and homocystinuria show lower concentrations of methylmalonate in urine and blood and generally low levels of propionyl CoA metabolites, if at all. However, these patients are severely affected clinically with moderate to severe mental retardation associated with lethargy, seizures, megaloblastic anaemia and cerebellar dysfunction, but without ketosis. Abnormalities of the brain are seen post mortem similar to those in the subacute combined degeneration of pernicious anaemia and accumulation of abnormal brain lipids containing odd-carbon number and methylbranched fatty acids. These patients do not appear to respond to vitamin B_{12} (cyanocobalamin) therapy although in vitro responsiveness to methylcobalamin suggests the need for more specific cofactor therapy.

Patients with methylmalonic aciduria show greatly increased ratios of acylcarnitine concentrations to free carnitine concentrations in urine and blood in which the predominant acylcarnitine is propionylcarnitine providing direct evidence for the accumulation of propionyl CoA and for secondary carnitine insufficiency in this disorder. Patients show favourable biochemical and clinical responses to administration of L-carnitine, both under basal metabolic conditions and during severe acute episodes, with reduced organic acid excretion associated with increased propionyl carnitine excretion. L-carnitine should prove of value in the treatment of these patients.

It is obviously of importance to exclude vitamin B_{12} deficiency in the diagnosis of methylmalonic aciduria: mild asymptomatic methylmalonic aciduria may be observed during 'well-baby' screening programmes. Transient neonatal acidosis associated with methylmalonic aciduria and B_{12} deficiency has also been recorded, and severe megaloblastic anaemia with combined methylmalonic aciduria and homocystinuria has been reported in the breast-fed infant of a strictly vegetarian mother. Rapid responses to single dose B_{12} therapy are recorded in these cases, with complete abolition of the metabolic abnormalities and no recurrence with adequate dietary intake.

Treatment and prognosis

The treatment of methylmalonic aciduria is similar to that of patients with propionic acidaemia, with reduced dietary protein intake to reduce isoleucine, valine, threonine and methionine, and supplemented with other essential amino acids including leucine and alanine. Some patients respond well to vitamin B_{12} treatment (1 mg/24 h intramuscularly initially, with 10 mg/24 h orally being suitable for maintenance therapy) and this should always be initiated early in the evaluation of the patient with methylmalonic aciduria. Care must be taken, however, to establish true responsiveness either by temporary withdrawal of the vitamin (for some weeks if necessary) or by L-leucine loading tests. In cases unresponsive to cyanocobalamin, hydroxocobalamin may be preferred as the usually administered (and natural) form of the vitamin. Vitamin B_{12} responsive cases generally require only minimal dietary restriction. In unresponsive cases increased carbohydrate is important with frequent feeding and use of naso-gastric feeding as necessary to overcome the severe anorexia associated with these forms of methylmalonic aciduria. Regular monitoring and rapid response to acute episodes is essential but failure to thrive and to grow are continuing problems in methylmalonic aciduria, with developmental retardation being a consistent feature of the disorder. Osteoporosis may occur and hyperuricaemia with impairment of renal function is often evident and requires appropriate treatment. L-Carnitine therapy has proved of value both during acute episodes and for regular treatment and should form a necessary adjunct to other treatments. Propionate produced by gut bacteria may form an important precursor to methylmalonate and other metabolites in this disorder and the use of neomycin,[23] amoxycillin and metronidazole[24] have proved very effective in some patients in greatly reducing the abnormal organic aciduria and improving clinical progress and prognosis.

The prognosis of patients with methylmalonic aciduria is variable and with improvements in therapy, particularly L-carnitine and the use of specific antibiotics to reduce gut bacterial propionate synthesis, it is improving. Similarly, the prognosis of the B_{12} responsive patient is good and such patients may have an unrestricted or moderately restricted protein intake with normal growth and development. Treatment appears necessary for life however with clinical deterioration associated with withdrawl of vitamin B_{12} therapy. The difficulty of management of the majority of patients with methylmalonic aciduria (i.e. the B_{12} unresponsive patients) and the severity of acute episodes, with associated developmental retardation, make the prognosis for many patients poor, however.

Genetics, enzymology and prenatal diagnosis

Willard and Rosenberg[25] define six classes of methylmalonic aciduria on the basis of fibroblast enzyme and complementation studies. About one-half to three-quarters of all patients with methylmalonic aciduria have mutase apoenzyme defects, subdivided into mut°, that show no increase in enzyme activity when cells are cultured in the presence of cobalamin, and mut⁻ in which a structurally-altered apoenzyme apparently exists with reduced cofactor affinity. The remainder of the patients have cobalamin synthetic defects, classified on the basis of complementation studies into Cbl A, B, C and D groups: Cbl A variants have defects in the mitochondrial cobalamin reductases (Fig. 5.10), Cbl B have deoxyadenosyltransferase deficiency and Cbl C and Cbl D have defects in the early cytosolic processing of hydroxocobalamin associated with combined methylmalonic aciduria and homocystinuria[3,25] (Table 5.4).

Each variant form of methylmalonic aciduria appears to be inherited in an autosomal recessive mode with an overall incidence of around 1 in 50 000 live births. The enzyme defects are expressed in cultured skin fibroblasts and amniocytes and are relatively simply detectable by measurement of

Table 5.4 Methylmalonic aciduria complementation groups

Enzyme activities in cell extracts	Cobalamin disorders			Apomutase disorders	
	Cbl A	Cbl B	Cbl C/D	mut°	mut⁻
Holo-mutase	−	−	−	−	−
Total mutase	+	+	+	−	±
Holo-methyltransferase	+	+	−	+	+
Total methyltransferase	+	+	±	+	+
Adenosyltransferase	+	−	+	+	+
Cobalamin metabolism in intact cells:					
Ado Cbl synthesis	−	−	−	+	+
Me Cbl synthesis	+	+	−	+	+

(Data from Willard and Rosenberg;[25] after Chalmers and Lawson[3])
+ = normal; − = markedly deficient or undetectable.
± = partially deficient.
Total enzyme activity, in presence of saturating cofactor concentrations

incorporation of [1-^{14}C] propionate into protein (acid-insoluble material) in cultured fibroblasts in sub-confluent culture. Prenatal diagnosis using enzymology is usually carried out using this approach which requires relatively few cells and is rapid to perform. Prenatal diagnosis is also carried out by direct analysis of amniotic fluid supernatant for methylmalonic acid and for methylcitric acids by quantitative selected ion monitoring GC-MS using either stable isotope dilution analysis or by comparison to chemically-related internal standards, for example, methylsuccinic acid and homocitric acids respectively. Prenatal diagnosis using chorionic biopsy material obtained at around 9 weeks' gestation should also be possible in the future.

Malonyl CoA decarboxylase deficiency

Two patients have been described with differing clinical presentations, who have been shown to have a deficiency of mitochondrial malonyl CoA decarboxylase in cultured skin fibroblasts. The first patient who presented with delayed development and persistent vomiting excreted increased amounts of malonic acid and methylmalonic acid into the urine (240 mmol/mol creatinine and 210 mmol/mol creatinine respectively), the former increasing with carbohydrate loading but falling after protein loading. The second patient, who had convulsions, had a malonate excretion of 308 mmol/mol creatinine with only minor increase in methylmalonate excretion. The relationship of the observed symptoms with the mild organic aciduria and enzyme deficiency (about 14% of normal activities) is unclear.[26]

Multicarboxylase deficiencies (McKusick 25327)

Introduction

As stated earlier, the three mitochondrial carboxylase enzymes, 3-methylcrotonyl CoA carboxylase, propionyl CoA carboxylase and pyruvate carboxylase, and the cytosolic acetyl CoA carboxylase are all dependent upon D-biotin for their activity, D-biotin being attached to the apoenzyme to form the active holo-enzyme by the action of a fifth enzyme, holocarboxylase synthetase.[3] A deficiency of the latter enzyme in the mitochondria results in deficient activity of all three mitochondrial carboxylases with clinical symptoms and biochemical findings associated with deficiencies of each of the individual carboxylases. Following the turnover and degradation of the holocarboxylases, the biotin-containing residue biocytin, composed simply of biotin attached to the ε-lysyl residue of the enzyme, is degraded further to release free D-biotin for re-utilisation, through the action of a further enzyme biotinidase. D-biotin is also made available from intestinal bacteria as an important source to man but this is also probably presented in the form of biocytin. Thus although D-biotin is also available from the diet, deficiency of biotinidase results in a severe deficiency of D-biotin with the activities of both mitochondrial and cytosolic carboxylases being affected and consequent severe clinical and biochemical results. Similar features are also observed in patients with severe dietary biotin deficiency and the multicarboxylase deficiencies, both inherited and acquired, are important metabolic disorders of children. Since they are readily treatable with oral D-biotin but may be fatal or be associated with severe neurological sequelae if left untreated, their early diagnosis is most important. Holocarboxylase synthetase deficient patients present early and acutely with severe acidosis whereas biotinidase deficient patients present later in infancy with neurological and other abnormalities. The long-term prognosis may be different between the two disorders and differential diagnosis remains important. A further complication is introduced by the relatively minor abnormal or absent organic aciduria in patients with biotinidase deficiency, and careful evaluation is required.

Presentation and diagnosis

The majority of patients with holocarboxylase synthetase deficiency (*early onset multicarboxylase deficiency*) present in the neonatal period with vomiting, ketoacidosis, hyperammonaemia, lactic acidosis, convulsions and profound hypotonia, leading to coma and death in most cases. Patients presenting later also show features associated with dietary biotin deficiency, including alopecia and an erythematous rash similar to those seen in patients with biotinidase deficiency. Infants with biotinidase deficiency (*late onset or juvenile multicarboxylase deficiency*) show these features, again associated with hypotonia, metabolic acidosis and with seizures, developmental delay, ataxia, kerato-conjunctivitis, optic nerve atrophy and severe deafness. Both types of multicarboxylase deficiency are generally fatal without treatment, with survivors suffering severe neurological damage, but both respond dramatically to treatment with D-biotin (10 mg/24 h, orally). Some holocarboxylase synthetase deficient patients may be only partially responsive to D-biotin and patients with biotinidase may progress to show features of nerve degeneration despite treatment, suggesting the latter features may be connected with biocytin toxicity.[27]

The first patient who was originally reported to have biotin-responsive 3-methylcrotonylglycinuria was shown to excrete, in addition to 3-hydroxyisovalerate and 3-methylcrotonylglycine, 3-hydroxypropionate, methylcitrate and lactate[3], providing the basis for subsequent demonstration of multicarboxylase deficiency[28] due to holocarboxylase synthetase deficiency. All patients described with holocarboxylase synthetase deficiency have this characteristic organic aciduria but only a moderate abnormal organic aciduria may be observed in patients with biotinidase deficiency with low but increased levels of some metabolites, particularly 3-hydroxyisovalerate and lactate but very low levels of other characteristic metabolites, for example, the methylcitrates and 3-methylcrotonylglycine. Thus biotinidase deficiency is more difficult to diagnose from the organic aciduria and careful and quantitative analytical methods are required. The abnormal organic aciduria is rapidly abolished on D-biotin treatment in patients with both biotinidase deficiency and holocarboxylase synthetase deficiency and hence diagnosis needs to be established prior to institution of vitamin therapy.

Biotinidase deficiency can be demonstrated in plasma, leucocytes and cultured skin fibroblasts and is most simply determined using blood plasma.[29] Carboxylase enzyme activities in cultured skin fibroblasts are reduced when the cells are cultured in biotin-deficient medium, but normal when biotin-containing medium (ie with fetal calf serum) is used. This distinguishes biotinidase-deficient patients from those with holocarboxylase synthetase deficiency where marked deficiency of all three mitochondrial carboxylases occurs, responding in vitro only to supplemental biotin concentrations in excess of 1 μmol/l. Direct assay of holocarboxylase synthetase is more complex requiring an apocarboxylase as substrate and generally patients with a deficiency of this enzyme are diagnosed on the basis of their multi-carboxylase deficiencies.

Treatment, genetics and prognosis

As stated above, treatment of both conditions is simple, with supplemental D-biotin, 10–50 mg/24 h orally. Response, both clinical and biochemical is dramatic and rapid but regular maintenance therapy with D-biotin is required since within a few days of cessation of therapy, abnormal signs return. Plasma and urine biotin concentrations pretreatment are normal in patients with holocarboxylase deficiency but reduced in biotinidase deficient patients but both groups require biotin therapy. A minority of patients with severe holocarboxylase synthetase deficiency show only a moderate response to biotin and it would be expected that a total deficiency of this enzyme would be incompatible with life. Prognosis for treated patients is very good with the original patient being a normal 15-year-old boy, still on biotin therapy. Some patients with biotinidase deficiency have developed optic atrophy and nerve deafness despite biotin therapy,[27] whereas these complications have not been reported in patients with holocarboxylase synthetase deficiency. It is possible that these complications relate to biocytin toxicity and alternative, and additional, forms of treatment may be required in the future.

Both conditions appear to be inherited in an autosomal recessive mode and although prenatal diagnosis is possible (Table 5.2), the ease of treatment and good prognoses of these conditions may make it unnecessary.

DISORDERS OF L-LYSINE (AND L-TRYTOPHAN) METABOLISM

Introduction

L-lysine is primarily metabolised in mammals via saccharopine and thence to 2-amino adipic acid (Fig. 5.11). 2-Amino adipic acid is transaminated to 2-ketoadipic acid, which is also an intermediate in the catabolism of tryptophan and of hydroxylysine. 2-Oxoadipic acid or 2-keto adipic acid is dehydrogenated (decarboxylated) via a reaction similar to pyruvate and 2-oxoglutarate dehydrogenation (see Fig. 5.4) to form glutaryl CoA which is itself dehydrogenated to glutaconyl CoA followed by decarboxylation to crotonyl CoA and thence β-oxidation to finally yield acetyl CoA. Deficiencies in the metabolism of 2-oxoadipic acid and of glutaryl CoA have been identified, leading to 2-oxoadipic aciduria and glutaric aciduria (Type I) respectively. The alternative and minor pathway for lysine metabolism, probably also involved in D-lysine metabolism, occurs via pipecolic acid (Fig. 5.11) and appears to occur in the peroxisome. Pipecolic acidaemia occurs in Zellweger's syndrome (hepatocerebrorenal disease) together with other abnormalities associated with peroxisomal dysfunction, including a moderate dicarboxylic aciduria and this is referred to in more detail below.

2-Oxoadipic aciduria (McKusick 24513)

2-Oxoadipic aciduria has been reported in a number of patients, being variously associated with psychomotor retardation in a *collodion baby* and mental retardation, but also occurring in the mentally and physically normal sister of one patient. Isolated 2-aminoadipic aciduria has also been reported in both mentally subnormal and normal patients and their affected siblings and the association of 2-oxoadipic aciduria and 2-amino adipic aciduria with mental retardation may be fortuitous, with these metabolic disorders being essentially benign. Patients with 2-oxoadipic aciduria show increased excretion of the ketoacid (500–1500 μmol/24 h or about 200–1000 mmol/mol creatinine) and of 2-hydroxyadipic acid, and increased excretion of 1,2-butene dicarboxylic acid, glutaric acid and 3-hydroxybutyric acid have also been observed. The enzyme deficiency has been demonstrated by reduced

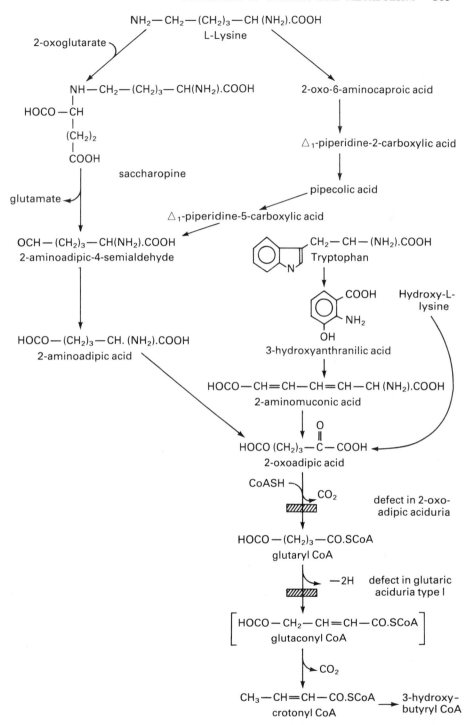

Fig. 5.11 Catabolism of L-lysine and L-tryptophan with positions of defects in 2-oxoadipic aciduria and glutaric aciduria Type I.

oxidation of 2-(D,L) [1-^{14}C]aminoadipic acid and of 2-[1-^{14}C]oxoadipic acid in cultured skin fibroblasts. The disorder is probably inherited in an autosomal recessive mode and prenatal diagnosis should be possible if ever required.

Glutaric aciduria 'Type I' (glutaryl CoA dehydrogenase deficiency, McKusick 23167)

Introduction

Following the dehydrogenation of 3-oxoadipic acid to form glutaryl CoA (Fig. 5.11), the latter is first dehydrogenated to form glutaconyl CoA in an FAD-requiring reaction and then decarboxylated on the same enzyme protein to give crotonyl CoA. The crotonyl CoA is hydrated to 3-hydroxybutyryl CoA which is then metabolised to acetoacetyl CoA and thence to acetyl CoA. Deficient activity of the glutaryl CoA dehydrogenase enzyme that catalyses both stages of the metabolism of glutaryl CoA leads to glutaric aciduria. This disorder has been designated by most authors to be '*glutaric aciduria Type I*' since the identification of '*glutaric aciduria Type II*' caused by multiple acyl CoA dehydrogenase deficiency (see below).

Presentation, diagnosis and biochemistry

Patients with glutaric aciduria are characterised by severe progressive neurological deterioration, generalised dystonic cerebral palsy and choreoathetosis. Convulsions and ketoacidotic episodes may occur with death occurring associated with similarities to Reye's syndrome. The patients appear to be of normal intelligence although this may be difficult to assess because of the severely dysarthric speech and severe impairment of motor function that leads to almost total helplessness. The disorder is associated with greatly increased excretion of glutaric acid and of 3-hydroxyglutaric acid and increased concentrations of glutaconic acid may also be observed in acute episodes. Excretion of 2-oxoglutaric acid is always increased and there may be a moderate associated increase in 2-hydroxyglutarate excretion. It is thus important to distinguish the two hydroxyglutaric acids in the diagnosis of this condition since only the latter is increased in 'glutaric aciduria Type II'. The disorder is caused by deficient activity of the FAD-dependent glutaryl CoA dehydrogenase[30] with the abnormal metabolites occurring via alternative metabolism of the accumulating glutaryl CoA and glutarate. The defect has been demonstrated in cultured skin fibroblasts, leucocytes and other tissues.

Treatment and prognosis

Treatment with a diet low in lysine and in tryptophan has been of value in reducing the excretion of glutaric acid and other metabolites. Similarly, treatment with riboflavin, the precursor to the FAD cofactor for the enzyme, will also reduce glutarate[31] and a combination of the low protein, low lysine diet with high oral doses of riboflavin appears of potential benefit, especially in patients with some residual enzyme activity. However in most cases, after presentation with severe neurological symptoms, little clinical benefit appears to result and the dietary treatment is difficult to manage. Following suggestions that the neurological damage is due to defective function of the basal ganglia caused by inhibition of GABA (γ-aminobutyric acid) synthesis by glutarate and its metabolites, some patients have been treated with the GABA analogue, 4-amino-3-(4-chlorophenyl) butyric acid, with some improvement in clinical function.[31] However, the disorder is extremely severe and progressive and the prognosis is generally very poor except in cases detected early prior to severe neurological damage and treated vigorously with diet and riboflavin.

Genetics and prenatal diagnosis

The disorder is inherited in an autosomal recessive mode and, in view of the clinical severity and poor prognosis, prenatal diagnosis is indicated and possible (see Table 5.2).

DISORDERS OF FATTY ACID METABOLISM: THE DICARBOXYLIC ACIDURIAS

Introduction

Glutaryl CoA dehydrogenase, described briefly above, is one of at least six mitochondrial FAD-dependent acyl CoA dehydrogenases that include those involved in β-oxidation of fatty acyl CoA esters and those involved in branched-chain amino acid metabolism, also discussed earlier (isovaleryl CoA dehydrogenase and 2-methylbutyryl CoA dehydrogenase). Other FAD-dependent mitochondrial dehydrogenases include sarcosine dehydrogenase and dimethylglycine dehydrogenase, both specifically associated with the metabolism of choline and betaine. Deficient activity of the fatty acyl CoA dehydrogenases leads to accumulation of the intermediate acyl CoA esters and their metabolism elsewhere in the cell, one of the major processes involving deacylation of the CoA, followed by ω-1 oxidation of the free fatty acids on the microsomes to produce dicarboxylic acids that then accumulate in the blood and are excreted into the urine. Defects in the β-oxidative pathway are thus generally associated with an abnormal dicarboxylic aciduria although this may be intermittent, dependent upon the fatty acyl load presented to the mutant enzyme system.

The FAD cofactor associated with these dehydrogenases is reduced and passes its electrons to a common electron transfer flavoprotein (ETF) which in turn passes them to coenzyme Q in the electron transport chain via the action of electron transfer flavoprotein (ETF) dehydrogenase (Fig. 5.12).

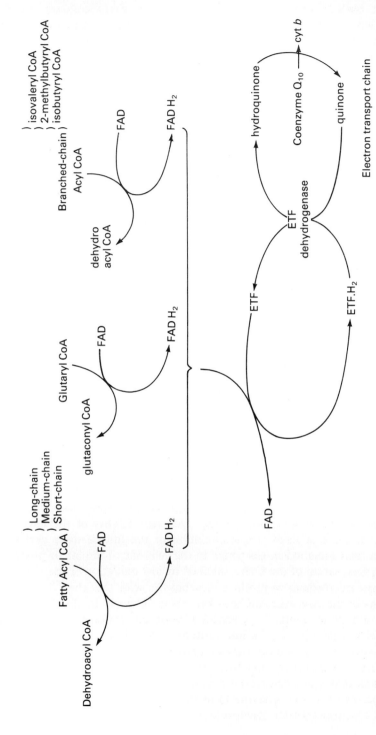

Fig. 5.12 Mitochondrial FAD and ETF-dependent Acyl CoA dehydrogenase. Deficiency of ETF (Electron-transfer flavoprotein) or ETF dehydrogenase will result in multiple deficiences of dependent (acyl CoA) dehydrogenases.

A defect in either ETF or ETF dehydrogenase will affect simultaneously all associated dehydrogenase systems to produce a multiple (acyl CoA) dehydrogenase deficiency in which other FAD/ETF dependent dehydrogenases are also affected.

Accumulating acyl CoA esters in patients with these dehydrogenase deficiencies are also converted into their corresponding acylcarnitine esters both for transport out of the mitochondria and within the cell and as a detoxification process for subsequent excretion into the urine. Systemic carnitine deficiency may occur, also associated with a moderate secondary dicarboxylic aciduria.

Finally, very long-chain fatty acids are metabolised initially in peroxisomes via the action of acyl CoA oxidases and defects in this vital processing for subsequent further β-oxidation in the mitochondria, or lack of the peroxisomes themselves, lead variously to adrenoleucodystrophy and to Zellweger's syndrome (hepatocerebro-renal disease). Similarly, the specific α-oxidation of phytanic acid is also a peroxisomal process and a deficiency of this process results in Refsum's disease.

Medium-chain acyl CoA dehydrogenase (MCAD) deficiency (McKusick 22274)

Presentation, biochemistry and diagnosis

Patients with medium-chain acyl CoA dehydrogenase (MCAD) deficiency present acutely with acidosis, hyperammonaemia, profound non-ketotic hypoglycaemia, encephalopathy, hepatomegaly and pathologically with severe microvesicular fatty infiltration of the liver. Features may thus closely resemble those of Reye's syndrome and the differential diagnosis is most important. The age of initial presentation varies widely with some patients presenting acutely in the early infantile period while others are diagnosed in later childhood although the clinical history often reveals milder episodes preceding the acute presentation.

Patients excrete large amounts of dicarboxylic acids during acute episodes in which suberic acid (C_8) predominates and suberylglycine is excreted as a characteristic and diagnostic metabolite. The enzyme deficiency leads to accumulation of medium-chain acyl CoA esters which are then converted into their corresponding acylcarnitine esters and excreted into the urine: the disorder is thus characterised also by low free carnitine levels associated with increased excretion of esterified carnitine into the urine with octanoylcarnitine and smaller amounts of hexanoylcarnitine. Evidence has also been obtained of excretion of octenoylcarnitine and decenoylcarnitine in the disorder, providing some evidence for the specificity of MCAD. Experience has shown that patients originally described in the literature with suberylglycinuria, dicarboxylic aciduria, and systemic carnitine deficiency with non-ketotic responses to fasting all probably had MCAD deficiency.

Although described as a non-ketotic disorder, some patients, with higher levels of residual enzyme activity, do show a moderate ketonuria in conjunction with the dicarboxylic aciduria and hence the suberylglycinuria and octanoylcarnitinuria are important diagnostic features of the acutely ill patient.

Diagnosis may not be easy since patients generally show no dicarboxylic aciduria when clinically well and careful assessment of patients with suspected MCAD deficiency is essential. Prolonged fasting however, and particularly the use of medium-chain triglyceride (MCT) loading, should be strictly avoided since this can precipitate acute and lethal attacks. Instead, loading with long-chain fats with careful analysis of urinary organic acids and acylcarnitines subsequent to the load should be employed, this representing a more physiological assessment of the ability of the patient to tolerate and metabolise fatty acids.[32] Medium-chain triglycerides will themselves provoke a dicarboxylic aciduria, even in normal subjects, in which the C_{10} acid predominates but no excretion of suberylglycine has been recorded.[33]

Accumulating evidence suggests that MCAD deficiency is relatively common with many cases probably remaining undiagnosed, and with a spectrum of clinical presentations dependent upon the level of residual enzyme activity present. The inheritance is autosomal recessive. The disorder is probably the underlying cause of at least some cases of apparent Reye's syndrome and has been indicated similarly as the cause of some cases of sudden infant death syndrome.

The enzyme deficiency is expressed in cultured skin fibroblasts[34] and other tissues and is demonstrable by measurement of [1-^{14}C] octanoate oxidation in intact fibroblasts in comparison to normal oxidation of butyrate and of oleate or palmitate. Varying levels of residual oxidative capacity have been recorded, from 15%–45% residual activities and it is of interest that some patients show such high residual activity but still present with severe clinical symptoms. Direct measurement of medium-chain acyl CoA dehydrogenase activity has confirmed the nature of the molecular defect in the disorder with relatively low activities of the enzyme being recorded:[35] thus much of the residual oxidative capacity of intact cells may represent variations in function of alternative pathways, for example in peroxisomes.

Treatment and prognosis

Acute management of patients with MCAD deficiency is directed towards rapid correction of the profound and potentially lethal hypoglycaemia. Carnitine may also be beneficial in acute episodes by promoting excretion of accumulating medium-chain acyl moieties as acylcarnitines. Regular maintenance treatment is simple with avoidance of fasting and with use of a diet with moderate reduction of fat intake and increased carbohydrate with, particularly, a carbohydrate-containing drink or snack before bedtime. Carnitine may be contraindicated for maintenance therapy since under basal conditions L-carnitine will increase mitochondrial uptake of fatty acids and hence β-oxidation. Since acute episodes may be induced by mild infections and after immunisations, care must be taken during such events to monitor the patient and maintain blood glucose levels. Prognosis of the correctly diagnosed and treated patient appears excellent.

Long-chain acyl CoA dehydrogenase (LCAD) deficiency

Presentation, biochemistry and diagnosis

Relatively few patients with proven long-chain acyl CoA dehydrogenase (LCAD) deficiency have been described, typical features including early presentation with hypoglycaemia without ketosis and a low plasma free carnitine and increased acylcarnitine concentration. Patients are hypotonic with lethargy, persistent vomiting, cardiomegaly, skeletal muscle weakness and pathologically with macrovesicular fatty infiltration of liver, heart and other tissues. Two patients have been microcephalic, both were severely retarded and a third patient died.[36] Conversely an older child with proven long-chain acyl CoA dehydrogenase deficiency presented with intermittent hypoglycaemia, lethargy and coma and a dicarboxylic aciduria and acidaemia with C_{12} and C_{14} dicarboxylic acids present but without suberylglycinuria. Long-chain acylcarnitines including palmitoylcarnitine have been reported as elevated in urine.

The enzyme deficiency is expressed in liver, leucocytes and cultured skin fibroblasts where oxidation of palmitic acid is greatly reduced in the presence of normal oxidation of octanoate and butyrate. Direct measurement of acyl CoA dehydrogenases shows a major deficiency of long-chain acyl CoA dehydrogenase in the presence of normal medium-chain and short-chain acyl CoA dehydrogenases.[36]

Treatment and prognosis

Treatment with a high carbohydrate, low fat diet and with medium-chain triglyceride supplementation has been used[36] and, although development continued to be slow, cardiac hypertrophy and hepatomegaly resolved. Carnitine therapy has also been used but might be expected to exacerbate the symptoms since carnitine will enhance the uptake of long-chain fats into the mitochondria with attempts to stimulate β-oxidation. It is apparent that, given the early presentation and severe clinical and neurological consequences of acute epidoses in some patients, the prognosis is poor, especially in patients in whom the diagnosis is made late. The disorder appears to be inherited in an autosomal recessive mode and prenatal diagnosis by enzymology on cultured amniocytes and possibly chorionic biopsy material should be possible.

Multiple acyl CoA dehydrogenase (MACD) deficiency (Glutaric aciduria Type II, McKusick 23168)

Presentation, biochemistry and diagnosis

Patients with the most severe form of multiple acyl CoA deficiency present in the neonatal period with severe hypoglycaemia, metabolic acidosis, hepatomegaly, hypotonia, hyperammonaemia, convulsions and neurological symptoms with death within the first months of life. Dysmorphic features are often observed with large head, depressed nasal bridge and other features and pathologically there is severe microvesicular fatty infiltration of the liver, heart and other organs and grossly enlarged polycystic kidneys.[37,38] In a less severe but neonatal form, dysmorphic features and polycystic kidneys may not be observed but these cases are also associated with similarly severe clinical features. Other patients with apparently 'milder' forms of the disease present later in infancy and childhood but acute episodes may occur with cardiomyopathy and death in some cases. The mildest cases with some features of the neonatal form have presented in adults and maternal multiple acyl CoA dehydrogenase deficiency[39] may be the cause of adverse effects in the fetus and newborn, although this is not invariable.

It is evident that these patients represent a spectrum of disease manifestations associated with a common cause or causes modified by residual enzyme activities and by the variable genetic phenotypes of individuals. The disorder is readily distinguished from other disorders of fatty acid metabolism and from isolated glutaryl CoA dehydrogenase deficiency by the characteristic organic aciduria observed in which glutaric acid is prominent but also with major increases in 3-hydroxyisovaleric acid, isovalerylglycine, 2-hydroxy-glutarate and C_6-C_{10} dicarboxylic acids and associated metabolites. Other glycine conjugates may also be observed including hexanoylglycine, isobutyrylglycine and 2-methylbutyrylglycine but *not* suberylglycine, and short-chain fatty acids are also elevated during acute attacks, providing the basis for the *sweaty feet* or *cheesy* odour associated with these episodes. Amino acids, particularly lysine, may also be elevated and there is a prominent sarcosinaemia and sarcosinuria in the neonatal patients without dysmorphic features or polycystic kidneys.

The spectrum of biochemical abnormalities observed in this organic aciduria is indicative of the inhibition, or loss of activity, of a variety of acyl CoA dehydrogenases including those involved in fatty acid β-oxidation at all levels, glutaryl CoA dehydrogenase, those involved in branched-chain amino acid metabolism (isovaleryl CoA dehydrogenase, 2-methylbutyryl CoA dehydrogenase and isobutyryl CoA dehydrogenase) with other mitochondrial FAD-dependent dehydrogenases also being affected, including sarcosine dehydrogenase and 2-hydroxyglutarate dehydrogenase. The common feature of these enzyme systems is their reliance upon FAD for electron transfer and subsequently upon ETF and ETF dehydrogenase for electron transfer into the electron transport chain (Fig. 5.12). Some patients have been shown to respond to riboflavin therapy and FAD synthesis from riboflavin has been shown to be normal in tissues from at least one patient.

Electron transfer flavoprotein (ETF) is an $\alpha\beta$ dimer containing one flavin which becomes reduced to its semiquinone on electron transfer from the dehydrogenases. ETF dehydrogenase (ETF: ubiquinone oxido reductase) also contains one flavin and one Fe_4S_4 iron-sulphur cluster per monomer with the sequence of electron transfer probably reducing first the flavin and the iron-sulphur complex and ultimately being transferred to ubiquinone (coenzyme Q_{10}). Studies using both electron paramagnetic resonance (epr) spectroscopy and using direct assays of ETF and ETF dehydrogenase have indicated that in patients with the severe neonatal disorder associated with dysmorphic features and polycystic kidneys the primary enzyme deficiency is in ETF dehydrogenase. In other patients, with slightly less severe neonatal forms of the disease, evidence suggests the primary defect may be in ETF itself resulting in a less complete metabolic block. The complexity of the electron transfer system, including the occurrence of different mito-chondrial coenzyme Q-binding proteins, provides the basis for a multi-plicity of defects as shown by the variant forms of multiple acyl CoA dehydrogenase deficiency that are observed.

The disorder may be diagnosed, in addition to the characteristic organic aciduria, by enzymology on cultured fibroblasts and other tissues in which the oxidation of fatty acid substrates, and incorporation of isovalerate and other substrates into acid-insoluble material, are greatly reduced. More direct dehydrogenase assays may also be used.

Treatment, prognosis and prenatal diagnosis

No really successful treatment of the severe neonatal cases has been reported although the milder cases may respond to moderate reduction of protein and fat intake with increased carbohydrate and particularly to riboflavin therapy, the latter also being of value in maternal cases.[39] The severity of the neonatal forms of the disease, with evidence in the form associated with polycystic kidney disease that the fetus is severely affected in utero even at 19 weeks' gestation,[40] makes prenatal diagnosis most important. Both neonatal forms appear to be inherited in an autosomal recessive mode, with both males and females being affected in the same sibship. Prenatal diagnosis has been made by direct analysis of amniotic fluid supernatant in which glutarate and 2-hydroxyglutarate concentrations are elevated and by enzymology on cultured amniocytes.[40] Dicarboxylic acids are not consistently elevated in amniotic fluid and analysis of these acids for prenatal diagnosis may be unreliable.[40]

Ethylmalonic-adipic aciduria (McKusick 22717)

Several patients have now been described who have presented with hypoglycaemic attacks leading to coma in early infancy. There is little or no ketosis but acidosis and hyperammonaemia may be observed. The disorder, if untreated, may be severe and several reports indicate death of affected children and their siblings. Analysis of urine for organic acids show increased concentrations of ethylmalonic acid, adipic acid and hexanoylglycine, but generally without evidence of the organic aciduria associated with multiple acyl CoA dehydrogenase deficiency. Butyric acid and butyrylglycine concentrations may also be increased and carnitine levels greatly reduced. During periods of remission the organic aciduria may be minimal or absent.

Ethylmalonic acid is formed as its CoA ester by carboxylation of butyryl CoA catalysed by propionyl CoA carboxylase and the presence of this metabolite and associated compounds in urine were believed to be indicative of a defect in short-chain acyl CoA dehydrogenase or possibly in electron transport affecting particularly this enzyme system. Oxidation of [1-^{14}C] butyrate is reduced in comparison to control values and residual activities ranging from 14% to around 45% have been recorded. Oxidation of lysine and leucine was reduced in one patient[41] suggesting again a defect associated with a common electron transport process.

Some cases appear to be clinically responsive to riboflavin therapy (200 mg/24 h) while others do not respond. Early treatment with a low fat, high carbohydrate diet suggests a good prognosis for patients with this autosomal recessively inherited disorder. However, the variability of presentation, and reports of the results of enzyme studies, leave the precise nature of this defect, and the prognosis of patients, unclear and more detailed studies, including those with direct dehydrogenase assays, are clearly needed to evaluate this condition further.

Disorders of peroxisomal fatty acid metabolism

Zellweger's syndrome (McKusick 21410)

Hepatocerebrorenal disease (Zellweger syndrome) is a rare, autosomal recessively-inherited, disorder associated clinically with cerebral dysgenesis, hepatic cirrhosis, polycystic kidney disease, psychomotor retardation, distinctive dysmorphic features and severe hypotonia, with death within the first year of life.[42] Biochemically there is a spectrum of metabolic disorders including abnormalities in glycogen storage, the metabolism of bile acids, pipecolic acid (see Fig. 5.11), plasmalogen biosynthesis and, in the present context, a dicarboxylic aciduria with defects in the metabolism of very long chain fatty acids. These defects are probably interlinked by the earlier discovery that peroxisomes are absent from liver and kidney of such patients and that their mitochondria are functionally abnormal. Studies of very long-chain fatty acid metabolism have shown that initial oxidation of these acids (C_{26}) occurs exclusively in the peroxisomes and that patients with Zellweger's syndrome and absent peroxisomes cannot therefore metabolise them for subsequent β-oxidation in the mitochondria. Patients show a characteristic pattern of fatty acids in plasma in which the $C_{26:0}$ and $C_{26:1}$ acids predominate and a defect in the oxidation of $C_{24:0}$ fatty acids occurs in fibroblasts. Study of the β-oxidative enzymes of peroxisomes of liver of patients has shown marked deficiencies of peroxisomal acyl-CoA oxidase, enoyl CoA hydratase/β-hydroxyacyl CoA dehydrogenase and 3-oxoacyl CoA thiolase activities, all of which can be ascribed to absence of peroxisomes. Not all peroxisomal enzymes are deficient, catalase activities for example being normal, but this enzyme is located in the matrix and major deficiences occur in those enzymes which are bound to the peroxisomal membrane. The defects in fatty acid metabolism and of plasmalogen biosynthesis have been valuable in the prenatal diagnosis of Zellweger's syndrome[43] and the further study of this and related disorders. The adverse clinical presentation and extremely poor prognosis of patients with Zellweger's syndrome make prenatal diagnosis an essential part of the management and care of the families concerned.

Other disorders of peroxisomal fatty acid and organic acid metabolism

Infantile adrenoleucodystrophy is a metabolic neuro-degenerative disease with a phenotypic resemblance to Zellweger's syndrome and is also characterised by accumulation of very long-chain fatty acids in plasma and tissues.[44] Peroxisomes are present in the tissues of such patients however it is apparent that the disorder is more specific than that in Zellweger's syndrome, with the defect probably occurring in the peroxisomal oxidative pathway of very long-chain fatty acids, either in the synthesis of the C_{24} and C_{26} long-chain fatty acyl CoA esters or in its subsequent processing and chain shortening. It is of interest that only saturated very-long-chain fatty acids accumulate, indicative of the specific nature of the defect involved. Infantile adrenoleucodystrophy is an X-linked disorder and prenatal diagnosis is possible on the basis of the accumulation of long-chain fatty acids in amniocytes and in the impaired oxidation of lignoceric ($C_{24:0}$) acid by cultured amniocytes and fibroblasts. Treatment with a diet restricted in saturated very long-chain fatty acids may be possible.

Pipecolic acidaemia (McKusick 23940) occurs in patients with Zellweger's syndrome and apparently as an isolated phenomenon in some patients with somewhat milder forms of degenerative neurological disease with hepatomegaly and features of Zellweger's syndrome.[45] It is probable that such patients represent part of the clinical spectrum of the latter syndrome and more detailed studies are required. Pipecolic acidaemia may also occur in patients with hyperlysinaemic syndromes, presumably as a secondary phenomenon.

Refsum's disease (McKusick 26650) or phytanic acid storage disease is a disorder characterised by peripheral polyneuropathy, cerebellar ataxia and retinitis pigmentosa. The disorder occurs in older children and adults, is of autosomal recessive inheritance, and is caused by accumulation of phytanic acid (3,7,11,15 tetramethylhexadecanoic acid) in tissues and blood, derived exclusively from dietary sources containing free phytol and phytanic acid (e.g. dairy products and ruminant meats). Phytanic acid is degraded normally in man by an exclusive α-oxidation pathway involving an initial α-hydroxylation followed by decarboxylation to form pristanic acid. This latter C_{19} fatty acid is then metabolised via normal β-oxidation to yield propionyl CoA, acetyl CoA and isobutyryl CoA. The defect is caused by deficiency of phytanic acid α-hydroxylase and is expressed in cultured skin fibroblasts. Treatment is by a diet low in phytol and phytanic acid and this may be combined with plasmapheresis, but for full success needs to be instituted prior to occurrence of permanent neurological damage.

Neonatal Refsum's disease has been reported in a number of patients who presented within the first month of life with jaundice, vomiting and diarrhoea and later with mental retardation with associated features including growth retardation, hepatomegaly, retinitis pigmentosa and nerve deafness and with increased amounts of phytanic acid in plasma. It is possible that such patients again represent the spectrum of disease associated with Refsum's syndrome with earlier detection occurring because of current awareness of such disorders. Refsum's disease is of interest in the present context because recent observations of increased concentrations of phytanic acid in plasma of patients with Zellweger's syndrome and neonatal adreno-leucodystrophy suggest this methyl-branched C_{20} acid is also metabolised in the peroxisomes and, indeed, that α-hydroxylation is a peroxisomal process. It is also of interest that very-long-chain fatty acids may be initially metabolised in the brain and neural tissue by α-hydroxylation giving rise to the high level of 2-hydroxy fatty acids and of odd-carbon number fatty acids in such tissues. The accumulation of phytanic acid and other very long chain fatty acids probably contributes significantly to the neurological symptoms observed and it is apparent that analysis of very-long-chain fatty acids should form part of the study of patients with progressive neuro-generative disorders.

Peroxisomal metabolism of organic acids and their derivatives is obviously of increasing interest with the peroxisome assuming much greater importance in intermediary metabolism than previously believed. In this context it is of particular interest that glyoxylate is metabolised by a peroxisomal alanine: glyoxylate aminotransferase[46] and deficiency of this enzyme is probably the true cause of many cases of primary hyperoxaluria Type I (see below).

HEREDITARY TYROSINAEMIAS AND RELATED ORGANIC ACIDURIAS

Introduction

L-tyrosine is a 'non-essential' amino acid derived both from the diet and from the metabolism (p-hydroxylation) of L-phenylalanine. It is metabol-

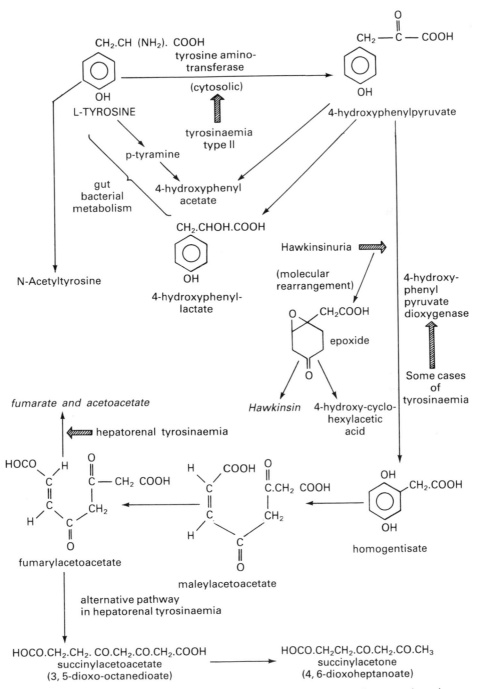

Fig. 5.13 Metabolism of L-tyrosine and site of the defects in the hereditary tyrosinaemias with origins of the metabolites observed.

ised in the cytosol by tyrosine aminotransferase to form 4-hydroxyphenyl-pyruvate which is further metabolised to homogentisic acid in an unusual reaction involving side chain transfer catalysed by 4-hydroxyphenylpyruvate dioxygenase. Homogentisic acid accumulates in alkaptonuria, due to a deficiency of homogentisate oxidase, and is the cause of the ochronosis observed. This enzyme normally cleaves the aromatic ring to give maleyl-acetoacetate which is isomerised to fumarylacetoacetate, the latter being cleaved by fumarylacetoacetase to form fumarate and acetoacetate (Fig. 5.13). The fumarate is converted into malate by the action of cytosolic fumarase for transport into the mitochondria and further metabolism in the tricarboxylic acid cycle.

Several disorders occur in which plasma tyrosine concentrations are increased and in which a tyrosyluria, urinary excretion of the metabolites of tyrosine, 4-hydroxyphenylpyruvate, 4-hydroxyphenyllactate and 4-hydroxyphenylacetate, occurs. Among these is transient neonatal tyrosi-naemia and tyrosyluria probably caused by delayed maturation of hepatic enzymes and usually responsive to a single dose of ascorbate (vitamin C), a required cofactor for the enzyme. More importantly, tyrosine aminotrans-ferase deficiency occurs causing tyrosinaemia Type II (Richner-Hanhart syndrome) and various causes, discussed below, lead to tyrosinaemia Type I (hepatorenal tyrosinaemia).

Tyrosinaemia also occurred in a patient with acidosis who excreted 2-L-cysteinyl-1,4-dihydroxycyclohexanylacetic acid ('Hawkinsin') and cis and trans 4-hydroxycyclohexylacetic acid. Other patients have also been iden-tified with this apparent metabolic disorder (Hawkinsinuria), including mothers and their infants and a father and son, implying an autosomal dominant inheritance. Hawkinsinuria (McKusick 14035) is postulated to be caused by a defect in 4-hydroxyphenylpyruvate dioxygenase in which an epoxy intermediate in the enzyme reaction is prevented from metabolism to homogentisate and is instead metabolised to 4-hydroxycyclohexylacetic acid and Hawkinsin. Asymptomatic family members have also been ident-ified and the precise cause of the disorder remains unproven since the enzyme activity has not been measured directly. 4-Hydroxycyclohexylacetic acid is also excreted by other children with suspected metabolic disorders and alternative dietary or bacterial origins remain possible. Oral tyrosine loading increased the excretion of the abnormal metabolites making the last more probable. The disorder appears responsive to ascorbate administration.[47]

Tyrosinaemia Type II (Oculocutaneous tyrosinaemia McKusick 27660)

Presentation

Tyrosinaemia Type II, oculocutaneous tyrosinaemia or Richner-Hanhart syndrome (keratosis palmoplantaris with corneal dystrophy) is caused by cytosolic tyrosine aminotransferase deficiency and presents with keratitis, skin and eye lesions, with mental retardation in some patients.[48] The features of this disorder are remarkable with ocular symptoms including lacrimation, photophobia with tyrosine crystals in the cornea and including dendritic keratitis and ulcers.[48] Thus such patients may often present initially to an ophthalmologist and, since the eye lesions in particular are often evident at an early age, it is important to determine blood tyrosine levels in any patient with unexplained keratitis. Similarly the skin lesions may lead to first presentation to a dermatologist. It is of interest that there is no liver or kidney disease in tyrosinaemia Type II and the lesions that occur are caused by tyrosine toxicity.

Diagnosis

The diagnosis is made on the basis of elevated plasma tyrosine (1–3 mmol/l) and of urinary tyrosine. Tyrosyluria also occurs in which 4-hydroxyphenyl-acetic acid is quite prominent and N-acetyltyrosine is also excreted in large amounts as a result of the very high tyrosine levels and probably reduced hepatic formation of other tyrosine metabolites. The formation of the other metabolites of tyrosine has been explained on the basis of tran-samination of tyrosine in extra-hepatic tissues by mitochondrial tyrosine (aspartate) aminotransferase to give 4-hydroxyphenylpyruvate which is readily reduced to 4-hydroxyphenyllactate and decarboxylated to 4-hydroxy-phenylacetate. The latter is probably further increased by bacterial metab-olism of tyrosine secreted into the small intestine where it is converted into p-tyramine and subsequently oxidised.

Treatment

Treatment is by protein restriction, or where necessary by a diet low in phenylalanine and tyrosine[48] to bring plasma tyrosine levels towards 1 mmol/l. Early therapy may prevent the possible neurological damage and in all cases dietary treatment will relieve the other symptoms, although residual corneal scarring may occur. Symptoms may recur on relaxation of treatment. Prognosis on such a diet is good and several adult female patients have had normal children. The disorder is inherited by an autosomal recess-ive mode. Many of the cases reported are of Mediterranean origin, particu-larly Italian.

Tyrosinaemia Type I (Hepatorenal tyrosinaemia, McKusick 27670)

Presentation and diagnosis

Patients with tyrosinaemia Type I or hepatorenal tyrosinaemia usually present acutely in early infancy with failure to thrive, vomiting, diarrhoea, hepatomegaly with early death occurring due to hepatic failure. Patients show hypertyrosinaemia and hypermethioninaemia, the latter often manifesting before the tyrosinaemia, and there is a profound tyrosyluria in which, however, excretion of 4-hydroxyphenylacetate is not particularly prominent. Excretion of N-acetyltyrosine may also occur when plasma tyrosine levels are particularly elevated. Hypoglycaemia is common and there may be a more generalised aminoacidaemia in which cystathionine, proline and hydroxyproline are prominent. Increased excretion of catecholamines, δ-aminolaevulinic acid and sugars (glucose, fructose and galactose) may occur. These latter features and renal tubular dysfunction are particularly evident in patients with an apparently more chronic presentation, who develop rickets and also hepatic cirrhosis. Mental retardation may also occur and these children die in the first decade. Diagnosis may be confirmed by demonstration of succinylacetone (4,6-dioxo-heptanoic acid) and succinylacetoacetate (3,5-dioxo-octanedioic acid) in urine (see below), generally with use of special analytical methods because of the relatively low levels observed.[49]

Biochemistry and pathogenesis

The nature of the primary defect in hepatorenal tyrosinaemia has long been a major interest. It has been considered by most workers that the primary defect does not occur in 4-hydroxyphenylpyruvate dioxygenase, although the activity of this enzyme is always reduced in liver of patients, but that this deficiency is caused secondarily to the liver malfunction, renal defects, and other multiple biochemical abnormalities including the hypermethioninaemia. This is supported by the report of a patient with chronic tyrosinaemia and tyrosyluria associated with acute intermittent ataxia and total absence of activity of hepatic 4-hydroxyphenylpyruvate dioxygenase without other features of tyrosinaemia Type I.[50] Similarly, by comparison with tyrosinaemia Type II, the disorder cannot be caused by tyrosine toxicity.

The hepatorenal disease, with multiple biochemical abnormalities, have been ascribed to inhibition of multiple systems by sulphydryl group inhibitors. Succinylacetone and succinylacetoacetate are found in the urine of patients with hepatorenal tyrosinaemia, these metabolites occurring presumably due to deficient activity of fumarylacetoacetase in the tyrosine metabolic pathway (Fig. 5.13) and with accumulation of fumarylacetoacetate and its metabolic precursor maleylacetoacetate acting as sulphydryl group inhibitors to produce the effects observed. This has been confirmed by demonstration in liver, kidney, skin fibroblasts and other tissues of deficient activity of fumarylacetoacetase, and deficient activity of this enzyme together with succinylacetone excretion in urine has been taken as diagnostic of hepatorenal tyrosinaemia, distinguishing it from other causes of similar symptoms. However, these observations do not explain the profound deficiency of 4-hydroxyphenylpyruvate dioxygenase in the disorder and, similarly, are to some extent contradicted by the observation of a case of hereditary fumarylacetoacetase deficiency with no tyrosinaemia or any clinical abnormalities and without succinylacetone excretion, even after tyrosine loading,[51] although the enzyme defect could have been confined to lymphocytes. Similarly, a patient receiving liver transplantation as a method of enzyme replacement in tyrosinaemia Type I continued to excrete succinylacetone at pretransplant levels after transplantation and this was ascribed to continuation of the deficiency in extrahepatic tissues.

Finally, a patient has also been reported who showed hepatic, kidney and fibroblast fumarylacetoacetase deficiency with profound tyrosyluria but without succinylacetone excretion into the urine. These studies have generally been troubled by the determination of only one or two of the various parameters in each patient studied, rather than the full spectrum of urinary metabolites both aromatic and aliphatic, and of enzyme activities of fumarylacetoacetase in fibroblasts and of fumarylacetoacetase and 4-hydroxyphenylpyruvate dioxygenase in liver, and much of the data remains contradictory. The case with fumarylacetoacetase deficiency in liver, kidney and fibroblasts without succinylacetone excretion and a patient with partial deficiencies of both fumarylacetoacetase and 4-hydroxyphenylpyruvate dioxygenase[52] serve to illustrate the continuing problem of elucidation of the true primary defect in hepatorenal tyrosinaemia, although deficient activity of fumarylacetoacetase may play a significant role in the pathogenesis of this disorder.

Prognosis, genetics and prenatal diagnosis

Patients with hepatorenal tyrosinaemia are difficult to treat although use of diets low in phenylalanine and tyrosine have been of apparent benefit. Treatment needs to be started as early in life as possible and results in improvement of renal tubular dysfunction, although varied effects on hepatic dysfunction have been reported. Administration of compounds containing sulphydryl groups may possibly be of benefit and liver transplantation has been used as a means of enzyme replacement therapy although succinylacetone excretion continues after transplantation. In general however, the prognosis, especially of the late treated patient, is poor and prenatal diagnosis may be of importance in the management of the families concerned. The disorder is apparently inherited in an autosomal recessive mode with an overall incidence, from neonatal well-baby screening programmes, of around 1 per 100 000 live births. Despite the continuing research into the primary defect in hepatorenal tyrosinaemia and the occurrence of patients with fumarylacetoacetase deficiency without succinylacetone excretion, prenatal diagnosis has been made on the basis of the succinylacetone concentrations in amniotic fluid supernatant[53] and also from measurement of the activity of fumarylacetoacetase in cultured amniocytes.[54]

DISORDERS OF PYRUVATE METABOLISM, THE TRICARBOXYLIC ACID CYCLE AND OF THE RESPIRATORY CHAIN

Introduction

Pyruvate has a central role in intermediary metabolism, being utilised in both lipogenesis and gluconeogenesis and in energy production via oxidation. It is metabolised by oxidative decarboxylation via the thiamine pyrophosphate, lipoate and coenzyme A dependent pyruvate dehydrogenase (PDH) complex to form acetyl CoA (Fig. 5.14), which becomes available for citrate synthesis and fatty acid biosynthesis, and is utilised for gluconeogenesis via conversion to oxaloacetate through the action of biotin-dependent pyruvate carboxylase and thence to phosphoenolpyruvate via GTP-dependent phosphoenol-pyruvate carboxykinase (PEPCK). Pyruvate dehydrogenase activity is regulated via the action of an activating phosphatase and an inactivating kinase, and the ratios of acetyl CoA to free CoA and of NADH to NAD$^+$. Pyruvate carboxylase activity and pyruvate initiated gluconeogenesis is regulated by the mitochondrial malate translocase, necessary for oxaloacetate transport via conversion to malate.

Pyruvate is also converted by transamination into alanine and is reduced by lactate dehydrogenase to L-lactate, the latter being the end product of the glycolytic pathway that is essential for ATP generation in several tissues, and also the predominant and characteristic metabolite observed in disorders of pyruvate metabolism, of gluconeogenesis, of tricarboxylic acid cycle turnover and of the electron transport chain. These disorders include deficient activity of the PDH complex, of pyruvate carboxylase (and multicarboxylase deficiency) and PEPCK, glycogenosis Type I and fructose-1,6-diphosphatase deficiency and of cytochromes and other elements of the respiratory chain which are collectively termed the congenital lactic acidoses or lactic acidaemias (Fig. 5.14).

Secondary lactic acidosis and lactic aciduria also occur in a number of other inherited disorders of organic acid metabolism including methylmalonic aciduria and propionic acidaemia.[3] Lactate concentrations in body fluids depend upon the pyruvate concentrations and upon the relative amounts of reduced and oxidised cytosolic NAD:

$$\frac{[\text{lactate}]\ [\text{NAD}^+]}{[\text{pyruvate}]\ [\text{NADH}]\ [\text{H}^+]} = K$$

and thus when the ratios of NAD/NADH are constant, changes in lactate concentration depend upon the pyruvate concentration and rate of pyruvate formation and conversely, lowering of the NAD/NADH ratio will also lead to a rise in lactate concentration, with lactic acidosis resulting from a variety of different causes[3], including a variety of uninherited conditions.

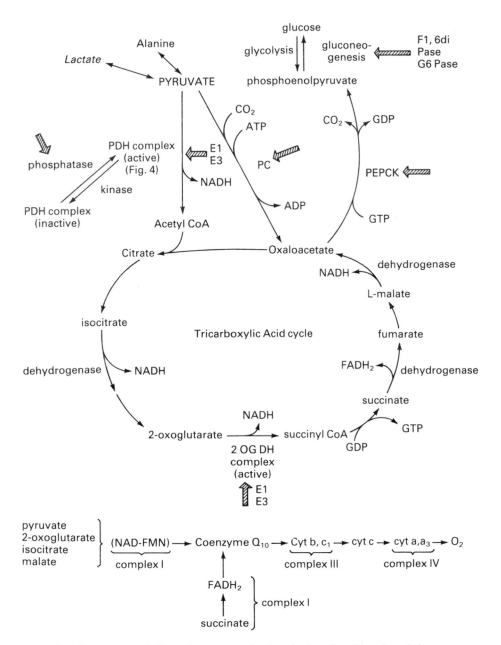

Fig. 5.14 Pyruvate metabolism, gluconeogenesis, the tricarboxylic acid cycle and the respiratory chain, arrows showing identified causes of congenital lactic acidosis. PDH, pyruvate dehydrogenase; PC, pyruvate carboxylase; PEPCK, phosphoenolpyruvate carboxykinase; 2OGDH, 2-oxoglutarate dehydrogenase; cyt, cytochromes.

Congenital lactic acidoses

Disorders of the pyruvate dehydrogenase complex (McKusick 20880)

Patients with disorders of the pyruvate dehydrogenase complex may present acutely in neonatal and early infantile life with severe acidosis and a rapidly progressive fatal illness or in later infancy and childhood with delayed motor and neurological development and ataxia and with features of Leigh's encephalomyelopathy in fatal cases. The severity of presentation is dependent upon the level of residual enzyme activity which may range from 2% of normal activity in fibroblasts in the severe neonatal cases to above 40% in less severely affected patients, but a strict correlation between the degree of enzyme deficiency and the lactate concentrations in body fluids does not occur, although there is a general trend from blood lactates of over 20 mmol/l in the neonatal cases to 3–5 mmol/l in others. Patients may show characteristic dysmorphic features with a narrowed head, wide nasal bridge with associated microcephaly and agenesis of the corpus callosum has been observed in some patients[55] with cystic lesions and demyelination in others.

Identified enzyme deficiencies include those of pyruvate decarboxylase, the E1 enzyme of the complex[56] (see Fig. 5.4) and of lipoamide dehydrogenase, the E3 enzyme, the latter being associated with combined deficiencies of PDH, 2-oxoglutarate dehydrogenase and of branched-chain ketoacid dehydrogenase, all three enzyme complexes sharing the same E3 enzyme.[57] (Fig. 5.4). These latter patients present within the first few months of life with delayed physical and mental development and death in the first years of life from overwhelming acidosis. Few reports have appeared consistent with a deficiency of the E2 enzyme of the complex, dihydrolipoyl transacetylase, and none have been demonstrated to have this defect, but one case has been recorded with apparent combined deficiencies of the E1 enzymes of both PDH and 2-oxoglutarate dehydrogenase, apparently caused by altered binding of thiamine pyrophosphate. Patients with defects in activation of the PDH complex, caused by deficient activity of PDH phosphate phosphatase, have also been recorded, and the possibility of other regulatory disorders may explain the majority of patients with lactic acidoses without demonstrable enzyme deficiencies.

Patients with the E1, pyruvate decarboxylase, deficiency are characterised by an organic aciduria in which concentrations of both lactate and pyruvate are greatly increased with a normal L/P ratio, reduced citrate excretion and increased 2-oxoglutarate excretion. Patients with the E3 deficiency show a less marked lactate and pyruvate excretion but increased concentrations of 2-oxoglutarate and of branched-chain keto and hydroxy acids. Branched-chain amino acids are also increased in the plasma of the latter patients but not to the concentrations observed in 'classical' branched-chain ketoaciduria. The disorders appear to be of autosomal recessive inheritance and attempts at treatment, including use of high fat, low carbohydrate diets, lipoic acid, thiamine, biotin and citrate, have been universally unsuccessful.

The defects are demonstrable in cultured skin fibroblasts and prenatal diagnosis should be possible although no cases have yet been recorded.

Disorders of gluconeogenesis

These disorders include fructose-1,6-disphosphatase deficiency (see p. 50), glucose-6-phosphatase deficiency (glycogenosis Type I, p. 22), glucose-6-phosphate translocase deficiency (glycogenosis Type IB, p. 23) and phosphoenolpyruvate carboxykinase (PEPCK) deficiency. The former disorders are characterised by fasting hypoglycaemia with hepatomegaly and by greatly increased concentrations of lactate and 2-oxoglutarate in urine. They are described in detail elsewhere in this book as indicated. PEPCK deficiency (McKusick 26165) has only been reported in a few patients, who were characterised by non-ketotic hypoglycaemia, hypotonia and moderate lactic acidosis, with fatty deposits in liver and other tissues. The PEPCK enzyme occurs in both cytosol and mitochondria and in one series of patients the defect appeared localised to the cytosolic enzyme while in another patient the mitochondrial enzyme was clearly deficient.[55]

Pyruvate carboxylase deficiency (McKusick 26615)

Pyruvate carboxylase deficiency has been described in more than 20 patients who were generally characterised by acidosis, hypotonia, seizures and retarded development. Fasting hypoglycaemia is rarely recorded and the age of presentation and symptoms observed are very variable, as is the degree of enzyme deficiency in individual patients. The patients may be divided into two groups, one associated with early infantile presentation and longer term survival (for several years of life), but with gross retardation, and with an organic aciduria in which lactate concentrations greatly exceed those of pyruvate, citrate excretion is normal but increased excretion of fumarate, malate and 2-oxoglutarate occurs.[58,59] The second group is associated with neonatal presentation with hepatomegaly, ketosis, hyperammonaemia and citrullinaemia and death within three months of birth.[55] The former patients have been shown to have enzyme protein present (cross-reacting material positive, CRM +ve), but with greatly reduced activity, whereas the latter group are CRM −ve[55], with no residual enzyme activity present. The CRM −ve patients are unable to synthesise oxaloacetate from pyruvate at all and utilise aspartate, glutamate and glutamine. This results in reduced availability of aspartate, affecting the urea cycle and the equilibration of cytosolic and mitochondrial redox states and produces the hyperammonaemia, citrullinaemia and ketosis observed.

Treatment of patients has included dietary supplementation with L-glutamine and aspartate to increase availability of oxaloacetate, and thiamine has also been used. D-biotin has no effect in the absence of much residual enzyme activity, unlike the response observed in patients with multi-carboxylase deficiency. Both groups of pyruvate carboxylase deficiency show apparent autosomal recessive inheritance and the enzyme deficiency is demonstrable in cultured fibroblasts as well as other tissues and in lymphocytes. Prenatal diagnosis should be possible.

Disorders of the respiratory chain

Several patients have now been described with mitochondrial myopathies, severe lactic acidosis, particularly on exercise, a progressive illness and with defects in the respiratory chain and energy transduction in muscle mitochondria.[60] Many of these patients present initially in adult life with marked progressive fatiguability and the aetiologies of their conditions including their inheritance, if at all, is unclear. However, acute neonatal lactic acidosis associated with feeding difficulties, severe hypotonia, mitochondrial myopathy, Fanconi syndrome and massive lactic aciduria and respiratory insufficiency and early death has been reported in a number of patients including sibships, and with apparent autosomal recessive inheritance.[3] These patients have all been shown to have deficiencies associated with cytochrome c oxidase (McKusick 22011) or with cytochrome aa$_3$ and are illustrative of the severity of true inherited generalised respiratory chain defects. Inherited defects isolated to skeletal muscle may be much less severe, especially in childhood, and may explain some of the adult cases reported.

DISORDERS OF OXALATE, GLYOXYLATE AND GLYCERATE METABOLISM

The metabolism of glyoxylate, oxalate and glycerate is interconnected through glycine and serine and by the occurrence of two forms of primary hyperoxaluria associated with glycolic aciduria and with L-glyceric aciduria respectively. Glyoxylate may be produced from glycine by oxidation and transamination and also to some extent from glycolate and is further metabolised by oxidation to oxalate, mediated by lactate dehydrogenase. Glyoxylate may also be metabolised via glyoxylate: 2-oxoglutarate carboligase, an enzyme closely associated with 2-oxoglutarate dehydrogenase. Glycine is interconverted into serine which is further metabolised to hydroxypyruvate and thence to D-glycerate. The latter is also produced from D-glyceraldehyde and is metabolised to 2-phosphoglycerate in the glycolytic and gluconeogenic pathways. Disorders of glyoxylate metabolism result in increased oxidation of glyoxylate to oxalate, giving rise to hyperoxaluria, defective D-glycerate dehydrogenase activity gives rise to L-glyceric aciduria and hyperoxaluria and isolated D-glyceric aciduria also occurs (Fig. 5.15).

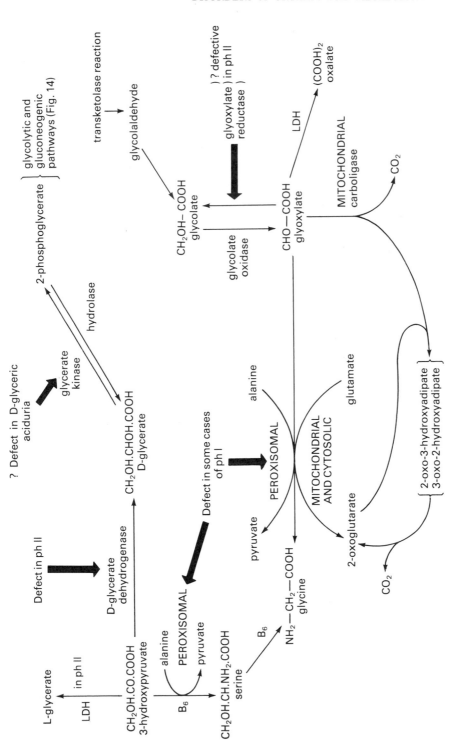

Fig. 5.15 Metabolism of glyoxylate, glycerate and oxalate showing the positions of defects in primary hyperoxaluria (ph) Type I (some cases), Type II and the possible defect in D-glyceric aciduria.

Primary hyperoxaluria Type I (Glycolic aciduria, McKusick 25990)

Primary hyperoxaluria Type I is a rare autosomal recessively inherited disorder in which patients present during the first decade of life with recurrent calcium oxalate nephrolithiasis. The disease is associated with progressive renal damage, renal failure, extra-renal oxalosis in tissues in which a high calcium flux occurs, heart block and with death, usually in the second decade of life. There is considerable variation in presentation, with some adult variants occurring with less severe renal damage and an acute neonatal form associated with rapid progressive oxalosis and renal failure and death in the first year of life.[3] The disorder is also associated with excessive excretion of glycolate and has been ascribed to a defect in glyoxylate metabolism. Originally it was suggested that the defect occurred in mitochondrial glyoxylate: 2-oxoglutarate carboligase but subsequent work has thrown some doubt on this. Alanine:glyoxylate aminotransferase has recently been shown to occur in hepatic peroxisomes[46] and has been shown to be grossly deficient in the liver of a patient with pyridoxine-unresponsive juvenile-presenting Type I primary hyperoxaluria[61], demonstrating the true metabolic lesions in at least some of these patients. Biochemically and clinically, any disorder in which glyoxylate accumulates will present as primary hyperoxaluria Type I and detailed studies on more patients, especially on patients with the acute neonatal form of the disease, will be valuable.

Some patients with primary hyperoxaluria Type I respond clinically and biochemically to the administration of large doses of pyridoxine, the cofactor for the transaminases, suggesting some residual enzyme activity may be present in these patients, or that an alternative pathway for glyoxylate transamination may be activated. The prognosis in these latter patients is more favourable than those with the pyridoxine-unresponsive form of the disease. The latter are treated generally with magnesium oxide to increase calcium oxalate solubility in urine and with high fluid intake. Renal and hepatic transplantation has been attempted with little success, especially in the longer term.

Primary hyperoxaluria Type II (L-glyceric aciduria, McKusick 26000).

L-glyceric aciduria with primary hyperoxaluria was originally reported in four patients, three of whom were siblings. The disorder was shown to be caused by deficient activity of D-glycerate dehydrogenase, the lack of this enzyme causing accumulation of its metabolic precursor hydroxypyruvate which was then reduced to L-glycerate by L-lactate dehydrogenase. The hyperoxaluria was believed to be a result of recycling of the NAD^+ produced by reduction of hydroxypyruvate to L-glycerate, with concomitant oxidation of glyoxylate to oxalate. However, the possible identity of D-glycerate dehydrogenase with glyoxylate reductase may result in accumulation of glyoxylate in the disorder with subsequent oxidation to oxalate and normal or reduced glycolate excretion.[3] Four further cases of L-glyceric aciduria have since been reported, in two sibships, with the configuration of the L-glycerate being confirmed by capillary gas chromatography of the O-acetyl-L-methyl esters of the acids and reduced activity of D-glycerate dehydrogenase being demonstrated in leucocytes. The observation of additional cases of primary hyperoxaluria Type II indicates the necessity for careful classification of patients with oxalate renal calculi since the prognosis and treatment of the different forms of the disease may differ, patients with L-glyceric aciduria not showing features of extra-renal oxalosis and surviving into their fourth and fifth decades of life.

D-glyceric aciduria

Three patients with D-glyceric aciduria have been described in the literature, presenting with severe hypotonia, choreoathetosis and fits or with severe metabolic acidosis and retardation. Greatly increased concentrations of D-glyceric acid were characterised in urine, using enzymic, optical rotatory dispersive and GC methods, with the excretion of other organic acids being normal. A loading test with fructose in the second patient showed a normal response whereas loading with L-serine produced a rise in D-glycerate excretion. The nature of the primary defect in these patients is unproven but the data is consistent with a defect in the metabolism of D-glycerate to 2-phospho-glycerate, at the D-glycerate kinase step. The rare disorder, which is probably of autosomal recessive inheritance, requires further study for characterisation of the molecular defect involved.

DISORDERS OF GLUTAMIC ACID AND GAMMA AMINO BUTYRIC ACID (GABA) METABOLISM

5-oxo-L-prolinuria (Pyroglutamic aciduria, McKusick 26613)

5-oxo-L-prolinuria was first reported in a 19-year-old mentally subnormal man with cerebellar ataxia who excreted 24–35 g of pyroglutamic acid per 24 h with increased concentrations in blood and cerebrospinal fluid. Several patients have now been described with the consistent features of a chronic metabolic acidosis of neonatal presentation and progressive haemolytic anaemia, with untreated patients showing psychomotor retardation and others dying within the first year of life with pronounced cerebellar damage. Pyroglutamic acid (5-oxoproline) occurs as an intermediate in the γ-glutamyl pathway (Fig. 5.16) and accumulates in the disorder as a result of a generalised deficiency of glutathione synthetase[62] due in part to increased synthesis and in part to loss of feed-back inhibition of γ-glutamyl synthetase. Increased pyroglutamate excretion may occur as a secondary phenomenon in other organic acidurias associated with hyperammonaemia

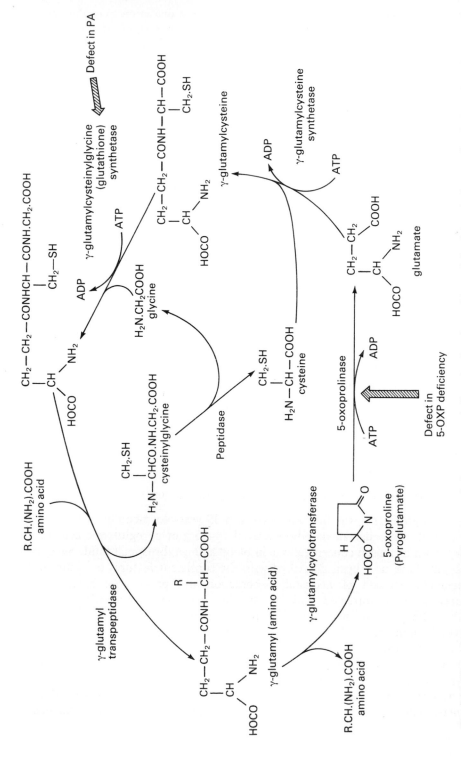

Fig. 5.16 The γ-glutamyl cycle, pyroglutamate and glutamate metabolism showing the positions of the defects in 5-oxoprolinuria (pyroglutamic aciduria) (PA) and 5-oxoprolidase deficiency (5OXP)

and from dietary sources[3] and diagnosis is dependent upon erythrocyte glutathione and glutathione synthetase determinations to avoid ambiguity. Treatment involves correction of the acidosis with bicarbonate and citrate. The disorder is of autosomal recessive inheritance.

Glutathione synthetase deficiency without pyroglutamic aciduria may occur in patients with haemolytic anaemia with an isolated enzyme deficiency in erythrocytes. Pyroglutamic aciduria without haemolytic anaemia or neurological abnormalities has been reported in two brothers with enterocolitis, calcium oxalate renal stones and 5-oxoprolinase deficiency in fibroblasts and leucocytes.[63]

4-hydroxybutyric aciduria

4-hydroxybutyric aciduria has been reported in four patients with marked hypotonia, non-progressive ataxia, ocular dyspraxia and mental retardation.[64] Succinic semialdehyde excretion was also increased and study of lymphocytes showed the primary defect to be in succinic semialdehyde dehydrogenase, a key enzyme in 4-aminobutyric acid (GABA) metabolism. Attempts at treatment were essentially unsuccessful but improvement in the cerebellar symptoms occurred over several years. The disorder appears to be of autosomal recessive inheritance and intermediate levels of enzyme activity were recorded in cells from parents and siblings of the patients. Prenatal diagnosis should be possible.

REFERENCES

1 Sweetman L 1984 Qualitative and quantitative analysis of organic acids in physiologic fluids for diagnosis of the organic acidurias. In: Nyhan W L (ed) Abnormalities in amino acid metabolism in clinical medicine. Appleton-Century-Crofts, Norwalk, Connecticut, Ch 45, p 419–453
2 Iles R A, Hind A J, Chalmers R A 1985 Use of proton nuclear magnetic resonance spectroscopy in detection and study of organic acidurias. Clinical Chemistry 31: 1795–1801
3 Chalmers R A, Lawson A M 1982 Organic acids in man. Analytical chemistry, biochemistry and diagnosis of the organic acidurias. Chapman and Hall, London
4 Tuchman M, Bowers L D, Fregien K D, Crippin P J, Krivit W 1984 Capillary gas chromatographic separation of urinary organic acids. Retention indices of 101 urinary acids on a 5% phenylmethyl silicone capillary column. Journal of Chromatographic Science 22: 198–202
5 Chalmers R A, Watts R W E 1972 The quantitative extraction and gas-liquid chromatographic determination of organic acids in urine. Analyst 97: 958–967
6 Dalgliesh C E, Horning E C, Horning M G, Knox K L, Yarger K 1966 A gas-liquid chromatographic procedure for separating a wide range of metabolites occurring in urine or tissue extract. Biochemical Journal 101: 792–810
7 Tanaka K, Hine D G 1982 Compilation of gas chromatographic retention indices of 163 metabolically-important organic acids and their use in detection of patients with organic acidurias. Journal of Chromatography 239: 301–322
8 Saudubray J-M, Ogier H, Charpentier C et al 1984 Neonatal management of organic acidurias. Clinical update. Journal of Inherited Metabolic Disease 7(suppl 1): 2–9
9 de Sousa C, Chalmers R A, Stacey T E, Tracey B M, Weaver C M, Bradley D 1986

The response to L-carnitine and glycine therapy in isovaleric acidaemia. European Journal of Pediatrics 144: 451–456

10 Sweetman L 1984 Prenatal diagnosis of the organic acidurias. Journal of Inherited Metabolic Disease 7 (suppl 1): 18–22

11 Nyhan W L 1984 Maple syrup urine disease. In: Nyhan W L (ed) Abnormalities in amino acid metabolism in clinical medicine. Appleton-Century-Crofts, Norwalk, Connecticut, Ch 2, p 21–35

12 Krieger I, Tanaka K 1976 Therapeutic effects of glycine in isovaleric acidaemia. Pediatric Research 10: 25–29

13 Bartlett K, Bennet M J, Hill R P, Lashford L S, Pollitt R J, Worth H G J 1984 Isolated biotin-resistant 3-methylcrotonyl CoA carboxylase deficiency presenting with life-threatening hypoglycaemia. Journal of Inherited Metabolic Disease 7:182

14 Stacey T E, de Sousa C, Tracey B M et al 1985 Dizygotic twins with 3-hydroxy-3-methylglutaric aciduria; unusual presentation, family studies and dietary management. European Journal of Pediatrics 144: 177–181

15 Norman E J, Denton M E, Berry H K 1982 Gas-chromatographic/mass spectrometric detection of 3-hydroxy-3-methylglutaryl CoA lyase deficiency in double first cousins. Clinical Chemistry 28: 137–140

16 Middleton B, Bartlett K 1983 Synthesis and characterisation of 2-methylacetoacetyl-CoA and its use in the identification of the site of defect in 2-methylacetoacetic and 2-methyl-3-hydroxybutyric aciduria. Clinica Chimica Acta 128: 291–305

17 de Groot C J, Luit-de Haan G, Hulstaert C E, Hommes F A 1977 A patient with severe neurological symptoms and acetoacetyl-CoA thiolase deficiency. Pediatric Research 11: 1112–1116

18 Tildon J T, Cornblath M 1972 Succinyl-CoA: 3-ketoacid CoA-transferase deficiency. A cause for ketoacidosis in infancy. Journal of Clinical Investigation 51: 493–495

19 Brown G K, Hunt S M, Scholem R et al 1982 β-hydroxy-isobutyryl coenzyme A deacylase deficiency: A defect in valine metabolism associated with physical malformations. Pediatrics 70: 532–538

20 Wolf B, Hsia Y E, Sweetman L, Gravel R, Harris D J, Nyhan W L 1981 Propionic acidaemia: A clinical update. Journal of Pediatrics 99: 835–846

21 Brandänge S, Josephson S, Måhlen A, Mörch L 1984 Characterisation of the citrate synthase reaction with propionyl CoA. Acta Chemica Scandinavica B38: 695–700

22 Chalmers R A, Roe C R, Stacey T E, Hoppel C L 1984 Urinary excretion of L-carnitine and acyl-carnitines by patients with disorders of organic acid metabolism: evidence for secondary insufficiency of L-carnitine. Pediatric Research 18: 1325–1328

23 Snyderman S E, Sansarico C, Norton P, Phansalkar S V 1972 The use of neomycin in the treatment of methylmalonic aciduria. Pediatrics 50: 925–927

24 Bain M, Borriello S P, Reed P J et al 1985 Therapeutic potential of antibiotics in methyl-malonic acidaemia. Pediatric Research 19:1083

25 Willard H P, Rosenberg L E 1979 Inherited deficiencies of methylmalonyl CoA mutase activity: biochemical and genetic studies in cultured skin fibroblasts. In: Hommes F A (ed) Models for the study of inborn errors of metabolism, Elsevier/North Holland Biomedical Press, Amsterdam, p 297–311

26 Brown G K, Scholem R D, Bankier A, Danks D M 1984 Malonyl coenzyme A decarboxylase deficiency. Journal of Inherited Metabolic Disease 7: 21–26

27 Taitz L S, Green A, Strachan I, Bartlett K, Bennett M 1983 Biotinidase deficiency and the eye and the ear. Lancet 2:918

28 Weyler W, Sweetman L, Maggio D C, Nyhan W L 1977 Deficiency of propionyl CoA carboxylase and methylcrotonyl CoA carboxylase in a patient with methylcrotonylglycinuria. Clinical Chimica Acta 76: 321–328

29 Wolf B, Grier R E, Allen R J, Goodman S I, Kien C L 1983 Biotinidase deficiency: the enzymatic defect in late-onset multiple carboxylase deficiency. Clinica Chimica Acta 131: 273–281

30 Hyman D B, Tanaka K 1984 Specific glutaryl-CoA dehydrogenating activity is deficient in cultured fibroblasts from glutaric aciduria patients. Journal of Clinical Investigation 73: 778–784

31 Brandt N J, Gregersen N, Christensen E, Grøn I H, Rasmussen K 1979 Treatment of glutaryl CoA dehydrogenase deficiency (Glutaric aciduria)—Experience with diet, riboflavin and GABA analogues. Journal of Pediatrics 94: 669–673

32 Tracey B M, Chalmers R A, Rosankiewicz J R, de Sousa C, Stacey T E 1986 Acylcarnitines in urine in medium-chain acyl-CoA dehydrogenase deficiency (MCADD) measured by quantitative HPLC. Biochemical Society Transactions 14: 700–701

33 Whyte R K, Whelan D, Hill R, McClorry S 1986 Excretion of dicarboxylic and ω-1 hydroxy fatty acids by low birth weight infants fed with medium-chain triglycerides. Pediatric Research 20: 122–125

34 Rhead W J, Amandt B A, Fritchman K S, Felts J J 1983 Dicarboxylic aciduria: deficient [1-^{14}C] octanoate oxidation and medium-chain acyl CoA dehydrogenase in fibroblasts. Science 221: 73–75

35 Coates P M, Hale D E, Stanley C A, Corkey B E, Cortner J A 1985 Genetic deficiency of medium-chain acyl Coenzyme A dehydrogenase: Studies in cultured skin fibroblasts and peripheral mononuclear leucocytes. Pediatric Research 19: 671–676

36 Hale D E, Batshaw M L, Coates P M, Frerman F E, Goodman S I, Singh I, Stanley C A 1985 Long-chain acyl Coenzyme A dehydrogenase deficiency: an inherited cause of non-ketotic hypoglycaemia. Pediatric Research 19: 666–670

37 Lehnert W, Wendel U, Lindenmaier S, Böhm N 1982 Multiple acyl-CoA dehydrogenation deficiency (Glutaric aciduria Type II), congenital polycystic kidneys, and symmetric warty dysplasia of the cerebral cortex in two brothers I: Clinical, metabolical, and biochemical findings. European Journal of Pediatrics 139: 56–59

38 Böhm N, Uy J, Kiessling M, Lehnert W 1982 Multiple acyl-CoA dehydrogenation deficiency (Glutaric aciduria Type II), congenital polycystic kidneys, and symmetric warty dysplasia of the cerebral cortex in two newborn brothers II: Morphology and pathogenesis. European Journal of Pediatrics 139: 60–65

39 Harpey J-P, Charpentier C, Goodman S I, Darbois Y, Lefèbvre G, Sebbah J 1983 Multiple acyl-CoA dehydrogenase deficiency occurring in pregnancy and caused by a defect in riboflavin metabolism in the mother. Journal of Pediatrics 103: 394–398

40 Chalmers R A, Tracey B M, King G S et al 1985 The prenatal diagnosis of glutaric aciduria Type II, using quantitative GC-MS. Journal of Inherited Metabolic Disease 8: (suppl 2): 145–146

41 Mantagos S, Genel M, Tanaka K 1979 Ethylmalonic-adipic aciduria: in vivo and in vitro studies indicating deficiency of activities of multiple acyl-CoA dehydrogenases. Journal of Clinical Investigation 64: 1580–1589

42 Kelley R I 1983 Review: the cerebrohepatorenal syndrome of Zellweger, morphologic and metabolic aspects. American Journal of Medical Genetics 16: 503–517

43 Roscher A, Molzer B, Bernheimer H, Stöckler S, Mutz I, Paltauf F 1985 The cerebrohepatorenal (Zellweger) syndrome: An improved method for the biochemical diagnosis and its potential value for prenatal detection. Pediatric Research 19: 930–933

44 Cohen S M Z, Brown F R, Martyn L et al 1983 Ocular histopathologic and biochemical studies of the cerebrohepatorenal syndrome (Zellweger's syndrome) and its relationship to neonatal adrenoleucodystrophy. American Journal of Ophthalmology 96: 488–501

45 Thomas G H, Haslam R H A, Batshaw M L, Capute A J, Neidegard L, Ransom J L 1975 Hyperpipecolic acidemia associated with hepatomegaly, mental retardation, optic nerve dysplasia and progressive neurological disease. Clinical Genetics 8: 376–382

46 Nakatani T, Kawasaki Y, Minatogawa Y, Okuno E, Kido R 1985 Peroxisome localised human hepatic alanine-glyoxylate amino-transferase and its application to clinical diagnosis. Clinical Biochemistry 18: 311–316

47 Wilcken B, Hammond J W, Howard N, Bohane T, Hocart C, Halpern B 1980 Hawkinsinuria: A dominantly inherited defect of tyrosine metabolism with severe effects in infancy. New England Journal of Medicine 305:865–869

48 Goldsmith L A, Kang E, Beinfang D C, Jimbow K, Gerald P, Baden H P 1973 Tyrosinaemia with plantar and palmar keratosis and keratitis. Journal of Pediatrics 83: 798–805

49 Tuchman M, Whitley C B, Ramnaraine M L, Bowers L D, Fregian K D, Krivit W 1984 Determination of urinary succinylacetone by capillary gas-chromatography. Journal of Chromatographic Science 22: 211–215

50 Giardini O, Cantani A, Kennaway N G, D'Eufemia P 1983 Chronic tyrosinaemia associated with 4-hydroxyphenylpyruvate dioxygenase deficiency with acute intermittent ataxia and without visceral and bone involvement. Pediatric Research 17: 25–29

51 Kvittingen E A, Børresen A L, Stokke O, Van der Hagen C B, Lie S O 1985

Deficiency of fumarylacetoacetase without hereditary tyrosinaemia. Clinical Genetics 27: 550–554

52 Furukawa N, Kinugasa A, Seo T et al 1984 Enzyme defect in a case of tyrosinaemia Type I, acute form. Pediatric Research 18: 463–466

53 Pettit B R, MacKenzie F, King G S, Leonard J V 1984 The antenatal diagnosis and aid to the management of hereditary tryosinaemia by the use of a specific and sensitive GC–MS assay for succinylacetone. Journal of Inherited Metabolic Disease 7 (suppl 2): 135–136

54 Kvittingen E A 1984 Prenatal diagnosis of hereditary tyrosinaemia by determination of fumarylacetoacetate fumarylhydrolase activity in cultured amniotic fluid cells. Pediatric Research 15: 94–98

55 Robinson B H 1985 The lactic acidaemias. In: Lloyd J K, Scriver C R (eds) Genetic and metabolic disease in pediatrics. Butterworths, London, p 111–139

56 Robinson B H, Sherwood W G 1984 Lactic acidaemia. Journal of Inherited Metabolic Disease 7 (suppl 1): 69–73

57 Munnich A, Saudubray J-M, Taylor J et al 1982 Congenital lactic acidosis, α-ketoglutaric aciduria and variant form of maple syrup urine disease due to a single enzyme defect: Dihydrolipoyl dehydrogenase deficiency. Acta Paediatrica Scandinavica 71: 167–171

58 Van Biervliet J P G M, Bruinvis L et al 1977 Report of a patient with severe, chronic lactic acidaemia and pyruvate carboxylase deficiency. Developmental Medicine and Child Neurology 19: 392–401

59 Chalmers R A 1984 Organic acids in urine of patients with congenital lactic acidoses: An aid to differential diagnosis. Journal of Inherited Metabolic Disease 7 (suppl 1): 79–89

60 Clark J B, Hayes D J, Morgan-Hughes J A, Byrne E 1984 Mitochondrial myopathies: disorders of the respiratory chain and oxidative phosphorylation. Journal of Inherited Metabolic Disease 7 (suppl 1): 62–68

61 Danpure C J, Jennings P 1986 Peroxisomal alanine: glyoxylate aminotransferase deficiency in primary hyperoxaluria Type I. FEBS Letters 201: 20–24

62 Larrson A 1981 5-oxoprolinuria and other inborn errors related to the γ-glutamyl cycle. In: Belton N R, Toothill C (eds) Transport and Inherited Disease. MTP Press, Lancaster, p 277–306

63 Larrson A, Mattsson B, Wauters E A K, Van Gool J D, Duran M, Wadman S K 1981 5-oxoprolinuria due to hereditary 5-oxoprolinase deficiency in two brothers—A new inborn error of the γ-glutamyl cycle. Acta Paediatrica Scandinavica 70: 301–305

64 Rating D, Hanefeld F, Siemes H et al 1984 A new disorder—4-hydroxybutyric aciduria. Clinical Review. Journal of Inherited Metabolic Disease 7 (suppl 1): 90–92

Purine and pyrimidine disorders

INTRODUCTION

Purines and pyrimidines are possibly best known as the basic constituents of the polynucleotides DNA and RNA. However, in addition to this, they serve equally vital but separate functions as integral components of many important intracellular mononucleotide pools such as ATP and GTP, or the pyrimidine diphosphate sugars, UDP glucose and CDP choline for example (Figs. 6.1 & 6.2). The function of purine and pyrimidine metabolism is to maintain the supply of basic components to these pools, as well as to remove the waste products of normal cell turnover.

The nephrotoxicity of purines has been known for more than a century. However, their potential cellular toxicity has only recently become evident from the differing clinical manifestations produced when one of the steps involved in the build-up and break-down of these pools is defective, or missing. The first inherited purine disorder, xanthine oxidase deficiency, was reported as a clinical entity as recently as 1954. The biochemical basis for the defect was identified in 1959. A total of eight inherited purine disorders are now known, six of them have been described since 1970. The first inherited pyrimidine disorder was also identified in 1959 and three defects have now been recognised.

Purine and pyrimidine metabolic pathways

Purine and pyrimidine mononucleotides may be synthesised de novo from simple molecules by energetically expensive, multi-step pathways. (Figs. 6.1 & 6.2). Alternatively, they may result from the recycling of basic components derived from nucleotide catabolism during the normal process of cell turnover — the so-called 'salvage' pathway. The latter is energetically less expensive and effectively exerts feedback control on the former, thus restricting de novo purine synthesis in man to the minimum required to replace purine irrevocably lost in the form of uric acid (2–3 mmol/24 h). Two-thirds of the uric acid produced daily from endogenous purine turnover is normally excreted by the kidney, the remainder by the gut.

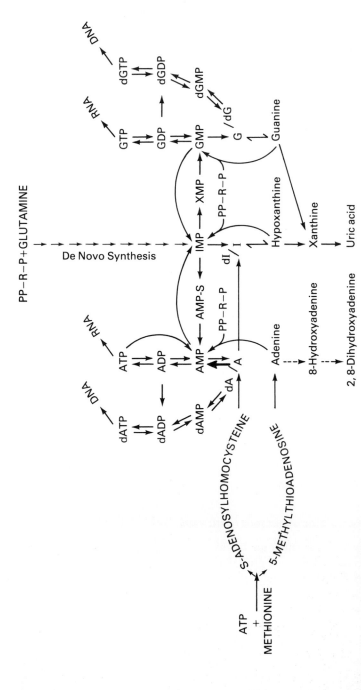

Fig. 6.1 Routes of synthesis, catabolism and salvage of the vital intracellular purine mono- and poly-nucleotides in man, indicating important associations with other metabolic pathways. Abbreviations: PP-R-P (phosphoribosylpyrophosphate); AMP, ADP, ATP (mono, di and triphosphate of adenosine); GMP, GDP, GTP (mono, di and triphosphate of guanosine); dAMP, dADP, dATP (mono, di and triphosphate of deoxyadenosine); dGMP, dGDP, dGTP (mono, di and triphosphate of deoxyguanosine); IMP (inosine monophosphate); dI (deoxyinosine); AMP-S (adenylosuccinic acid); XMP (xanthosine monophosphate).

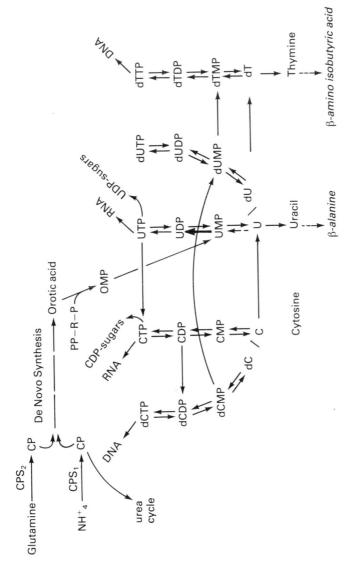

Fig. 6.2 Routes of synthesis, catabolism and salvage of the different intracellular pyrimidine nucleotides in man. The potential for stimulating the de novo pathway when the enzymes of the urea cycle are defective is evident, as is the importance of the pathway for the maintenance of the pyrimidine diphosphate sugars as well as the nucleic acids. Abbreviations: CPS₁ and CPS₂ (carbamoyl phosphate synthetases 1 and 2); U, UMP, UDP and UTP (uridine and its mono, di and triphosphates); dU, dUMP, dUDP and dUTP (deoxyuridine and its mono, di and triphosphates); C, CMP, CDP and CTP (cytidine and its mono, di and triphosphates); dC, dCMP, dCDP and dCTP (deoxycytidine and its mono, di and triphosphates); dT, dTMP, dTDP and dTTP (thymidine and its mono, di and triphosphates); OMP (orotidine monophosphate).

By contrast, pyrimidine metabolism lacks any defined metabolic end-product but turnover is considered to be of a similar order to that of purines. In man, purine salvage takes place at the base level whilst pyrimidine salvage occurs at the nucleoside (uridine) level; the reverse is true for micro-organisms. It is equally noteworthy that for both purine and pyrimidine metabolism, direct interconversions of the aminated nucleosides (adenosine, cytidine) with the corresponding bases (adenine, cytosine), or deamination at the base level, occurs only in micro-organisms and not in man.

Studies in the different inherited disorders have demonstrated that both purine and pyrimidine metabolism have equally crucial functions associated with the removal of metabolic waste from other pathways. It is now obvious that a considerable amount of adenosine is produced endogenously (14–23 mmol/24 h) as a by-product of the S-methylation pathway (Ch. 4, p. 112), a fraction of this being compartmentalised by protein binding. A small amount of adenine may also be produced via this route, but the bulk of adenine produced endogenously, about 1 mmol/24 h, arises as a by-product of another pathway, the polyamine pathway[1]. The same is true for pyrimidine metabolism where associations with the urea cycle are well documented (Ch. 4, p. 118).

Additionally, it has become apparent that the original concept of purine metabolism and its overall control does not apply to all cells, but is governed by a tissue or cell specific complement of enzymes and/or controls on them, depending on the function of that cell or tissue. For instance, unlike most cells, the human erythrocyte lacks adenylosuccinate synthetase and cannot use synthesis or salvage to maintain its ATP levels, requiring adenosine for this.[2] It also lacks guanase. The tissue-specific aspect of purine metabolism will be dealt with in more detail in the different inherited disorders.

Clinical and biochemical consequences of disorders of purine and pyrimidine metabolism

The importance of the normal recycling of purine bases in the feedback control of de novo purine synthesis is demonstrated by the gross purine overproduction found in three of the seven inherited disorders where this is defective. These are hypoxanthine-guanine phosphoribosyltransferase (HGPRT) deficiency, aberrant phosphoribosylpyrophosphate synthetase (PP-R-PS) activity, and purine nucleoside phosphorylase (PNP) deficiency. In their severest form, all three are also characterised by retarded development and generalised muscular hypotonia. Patients with the aberrant synthetase and HGPRT deficiency may also develop gout, uric acid stones or renal failure. Both are X-linked disorders (Table 6.1).

The potential nephrotoxicity resulting from the relative insolubility of most purine bases is also demonstrated in xanthine oxidase (XOD) and

Table 6.1 Characteristic clinical signs relative to the importance of early diagnosis in the ten different inherited purine and pyrimidine disorders

Defect	Early diagnosis	Clinical signs
XOD⁻	Generally benign	Mostly adults, hypouricaemia, radiolucent stones, ARF, myopathy.
APRT⁻	Essential—benign or lethal. Responds to treatment.	Birth ↑ —Crystalluria, recurrent UTI, haematuria, ARF, radiolucent stones.
*HGPRT⁻	Essential—benign or lethal.	Infant: Birth ↑ —Crystalluria, recurrent UTI, Haematuria. ARF, radiolucent stones, gout. Delayed motor development: 3 months ↑, CNS involvement: 8 months ↑ Adult: Gout, radiolucent stones.
PPRPS ↑	Essential—benign or lethal	Infant: Birth ↑ —Crystalluria, recurrent UTI, radiolucent stones. Head drops, nerve deafness. Delayed motor development: 3 months ↑. Adult: Gout, radiolucent stones.
*PNP⁻	Essential—generally lethal	Birth ↑ —Viral infections, lymphopenia, T-cell disfunction. Delayed motor development: 3 months ↑.
*ADA⁻	Essential—generally lethal.	Birth ↑ —Failure to thrive, diarrhoea, thrush, lymphopenia, SCID.
AMPDA⁻	? Benign	Infant: Hypotonia, cardiomyopathy. Adult: Exercise intolerance, myopathy.
OPRT⁻/ODC⁻	Essential—lethal. Responds to treatment.	Birth ↑ —Crystalluria, hypochromic, megaloblastic anaemia.
diHPyDH⁻	? Lethal	Birth ↑ —Currently undefined. Neurological abnormalities ? Other.
PyrNT	Benign	Non-spherocytic haemolytic anaemia with basophilic stippling, haemoglobinuria.

* Indicates defects for which prenatal diagnosis is essential/currently available.
UTI —Urinary Tract Infection
CNS —Central Nervous System
↑ —Can present at any time from birth upwards

ARF —Acute Renal Failure
? —Insufficient data currently available.

adenine phosphoribosyltransferase (APRT) deficiencies, which can present with kidney stones and/or renal failure. Additionally, in rare instances, xanthine oxidase deficiency may be associated with myopathy and this is the presenting symptom in myoadenylate deaminase (AMPDA) deficiency.

Patients with PNP deficiency present neonatally with immunodeficiency, as do homozygotes for adenosine deaminase (ADA) deficiency. Low lymphocyte ecto 5'-nucleotidase activity has also been reported in different immunodeficiency syndromes.[3] Since it is not certain whether this reflects a failure of lymphocyte maturation, or is the primary cause of the hypo-gammaglobulinaemia, it will not be discussed in this review. Patients with the other disorders are not immunodeficient.

The three pyrimidine disorders are associated with retarded growth and development. They are hereditary oroticaciduria or orotic acid phospho-ribosyltransferase/orotidylate decarboxylase (OPRT/ODC) deficiency, uraciluria and thymine-uraciluria or dihydropyrimidine dehydrogenase (diHPyDH) deficiency and pyrimidine 5'-nucleotidase (PyrNT) deficiency. OPRT/ODC deficiency is also characterised by hypochromic megaloblastic anaemia and the third defect, PyrNT deficiency, presents with chronic non-spherocytic haemolytic anaemia.

DISORDERS OF PURINE METABOLISM

Primary gout is the most prevalent of the purine disorders. Although it has been known since ancient times, as yet no underlying metabolic basis has been recognised. However, a total of eight inherited purine disorders have now been described in which a specific enzyme defect has been identified and only these will be described in greater detail in this review.

Gout

To date an hereditary defect has been found in less than one percent of patients presenting with gout. Two of these (HGPRT deficiency and PP-R-PS superactivity) are X-linked disorders and will be discussed in detail in the next sections. Gout is also a frequent complication of the recessively inherited disorder glycogenosis Type I (Ch. 2, p. 22).

Primary gout

Primary gout has been the subject of many excellent reviews.[4] It is a disease of plenty, associated generally with over-indulgence in dietary purine, and may involve other factors affecting the renal clearance of uric acid. It occurs predominantly in the middle-aged male. The basic problem lies in a mark-edly reduced ability of the gouty kidney to excrete uric acid, with a clear-ance of about 5 ml/min/100 mlGFR compared with healthy controls matched for age and sex of 8 ml/min/100 mlGFR. This is not due to reduced renal function per se. In the majority of patients with primary gout GFR is normal for age.

Secondary gout

This may be found in association with rapid tissue breakdown or accelerated cell turnover, often occurring spontaneously, or during aggressive therapy, in malignancy or haematological disorders. Gout may also be precipitated by any situation which effectively reduces the clearance of uric acid; for example, volume depletion, starvation, keto-acidosis or drug therapy for alternative condition. Thiazide diuretics now account for up to 50% of new patients presenting with gout.

Familial juvenile gout

This is now being recognised as a distinct entity. In the past decade it has become apparent that there may be at least three distinct varieties, designated here Types I, II and III. They are dealt with in more detail because of their relatively recent recognition and potentially fatal nature, although the biochemical defect is unknown. A summary of findings in the three types is shown in Table 6.2.

Clinical presentation

In all instances there is a strong family history, with at least one family member presenting with gout, generally in the big toe. The age of presentation is around puberty up to the third decade. Affected cases of Types I and II may be distinguished from primary gout, or the X-linked disorders, by the occurrence of gout in a young age group, usually affecting females as well as males, and frequently associated with a rapidly declining renal function leading to early death. Type III is characterised by a chronic compensated non-anaemic haemolytic syndrome of unknown aetiology.

Inheritance and incidence

These are rare sub-groups. Twelve families have been reported in Type I, two in Type II and eight patients in Type III. The inheritance appears dominant in Type I. Type II and III may be X-linked recessive disorders, strongly expressed in the heterozygous female in Type II.

Diagnosis

Hyperuricaemia with gout and impaired renal function before the age of 25, plus a strong family history involving both sexes, requires immediate investigation. In all instances plasma uric acid is disproportionately high for

Table 6.2 Summary of clinical and biochemical characteristics in three different types of gout presenting in adolescence, frequently affecting males and females alike

Familial juvenile gout	Type I	Type II	Type III
Clinical Details			
GFR	Rapid decline:	Dialysis in 3rd decade Rapid decline if untreated	N
Concentrating capacity	Reduced for GFR	Reduced for GFR	N
Blood pressure	Majority N	?	?
Other	—	—	Mild Jaundice
Prognosis	Potentially lethal	?	?
Inheritance	Dominant	?X-linked	?X-linked
Incidence	12 Families	2 Families	8 Cases
Purine Enzymes (red cells)			
HGPRT	N	?N	N
PP-R-PS	N	N	N
APRT	N	↑	N
Biochemical Defect	Unknown (? renal component)	Unknown (?HGPRT not fully active in vivo)	Unknown
Haemotology	N	N	(Compensated haemolytic syndrome) Reticulocytosis Low/absent Haptoglobin ↑ Bilirubin
Uric Acid excretion	?↑ Initially	2–4xN	2–4xN
Plasma uric acid	↑	↑	↑

N = Normal   ↑ = Increased

age, sex and GFR, three factors which must be taken into account in evaluating plasma uric acid levels. In Types II and III uric acid excretion is also grossly increased (7–14 mmol/24 h compared to the normal of 2–3 mmol/24 h).

A markedly reduced urinary concentrating capacity, disproportionately low for the reduction in GFR, is typical of Types I and II. Characteristic histological findings have been found at renal biopsy in Type I[5,6] and it has been argued that the basic defect may be primary renal disease in some. In Type III there may be mild jaundice, elevated indirect bilirubin, low to complete absence of haptoglobin, reticulocytosis, raised serum and urine iron levels or other associated abnormalities.[7]

In all three sub-groups activity of the purine enzymes HGPRT and PP-ribose-P synthetase is normal in lysed red cells (Table 6.2). APRT activity is raised exclusively in Type II and HGPRT activity may also not be fully active in intact cells in vivo in this type.

Treatment

Treatment involves the use of allopurinol at reduced dosage allowing for the degree of reduction in GFR. In Type I allopurinol appears to have halted the rapid decline in renal function in some family members. In Type II poor compliance initially was associated with a rapid decline in GFR which stabilised with improved compliance. The long-term prognosis in all remains to be determined.

Hereditary xanthinuria (McKusick 27830)

Biochemical disorder

The enzyme xanthine oxidase (EC 1.2.3.2) or, more correctly, xanthine dehydrogenase (EC 1.2.1.37), since in human tissue NAD^+ is the electron acceptor, catalyses the degradation of hypoxanthine and xanthine to uric acid (Fig. 6.3), the end-product of purine metabolism in man. It has an absolute requirement for molybdenum, FAD and iron. In man activity is concentrated mainly in the liver and intestinal mucosa.

In homozygotes for xanthine oxidase deficiency xanthine and, to a lesser extent, hypoxanthine accumulate in place of uric acid. The preferential excretion of xanthine is due to extensive normal recycling of hypoxanthine by the salvage pathway for which xanthine is not an effective substrate in vivo. Excess xanthine in the defect results from guanine nucleotide catabolism via guanase (Fig. 6.1).

Recently, combined xanthine oxidase/sulphite oxidase deficiency has been described due to a congenital absence of a molybdenum co-factor essential for both enzymes, in which the clinical features of sulphite oxidase deficiency overshadow those of the xanthine oxidase defect (p. 118 and 409).

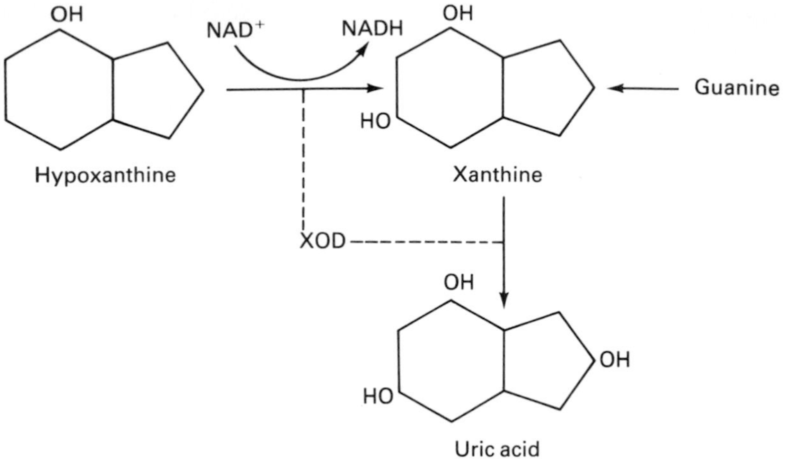

Fig. 6.3 The formation of uric acid from hypoxanthine and xanthine catalysed by xanthine oxidase (XOD).

Clinical presentation

More than 50% of homozygotes are asymptomatic. They are generally detected by finding a very low plasma uric acid level during routine screening for a presumably unrelated disorder. In four cases myopathy was reported associated with crystalline deposits of xanthine and hypoxanthine in skeletal muscle. A third have presented with symptoms which can be attributed directly to the defect—urinary tract infection, colic and/or xanthine calculi. Xanthine is an extremely insoluble purine. Unlike uric acid, its solubility in urine at pH 5.0 (0.5 mmol/l) is not greatly enhanced by alkalinisation of the urine (0.9 mmol/l at pH 7.0). In some cases, this has resulted in clubbing of the calyces of the kidney, hydronephrosis, nephrectomy, chronic renal failure, or death.

Xanthine nephropathy and acute renal failure can also be precipitated by aggressive therapy for malignant disorders treated concomitantly with the xanthine oxidase inhibitor allopurinol to reduce the risk of uric acid nephropathy.

Inheritance and incidence

Xanthine oxidase deficiency has been identified in more than fifty cases, including men and women, of Caucasian, Asian and Negroid descent. Studies in several kindreds are consistent with an autosomal recessive mode of inheritance. Genetic heterogeneity in the defect has been demonstrated by the fact that some xanthinurics can convert allopurinol to oxipurinol, whilst others do not.[8] This may be related to activity of the associated enzyme, aldehyde oxidase.

Diagnosis

The defect may be identified by the finding of low to undetectable levels of uric acid in plasma. On a purine-free diet uric acid is virtually undetectable in plasma or urine, being replaced in urine by xanthine and hypoxanthine in an approximate ratio of 5:1. Total oxypurine excretion on a low purine diet is generally reduced (1–2 mmol/24 h compared to the normal of 2–3 mmol/24 h). Sensitive methods have recently identified raised plasma levels of hypoxanthine and xanthine in the defect.[8,9] Renal clearances in homozygotes suggest that hypoxanthine clearance approximates to the GFR, but tubular secretion of xanthine also occurs.[9] Raised urinary levels of xanthine and hypoxanthine have been reported in some heterozygotes. The enzyme defect cannot be detected in red cells as xanthine oxidase is confined to the liver and intestinal mucosa. Biopsy of these tissues is necessary to confirm homozygosity for the deficiency.

Xanthine stones are generally brownish orange, smooth and oval. They are easily cut and have a laminated appearance inside. Except for those with a calcium oxalate core, the stones are radiolucent and give a positive murexide test. They can be distinguished from uric acid or 2,8-dihydroxyadenine stones by the UV spectrum at pH 2.0 and 10.0, by infra-red or mass spectrometry and by X-ray crystallography.

Treatment

Because of the poor solubility of xanthine at any pH, alkalinisation of the urine is ineffective and a high fluid intake is the only therapy. The importance of this is indicated by the nephropathy and the frequent necessity for nephrectomy in xanthinurics from arid climates.[8] The serious nephrotoxicity of xanthine is supported by experimental studies in the pig indicating that even short periods of crystal deposition could produce an acute nephropathy resulting in severe and permanent renal damage.

Adenine phosphoribosyltransferase deficiency (McKusick 10260)

Biochemical disorder

Adenine phosphoribosyltransferase (APRT, EC 2.4.2.7) catalyses the conversion of adenine to AMP, a reaction requiring PP-ribose-P (Fig. 6.4). The ubiquitous distribution of the enzyme in all human cells, with the highest concentration in nucleated cells, was at first puzzling, since adenine is not a normal consitituent of body fluids. Moreover, pathways in purine metabolism for its endogenous production appeared to to be lacking in man.

The finding of subjects homozygous for the defect, excreting 30% of total purine end-product in the form of adenine and its metabolites, 8-hydroxyadenine and 2,8-dihydroxyadenine, even on a purine-free diet, led to recognition of adenine as an endogenous by-product of the polyamine

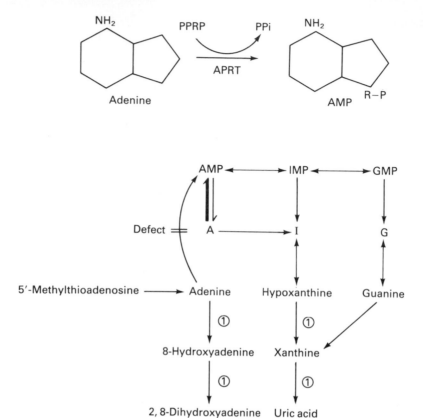

Fig. 6.4 The normal function of adenine phosphoribosyltransferase (APRT) in the removal of adenine derived as metabolic waste from the polyamine pathway and the alternative route of adenine metabolism to the extremely insoluble 2,8-dihydroxyadenine, which is operative when APRT is inactive. The alternative pathway is catalysed by xanthine oxidase 1.

pathway (Fig. 6.4). In APRT deficiency, adenine, unable to be salvaged normally, is catabolised by xanthine oxidase via 8-hydroxyadenine to the extremely insoluble 2,8-dihydroxyadenine.

Clinical presentation

The defect may be benign or life-threatening. When 2,8-dihydroxyadenine stones are formed as a consequence of the defect, the whole scale of symptoms associated with stone formation may be observed within the first two years of life.[1] These include fever from urinary tract infection, macroscopic haematuria, crystalluria, dysuria, urinary retention and abdominal colic. Several cases have presented in acute renal failure. However, the expression may be extremely variable with 25% of homozygotes remaining completely asymptomatic and only detected during family studies. Others have not presented until the fourth decade, indicating that homozygotes may remain asymptomatic for long periods. Purine production and excretion is otherwise normal, as is the general biochemistry and immunology. The occurrence of spontaneous abortions in one family may represent in utero expression of the defect.[2]

Inheritance and incidence

The gene for this autosomal recessive disorder is coded for on the long arm of chromosome 16. Detailed studies of the electrophoretic, catabolic and immunological properties of the mutant enzyme have shown less than one percent immunoreactive protein to APRT antibody in erythrocytes of homozygotes, while in heterozygotes the activity was generally 25% of normal. The latter finding has been attributed to the fact that the enzyme is a dimer and that protein-protein interaction of two normal sub-units is required for expression of normal activity.[10]

Lymphocytes and fibroblasts of homozygous subjects also lack APRT activity. Studies of the variant enzyme in heterozygotes have shown normal heat stability, kinetic parameters, end-product inhibition, substrate affinity and half-life in circulating erythrocytes. Immunoreactive protein ranged from 22–112% suggesting there are a variety of mutations in the structural gene coding for APRT.[10] 29 cases have been reported in the decade since the original diagnosis, 19 children and 10 adults. 11 of the cases are from Japan. Studies in five countries have indicated heterozygosity for the defect to be about 1%, suggesting homozygosity may be more frequent than is currently recognised.[1]

Diagnosis

The defect could be suspected in any case with a history of recurrent urinary tract infection and 'uric acid' crystalluria or lithiasis but normal uric acid levels. Renal ultrasound drew attention to the underlying nephropathy in a case presenting in coma. The stones are composed of 2,8-dihydroxy-adenine and have been erroneously diagnosed as uric acid in the past because of an identical reactivity in all colorimetric reactions, as well as in the murexide test and thermogravimetric analysis.[1] The stones are radiolucent, like uric acid and xanthine stones, but are soft, creamy-grey and crush with ease. They may also be distinguished by the UV spectrum at pH 2.0 and pH 10.0, infra-red and mass spectrometry, and the lack of action of uricase which degrades uric acid to allantoin. The defect is established by the finding of high levels of adenine, 8-hydroxyadenine and 2,8-dihydroxyadenine in the urine in the approximate ratio of 1:0.03:1.5. The combined excretion usually equals 20–30% of the total purines.

The diagnosis may be confirmed by the absence of APRT activity in intact or lysed red cells. However, APRT activity may be falsely raised if transfusion has been essential on admission and then it may take six months before homozygosity can be confirmed on erythrocytes. Significant APRT activity has been reported from Japan in some cases of 2,8-dihydroxy-adenine lithiasis. Previous transfusion was excluded and it has now been shown that these represent kinetic mutants with a reduced affinity for PP-ribose-P. Elevated APRT activity due to the high percentage of young red cells has been noted in new-borns, in renal failure, megaloblastic anaemia with reticulocytosis and in fetal blood.

Treatment

Dietary purine restriction, together with a high fluid is advised in asymptomatic homozygotes. In stone formers allopurinol (5–10 mg/kg, depending on age and renal function), but without alkali, will prevent further stone formation. Unlike uric acid, 2-8-dihydroxyadenine solubility is not improved by alkali, and in at least three cases stone formation was actually increased, suggesting its use is contra-indicated.

Allopurinol inhibits conversion of adenine to 2,8-dihydroxyadenine, but adenine does not normally accumulate because it is secreted and cleared rapidly by the human kidney. The possibility of long-term toxicity developing, particularly in renal failure, requires careful monitoring. Early diagnosis is important because this is a treatable disorder. Three cases have required chronic haemodialysis, but such serious complications should be avoidable in the future.

Hypoxanthine-guanine phosphoribosyltransferase deficiency (McKusick 30800)

Biochemical disorder

Hypoxanthine-guanine phosphoribosyltransferase (HGPRT, EC 2.4.2.8) catalyses the salvage of the purine bases hypoxanthine and guanine to IMP and GMP respectively, and requires PP-ribose-P (Fig. 6.5). The enzyme does not react with xanthine in vivo in man. The nucleotides so formed exert strong feed-back control on de novo synthesis and salvage will normally predominate over de novo synthesis. This effectively restricts endogenous purine loss in the form of uric acid to 2–3 mmol/24 h in adults.

The importance of HGPRT in the normal interplay between synthesis and salvage is demonstrated by the biochemical and clinical consequences of the defect.[11] Gross uric acid over-production results from the inability to recycle either hypoxanthine or gaunine, with a resultant lack of feed-back control of synthesis and rapid catabolism of these bases to uric acid (Fig. 6.1). PP-ribose-P not utilised in the salvage reaction is considered to provide an additional stimulus to de novo synthesis and uric acid over-production.[12]

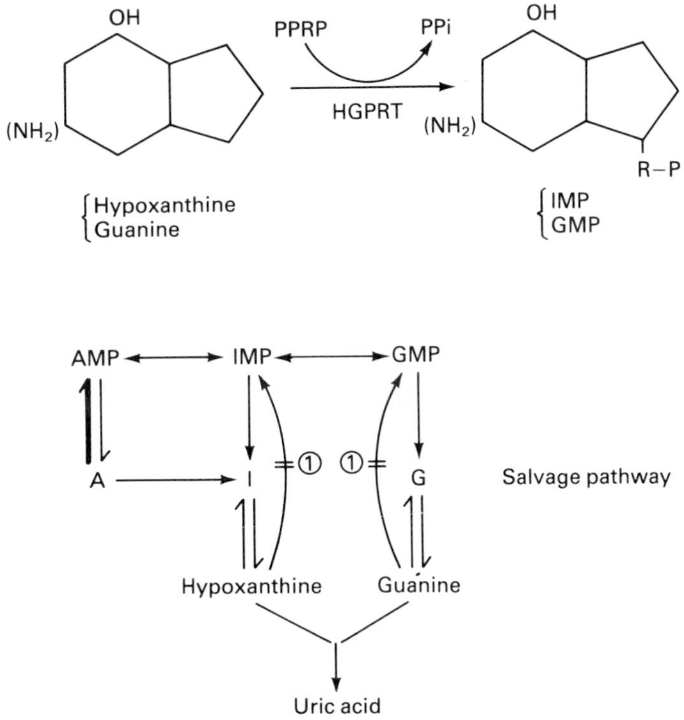

Fig. 6.5 The salvage pathway of the purine bases, hypoxanthine and guanine, to IMP and GMP, respectively, catalysed by HGPRT (1) in the presence of PP-R-P. The defect in HGPRT is shown.

Clinical presentation

There is a broad spectrum of clinical presentation depending on the severity of the enzyme defect. In the most severe form (the Lesch-Nyhan syndrome), affected subjects may present in the first week of life with crystalluria, acute renal failure and gout if renal function is severely impaired. Severe cases are characterised by spasticity, with pyramidal tract signs, compulsive self-mutilation, choreoathetosis and mental retardation.[11] The full gamut of expression may take years to manifest. Some workers consider the pyramidal tract lesion may be the consequence of cervical cord compression and that the basic motor abnormality is generalised muscular hypotonia. Moreover, the apparent mental handicap may be complicated by a variety of factors including lack of educational opportunities or suitable intelligence tests.

Some patients have also shown megaloblastic anaemia. It was originally reported, but subsequently disputed, that immunodeficiency due to a B cell lymphocytopenia with reduced IgG levels, was characteristic of the Lesch-Nyhan syndrome. However, although lung and urinary tract infections are frequent, they can be secondary to aspiration or nephropathy.[11]

A partial defect of HGPRT is found in patients who lack the severe manifestations of the Lesch-Nyhan syndrome and usually present in their teens or early adulthood with hyperuricaemia, gout, renal failure, or kidney stones.[11,13,14]

Inheritance and incidence

HGPRT deficiency is an X-linked recessive disorder. Although rare, the incidence is higher than for the other purine disorders. It has been estimated that one-third of cases may be new mutations. The enzyme defect has recently been reported in a girl with classic Lesch-Nyhan symptoms. The possibility that she has inherited structural gene mutations on both parental X chromosomes was proposed.

The complete amino acid sequence for human erythrocyte HGPRT has been established recently. A nucleotide-binding domain has been identified and single amino acid substitutions characterised in structural variants in several cases of partial HGPRT deficiency.[15] HGPRT is a cytoplasmic enzyme with highest activity in brain and rapidly dividing tissues. A variety of studies have demonstrated altered kinetic, catalytic, electrophoretic and immunochemical properties, as well as in vitro or in vivo stability, in different mutants.[15]

Diagnosis

All patients with either partial or complete HGPRT deficiency exhibit gross uric acid over-production and excretion. In HGPRT deficient children plasma uric acid may not appear raised until puberty, but uric acid excretion on a creatinine basis is 2–4 times the normal which is less than 1.0 mmol/mmol creatinine. In adults the plasma uric acid is higher and the urine uric acid lower, but still raised on a creatinine basis, normal being less than 0.3 mmol/mmol creatinine. All patients also have high hypoxanthine levels in plasma and urine.

It is noteworthy that in both children and adults presenting in acute renal failure due to obstructive uropathy, excessive uric acid excretion will be masked if expressed on a creatinine basis.[14] The diagnostic criteria in this situation is a grossly raised plasma uric acid (in excess of 1 mmol/l) in any subject presenting in acute renal failure. Renal ultrasound provided the clue to the correct diagnosis in one such neonate. Uric acid stones may be the sole manifestation in some cases. They are radiolucent and generally yellowish, smooth, hard and crush with difficulty.

The defect may be confirmed by the finding of low to undetectable levels of HGPRT in lysed red cells. Lesch-Nyhan patients have no detectable enzyme in any cell type, intact or lysed, by immunochemical or conventional assay. Patients with the partial deficiency have variable amounts of activity in lysed red cells. However at least 12 cases have been described whose lysed red cells completely lacked enzyme, but who had no neurological complications. In such cases significant activity (5–25% of normal) has been found in intact red cells suggesting an unstable enzyme in vitro.[13,14]

Heterozygotes cannot be detected reliably from enzyme activity in lysed red cells, probably due to random Lyonisation of one X-chromosome (Ch. 1, p. 9). Most studies have relied on comparative HGPRT/APRT ratios in hair roots.[16] Heterozygote detection has also proved difficult using fibroblasts but recent developments using recombinant DNA technology and southern blotting have now made accurate diagnosis possible. The latter technique has recently been applied to much earlier prenatal diagnosis of HGPRT deficiency using chorionic biopsy material. Cultured amniotic fluid cells and also fetal blood may be used for prenatal diagnosis in the second trimester.[11,17]

APRT activity is raised, but only in lysed red cells, possibly due to stabilisation by the raised PP-ribose-P levels also found in all cell types. Altered pyrimidine nucleotide levels[18] and grossly raised NAD^+ levels, accompanied by severe GTP depletion,[19] have been reported in red cells in the Lesch-Nyhan syndrome, but GTP levels were normal in the partial deficiency.[19] Whether the latter are consistent findings, of use in determining prognosis or the understanding of the underlying CNS dysfunction in the Lesch-Nyhan syndrome, remains to be established.

Other findings in the Lesch-Nyhan syndrome include raised urinary excretion of imidazole carboxamide. Much lower concentrations of brain free-amino acids have also been reported. This may restrict precursors essential for neurotransmitter or protein synthesis as well as contributing to the decrease in catecholamine levels in basal ganglia noted by others.[20] However, the basic defect underlying the neurological complications remains undefined.

Treatment

Allopurinol, high fluid and alkali is the treatment of choice for either the complete or partial deficiency. Lesch-Nyhan patients appear exquisitely sensitive to allopurinol and both xanthine and oxipurinol calculi have been reported. In patients with renal failure the dose must also be carefully monitored and reduced to no more than 5 mg/kg in children, or 100 mg/24 h in adults, to prevent accumulation of oxipurinol, the active drug metabolite, with its attendant risk of bone marrow depression and other side effects.[21] Exchange transfusion as a source of enzyme replacement and pharmacological approaches to therapy with tryptophan, 5-hydroxytryptophan or glutamate, have failed to reverse the biochemical or neurological complications in the syndrome.[13,16] There is at present no successful treatment for the severe neurological complications.

Phosphoribosyl pyrophosphate synthetase superactivity (McKusick 31185)

Biochemical defect

Phosphoribosyl pyrophosphate synthetase (PP-ribose-P synthetase, EC 2.7.6.1) catalyses the transfer of the pyrophosphate group of ATP to ribose-5-phosphate to form PP-ribose-P (Fig. 6.6). The synthetase is activated by inorganic phosphate, and is subject to complex regulation by different nucleotide end products of the pathways for which PP-ribose-P is a substrate, particularly ADP and GDP.[22]

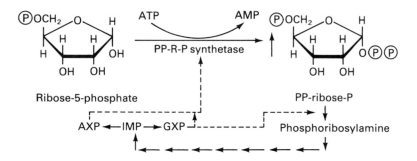

Fig. 6.6 The role of PP-R-P in the de novo synthesis of IMP and adenosine (AXP) and guanosine (GXP) nucleotides and the feed-back control normally exerted by these nucleotides on de novo purine synthesis.

PP-Ribose-P acts as an allosteric regulator of the first specific reaction of de novo purine biosynthesis (Fig. 6.1), in which the interaction of glutamine and PP-ribose-P is catalysed by amidophosphoribosyl transferase. PP-ribose-P produces a slow activation of the amidotransferase by changing it from a large, inactive dimer to an active monomer.[12] Purine nucleotides, on the other hand, can cause a rapid reversal of this process, towards the inactive form.

Thus, the de novo synthesis of purine nucleotides is normally under fine control. A reduction in nucleotide concentration enhances the synthetase and the increased level of PP-ribose-P, in turn, activates the amidotransferase and promotes purine synthesis. After a lag period, a build up of purine nucleotides occurs which will cut off further synthesis by inactivating amidotransferase.

Variant forms of PP-ribose-P synthetase have been described, insensitive to normal regulatory functions, or with a raised specific activity. This results in continuous PP-ribose-P synthesis which stimulates de novo purine production, resulting in accelerated uric acid formation and gross overexcretion.[22]

Clinical presentation

The majority of cases have presented with severe gout or kidney stones in adolescence or early adulthood.[22] However, in possibly 3 families a more severe form of presentation has been observed in which in addition to gross purine over-production, there was severe neurodevelopmental retardation, hypotonia, a left convergent squint and inherited nerve deafness. There was also a history of repeated attacks of bronchopneumonia and of previous siblings dying with identical symptoms in early infancy. Whether, as in HGPRT deficiency, these extremes of clinical expression merely reflect the degree of enzyme deficiency, remains to be determined. Female heterozygotes also show purine over-production and, in the severe form, sensorineural deafness.

Inheritance and incidence

This is an extremely rare X-linked disorder described in only 8 families to date.[23] Several different variant forms of the enzyme have been identified, which show either a reduced sensitivity to the nucleotide inhibitors ADP or GDP, increased specific activity per enzyme molecule, increased affinity for ribose-5-phosphate, or a combination of these.

The normal enzyme comprises a single sub-unit which undergoes reversible aggregation to forms containing 2,4,8,16 and 32 sub-units. Only the largest of these is compatible with normal enzyme function,[23] which may explain the variety of mutants observed.

Diagnosis

The defect should be suspected in any young adult of either sex with marked hyperuricaemia and/or hyperuricosuria which is 2–4 times normal, but with normal HGPRT and APRT activity in lysed red cells. Reported values for PP-ribose-P synthetase activity have varied widely. Improved methods for detection of activity in red cells have recently been published and patients with variant enzymes have been found to have activity 2–4 times the normal range.[23] Erythrocyte PP-ribose-P levels are also generally elevated but in the more severe form this may only be evident in the youngest red cells, due possibly to red cell enzyme instability. Raised PP-ribose-P levels have also been found in lymphoblasts and fibroblasts.[22] In the severe form another characteristic feature has been the inability of intact red cells to increase the incorporation of either hypoxanthine or adenine into the corresponding nucleotide at high phosphate concentrations, that is under PP-ribose-P stimulating conditions, as do normal red cells. Low red cell NAD and GTP levels have been reported in two cases with the severe form, but whether these observations are characteristic remains to be proven. Immune function is normal.

Treatment

Allopurinol at a level of 300 mg/24 h for adults and 10 mg/24 h for children, will control plasma and uric acid levels in patients with normal renal function and gout or kidney stones. The dose must be reduced in parallel with the degree of reduction in renal function in any case with associated gouty nephropathy.[21] A high fluid intake and alkalinisation of the urine may help. To date, no successful therapy for the associated neurological complications has been devised.

Purine nucleoside phosphorylase deficiency (McKusick 16405)

Biochemical defect

Purine nucleoside phosphorylase (PNP, EC 2.4.2.1) is responsible for the degradation of the nucleosides inosine, guanosine or their deoxy-analogues to the corresponding base. Although this is essentially a reversible reaction, base formation is favoured because intracellular phosphate levels normally exceed those of either ribose-, or deoxy-ribose-phosphate. The enzyme is a vital link in the purine salvage pathway (Fig. 6.7) and has a wide tissue distribution.

Homozygotes for PNP deficiency are unable to catabolise the above nucleosides or deoxnucleosides which consequently accumulate in body fluids. Enzyme deficient patients have in effect a double defect, since the

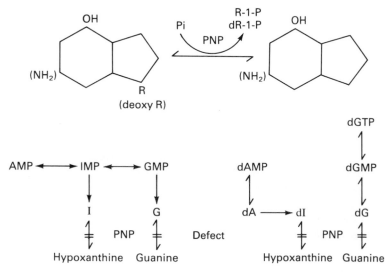

Fig. 6.7 The importance of purine nucleoside phosphorylase (PNP) for the normal catabolism and salvage of both nucleosides and deoxynucleosides resulting in the accumulation of dGTP, exclusively, in the absence of the enzyme, since kinases do not exist for the other nucleosides in man. The lack of functional HGPRT activity, through absence of substrate, in PNP deficiency is also apparent.

next step in the purine salvage cycle, involving HGPRT, is unable to operate due to absence of substrate. Gross purine over-production results, due to lack of nucleotide formation and of feed-back inhibition of de novo synthesis, as in the Lesch-Nyhan syndrome (Fig. 6.1).

Red cells and fibroblasts from PNP deficient patients incorporate hypo-xanthine and guanine into the nucleotide more rapidly than normal cells, indicating HGPRT is active though normally inoperative. However in contrast to normal cells, IMP and GMP are rapidly degraded to the nucleo-side, leading to the suggestion that the enzyme defect has unmasked a normal cyclic process.[24]

The cause of the toxicity to the immune system is unknown. It has been related to the conversion of deoxyguanosine to dGTP by either deoxycyti-dine kinase[25] or a specific kinase. Preferential accumulation of dGTP in T but not B cells[26] with subsequent inhibition of ribonucleotide reductase and DNA synthesis has been proposed. However this has been questioned by others who demonstrated growth inhibition at a later phase in the cell cycle than would have been anticipated.[27] The presence of some T-helper cell function is considered to explain the relatively normal B cell function. Kinases for the other three nucleosides accumulating in PNP deficiency do not exist in human cells.

Clinical presentation

The age of presentation of the defect has varied and in all but one instance has occurred by the first four years of life. The most severely affected present neonatally with lymphopenia and defective cell-mediated (T-cell) immunity: phytohaemagglutinin responses may be normal at birth but diminish rapidly. Although actual B-cell numbers may be low, as a percentage of total lymphocytes they are normal. Immunoglobulin levels are normal or increased, and some cases with the latter have developed autoim-mune disease. Some late presenters have been identified by the hypouri-caemia noted during screening for Coombes positive haemolytic anaemia; anaemia has been reported in 30% of cases. Three long-term survivors have some PNP activity in certain cell types.

Infections are less frequent than in ADA deficiency but otitis media is common. Patients become increasingly susceptible to varicella, vaccinia or cytomegalovirus and the majority have died from such viral infections. Many have been immunised prior to diagnosis with live vaccines, or given non-irradiated blood transfusions without effect, indicating some residual T-cell function. Histological changes in the thymus at autopsy have been considered consistent with involution rather than a congenital absence of the thymus.

Additional clinical symptoms include head-lag and excessive irritability noted as early as 3 months. Severely deficient patients have remained extremely hypotonic and developmentally retarded; some have manifest spastic tetraparesis. Such symptoms are undoubtedly due to the lack of a functional salvage cycle.

Inheritance and incidence

This is an extremely rare disorder which has been described in some 18 patients to date. The defect is inherited in an autosomal recessive manner and in some families there is evidence of consanguinity. The enzyme is coded for by a gene located on the long arm of chromosome 14. Studies in different families have demonstrated varying amount of immunologically reactive protein with varying kinetic parameters, isoelectric points and altered electrophoretic mobility. Such genetic heterogeneity confirms alterations on a structural gene coding for the enzyme.

Diagnosis

The presence of an extremely low blood and urine uric acid in a child with recurrent viral infection is suggestive of PNP deficiency. The biochemical abnormality may be established by the presence of grossly raised amounts of inosine, guanosine, deoxyinosine and deoxyguanosine in plasma, about 50, 10, 5 and 5 μmol/l respectively compared to normally undetectable levels. In urine the same compounds are excessively excreted, in about the same relative proportions. In severe cases no uric acid is detectable in any body fluid but significant levels are found in late presenters. Hypoxanthine or guanine may be found in urine in severe cases due to nucleoside degradation by bacterial contamination. Total purine excretion on a creatinine basis is increased 2–4 fold.

The defect may be confirmed by the finding of low to undetectable PNP activity in lysed erythrocytes. Heterozygotes have intermediate levels but are clinically normal. Red cell APRT activity is twice normal, possibly, as in HGPRT deficiency, due to stabilisation by the raised PP-ribose-P levels also found. Increased PP-ribose-P levels have likewise been noted in fibroblasts and lymphoblasts in severely affected cases. Prenatal diagnosis has recently been carried out using cultured amniotic fluid cells and fetal blood may also be used.[17]

Raised levels of dGTP have been found in red cells, accompanied in six developmentally retarded patients by severe GTP depletion and three times normal NAD$^+$ levels. Similar biochemical findings occur in HGPRT deficiency, but in neither condition is it established that these changes are causally related to the neurological abnormality.

Treatment

No satisfactory therapy has yet been found for any of these patients. Two cases have been supported for long periods by enzyme replacement using irradiated red cells, with only partial restoration of T-cell function in vitro and no neurological improvement.[28]

Different pharmacological approaches have been tried. Some have been based on in vitro studies demonstrating the reversal of lymphotoxicity by uridine or the pyrimidine deoxycytidine. The latter is the preferred substrate for the kinase considered responsible for the conversion of deoxyguanosine to the toxic intracellular deoxynucleotide dGTP.[26] However, parenteral deoxycytidine over a 12-month period together with tetrahydrouridine to inhibit the rapid in vivo deamination of the pyrimidine, produced no sustained improvement in biochemical, immunological or clinical parameters,[29] despite in vitro enhancement of T-cell function. Alternative approaches using hypoxanthine or guanine (alone or with allopurinol) proved equally ineffective, confirming that salvage of dietary purines is of little significance in man. A trial of human amnion implantation as an alternative source of enzyme replacement was also unsuccessful.[29]

Adenosine deaminase deficiency (McKusick 10270)

Biochemical disorder

Adenosine deaminase (ADA, EC 3.5.4.4) catalyses the deamination of adenosine and 2'-deoxyadenosine to inosine or 2'-deoxyinosine respectively (Fig. 6.8). However, most of the adenosine derived endogenously is normally phosphorylated rather than deaminated because the K_m for aden-

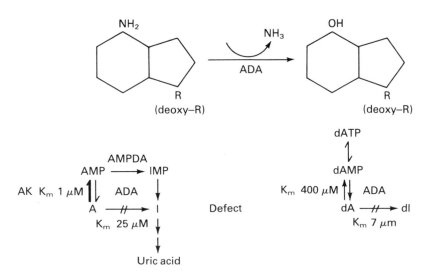

Fig. 6.8 The importance of adenosine deaminase (ADA) for the catabolism of dA, but not A, and the resultant accumulation of dATP when ADA is defective. A is normally salvaged by adenosine kinase (see Km values of A for ADA and the kinase, AK) and deficiency of ADA is not significant in this situation.

osine kinase (1 μM) is an order of magnitude lower than that for ADA (25 μM).[30] In contrast to micro-organisms, humans lack any significant ability to convert adenosine to adenine, or to deaminate the latter at the base level.[1] A series of rigorous controls normally ensures that adenine nucleotides are deaminated at the nucleotide level in most tissues by AMP deaminase. Consequently there should generally be little flux of adenosine nucleotides through the ADA degradative pathway (Fig. 6.1). By contrast $2'$-deoxy AMP (dAMP) is not a substrate for AMP deaminase and must be degraded via $2'$-deoxyadenosine and ADA. The importance of ADA for the catabolism of toxic deoxynucleotides thus becomes obvious.[30] Highest activity is found in the lymphoid tissues.

In patients homozygous for ADA deficiency $2'$-deoxyadenosine accumulates[30,31] and is converted back to dATP, either by adenosine kinase or deoxycytidine kinase.[26] Two main hypotheses have been put forward to explain the specific toxicity to the immune system in ADA deficiency.[27,31] One is based on the apparently selective accumulation of dATP in T but not B cells, with resultant inhibition of ribonucleotide reductase and DNA synthesis.[26,30] The other implicates 2-deoxyadenosine directly through its irreversible binding to S-adenosylhomocysteine hydrolase which is inhibited and leads to inactivation of methylation reactions equally vital to normal cell function. However, there is as yet no clear evidence in favour of either and the biochemical basis for the immunodeficiency remains undefined.[27]

Clinical presentation

Patients with ADA deficiency are subject to recurrent chronic, viral, fungal, protozoal, and bacterial infections and frequently present with persistent diarrhoea, failure to thrive and candidiasis.[31] The age of onset has varied but is usually within the first 2 years of life. Severely affected cases present neonatally with no detectable lymphocytes in peripheral blood or bone marrow and both cell mediated and humoral immunity is defective. T-cells are generally absent, agammaglobulinaemia is the rule and lymphocyte proliferative and specific antibody responses are lacking. In later presenters the defect may not be easily recognised; lymphocyte numbers are not reduced, cellular immunodeficiency may not be so profound and immunoglobulin levels are normal. Histopathological studies have shown the presence of Hassals corpuscles and other criteria suggesting involution of a previously differentiated thymus, but this has been disputed subsequently.[31] Some patients have had associated bony and hair growth abnormalities and occasionally non-specific neurological disorders.

Inheritance and incidence

This is an autosomal recessive disorder. The gene coding for ADA is on the long arm of chromosome 20. The enzyme is genetically polymorphic in the normal population and three phenotypes have been recognised on electrophoresis: ADA 1, ADA 2 and ADA 2/1, ADA 2 being much less common. Tissues other than red cells show more complex electrophoretic patterns due to a high molecular weight binding protein, one molecule of which binds two molecules of ADA.[32] Severely affected children have no detectable ADA isoenzymes in any tissues but binding protein is normal Late presenters have had low but detectable activity in mono-nuclear cells. More than 100 cases have now been identified. ADA deficiency has been found in 20–30% of cases with recessively inherited severe combined immunodeficiency (SCID). The defect has been described in Caucasians, Negroes and Asians.

Diagnosis

Because of the considerable variation in expression, ADA deficiency may not always be suspected as a cause of SCID, but should be considered in any child presenting with generalised candidiasis. The defect may be confirmed by the finding of undetectable ADA levels in lysed red cells. As ADA is unstable at $-20°C$, blood must be transported at room temperature and stored at $-70°C$. S-adenosylhomocysteine hydrolase activity is also grossly reduced in lysed red cells. 11 cases exist with complete red cell ADA deficiency who are not immunodeficient.[31] In these instances some ADA activity is detectable in lymphocytes, lymphoblasts and fibroblasts, presumably suffucent for immunocompetence. Heterozygosity for the defect is difficult to detect, most obligate heterozygotes have ADA levels at the lower limit of the normal range.[31]

Raised red cell dATP levels accompanied by ATP depletion will also reflect the severity of the genetic disorder. The same biochemical changes have also recently been found in platelets and may account for the in vitro functional abnormalities reported previously.[31]

The finding of 2'-deoxyadenosine in urine (0.04–0.16 mmol/mmol creatinine) is another characteristic feature[30,31] and it is also present in plasma in severely affected infants, whilst adenosine has been found in plasma and urine in some, but not all, cases.[31] Purine production as well as uric acid and other purine and pyrimidine levels are normal in the defect.

Prenatal diagnosis has been performed using cultured amniotic fluid cells[31] and more recently from enzyme and nucleotide levels in fetal blood.[17] It is of interest that in two affected cases diagnosed by the latter technique, the amniotic fluid cells failed to grow. In both cases there was already severe lymphopenia, with complete absence of T cells and T cell subsets, indicating the early onset of lymphocytotoxicity.

Treatment

There is no generally effective therapy in ADA deficiency. Many different regimes have been tried. These have included enzyme replacement with irradiated red cells, thymic hormone[31] and pharmacological approaches employing deoxycytidine, the preferred substrate for deoxycytidine kinase. All have had minimal success except in late presenters with residual ADA activity in mononuclear cells.[31] Thymic transplant has also been attempted. The only long-term successful therapy to date has been in those few cases where bone marrow from an HLA/MLR compatible sibling donor was available.[31] However, recent results using T cell depleted mis-matched sibling marrow have been encouraging.

Myoadenylate deaminase deficiency (McKusick 25475)

Biochemical disorder

Adenylate deaminase (AMPDA: EC 3.5.4.6) catalyses the deamination of AMP to IMP. The enzyme is normally under rigorous control, being inhibited by GTP and inorganic phosphate (P_1) and stimulated by ATP. In most tissues AMP is predominantly deaminated via this route, rather than dephosphorylated. Only when the adenylate energy charge has fallen below 0.6 does the latter route become significant.[33] There are a variety of isoenzymes of AMPDA which vary from tissue to tissue.

In muscle the enzyme is considered to form part of an important cycle—the purine nucleotide cycle.[34] This cycle involves two other enzymes, adenylosuccinate synthetase which requires GTP and aspartate, and adenylosuccinate lyase, which reconverts IMP to AMP (Fig. 6.9). There has been much debate about the significance of this cycle for normal muscle function. Following exercise AMPDA activity increases and this may increase local ammonia production which in turn would stimulate glycolysis. An alternative suggestion relates to an increase in fumarate during reconversion of IMP to AMP, which provides a mechanism whereby citric acid cycle intermediates, such as fumarate, would be replenished during muscle work, a period necessitating an increased demand for ATP.

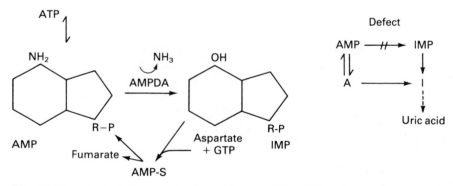

Fig. 6.9 The role of AMPDA in the deamination of AMP to IMP and the reconversion of the latter to AMP via AMP-S, thus completing the purine nucleotide cycle which is of particular importance in muscle.

In myoadenylate deficiency muscle AMPDA activity is less than 5% of normal. The limited amount of information currently available suggests that IMP or AMP do not accumulate after exercise, but that the defect results in a depletion of all adenine nucleotides in muscle.

Clinical presentation

The majority of patients have presented with muscle cramps or myalgias following exercise and 67% of them had their first symptoms in childhood or adolescence. Muscle weakness has been found in 27% of patients, but muscle wasting has not been reported. Hypotonia has developed in only 8%. In one family the defect was associated with progressive muscle weakness and fatal cardiomyopathy.

Inheritance and incidence

The defect is generally specific to skeletal muscle. AMPDA activity is normal in other tissues and cells, including erythrocytes, leucocytes and fibroblasts, suggesting there may be a separate genetic locus for the isoenzymes demonstrated in different tissues.

The defect has been described in more than 30 patients but, in addition, three separate studies of 770 muscle biopsies in all, from patients with muscle weakness or poor exercise tolerance, revealed histological and biochemically confirmed AMPDA deficiency in 2% of cases. Thus the condition may be more common than early work suggests.

AMPDA deficiency shows equal sex distribution and is usually considered to be autosomal recessive but in the family with the fatal cardiomyopathy it appeared to be dominant.

Diagnosis

A simple test is used in diagnosis—the lactate/ammonia exercise ratio during ischaemic exercise.[35] Exercise does not lead to NH_3 production, or deamination of AMP to IMP, as in normal subjects, and muscle ATP and total purine content fall following exercise to a greater extent than in control subjects. Increased serum creatine kinase has been found in some 60% of patients. As already stated, AMPDA activity (determined histochemically or enzymatically) is low to undetectable in muscle samples from all patients, but is normal in other types of cell. Intermediate levels have recently been reported in muscle biopsies from carriers for the defect. Levels of purine metabolites such as uric acid, xanthine and hypoxanthine have not generally been reported, so it is not known whether total purine production and excretion is altered in this defect. However, gout and/or hyperuricaemia has been noted in three patients.

Treatment

The prognosis in most instances is good, with no evidence of progressive debilitation or structural damage. At present there is no known treatment. Although ribose has successfully increased ATP synthesis in rat myocardium, it has had mixed success in man.[36]

Adenylosuccinase deficiency

Biochemical disorder

Adenylosuccinase (adenylosuccinate lyase: EC 4.3.2.2) is involved in two important steps in purine metabolism. It is the enzyme catalysing the eighth step in the ten-step de novo synthetic pathway, and also the second step in the formation of ATP from IMP (Fig. 6.10). The substrate for the first reaction is succinylaminoimidazole carboxamide ribotide (ribotide); the product is aminoimidazole carboxamide ribotide. In the second reaction the substrate is adenylosuccinic acid and the product is AMP, with fumarate also being released in both instances.

A defect of this enzyme results in the accumulation of the two

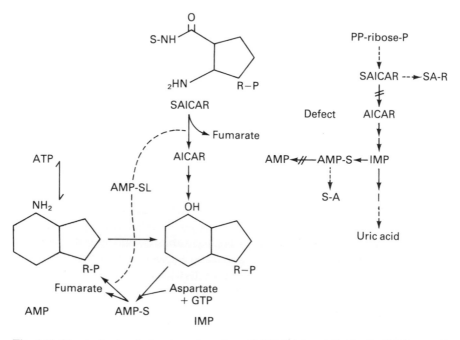

Fig. 6.10 The dual role of adenylosuccinate lyase (AMP-SL) in catalysing the eighth step of the de novo pathway, the conversion of succinylaminoimidazole carboxamide ribotide (SAICAR) to aminoimidazole carboxamide ribotide (AICAR), as well as the second step in the conversion of IMP to AMP via adenylsuccinic acid (AMP-S), with the release of fumarate. The formation of both succinylaminoimidazole carboxamide riboside (SA-R) and succinyl adenosine (S-A) occurs when AMP-SL is defective.

substrates for these enzymes in the form of their nucleoside derivatives[37]. The defect has been demonstrated in liver and kidney, but not red cells, granulocytes or skeletal muscle, suggesting that, as with AMP-deaminase deficiency, there may be several isoenzymes in human tissue.

Clinical presentation

To date only seven cases have been identified. Although the history at birth is unremarkable, psychomotor retardation has become evident within the first two years of life. All showed pronounced autistic features, were hypokinetic and could not maintain eye contact. There was axial hypotonia with normal tendon reflexes. There was also some evidence of self-mutilation. Routine biochemistry was normal. Cerebellar hypoplasia was visible on CT scan.

Inheritance and incidence

The occurrence of the defect in two children of different sex and belonging to related parents, suggests an autosomal recessive mode of inheritance.

Diagnosis

The diagnosis may be suspected from the presence of raised levels of aspartic acid and glycine detected in body fluids by TLC or GLC following acid hydrolysis. It may be confirmed using HPLC by the finding of two additional u.v. absorbing peaks in plasma, urine and CSF, with the characteristic retention times of succinyladenosine and succinoaminoimidazole carboxamide riboside. The absence of phosphate but presence of ribose on hydrolysis confirm that these components are present as the nucleosides, presumably derived from the corresponding nucleotides by the action of a cytoplasmic 5′-nucleotidase. Renal clearance of both nucleosides is in excess of the GFR. Uric acid in plasma and urine is normal but no further data on levels of other purine enzymes or levels in body fluids has yet been published.

Treatment

As yet, no treatment is available, but the finding of this defect in children with autism may open up new perspectives in this area.

DISORDERS OF PYRIMIDINE METABOLISM

Hereditary orotic aciduria (McKusick 25890)

Biochemical defect

Orotic acid is an intermediate in the six-step de novo pyrimidine synthetic pathway which commences with carbamoyl phosphate (CP). CP may be synthesised by a synthetase (CPS 1) present in the mitochrondria which is essential for the urea cycle (Ch. 4, p. 118). This enzyme is confined almost exclusively to the liver, with low activity in kidney, intestinal mucosa and leucocytes. CP may also be synthesised by CPS 2, a cytosolic enzyme. The latter is widely distributed throughout the body and apparently forms a multi-enzyme complex with the next two enzymes of pyrimidine biosynthesis, and is subject to complex feed-back regulatory processes (Fig. 6.2). However, CPS 1 may be a significant source of liver pyrimidines since, even at optimal conditions, a third of the CP synthesised by this route is reportedly exported to the cytosol, with 80% being incorporated into hepatic pyrimidines.

In hereditary orotic aciduria the last two enzymes of the pathway, orotic acid phosphoribosyltransferase (OPRT: EC 2.4.2.10) and orotidine-5′-monophosphate decarboxylase (ODC: EC 4.1.1.23), are defective or absent; orotic acid accumulates and is excreted in quantity.[38] These two enzymes catalyse the conversion of orotic acid to UMP and other pyrimidine nucleotides, the first step requiring PP-ribose-P (Fig. 6.11). They also exist as a complex, possibly associated in turn with the membrane bound mitochondrial enzyme responsible for orotic acid synthesis.[39]

Clinical presentation

The onset of symptoms usually occurs in the first few months of life. The common presenting symptoms are hypochromic anaemia with megaloblastosis, unresponsive to iron, folic acid and B_{12} therapy, and leucopenia. Failure to thrive, developmental retardation, bilateral strabismus, sparse hair, inability to sit unaided, and gross crystalluria, sometimes with ureteric obstruction, have been general findings. Immunodeficiency has been described in one family but it has been questioned whether this is a true facet of the defect. Renal function is normal. Heterozygotes show mild orotic aciduria but are otherwise unaffected.

Inheritance and incidence

The gene coding for the multi-functional protein carrying OPRT and ODC is located on the long arm of chromosome 3. The disorder has been identified in Caucasians and Polynesians and is inherited in an autosomal recessive fashion. The enzyme defect has been confirmed in liver, fibroblasts, lymphoblasts, red cells and leucocytes from affected individuals. There has been some debate as to whether homozygotes carry a structural or regulatory gene defect.[40] The defect is rare and the majority of patients lack both OPRT and ODC. Prenatal diagnosis has not been recorded.

Diagnosis

Homozygotes may be detected by the severe refractory megaloblastic anaemia and the high levels of orotic acid in the urine of up to 2 g or

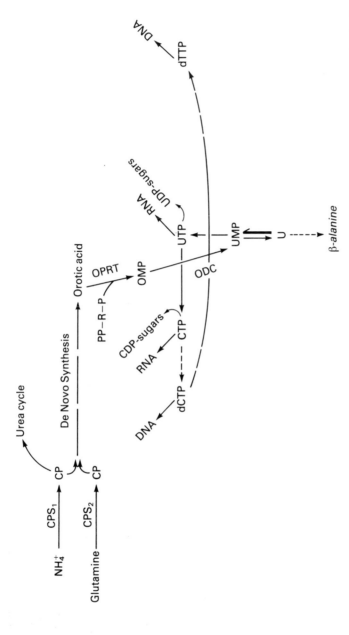

Fig. 6.11 The orotic acid phosphoribosyltransferase (OPRT) orotidine-5'-monophosphate decarboxylase (ODC) complex which is essential for the de novo synthesis of UMP. Over excretion of orotic acid results when the enzyme complex is defective.

10 mmol/24 h, with normal values of less than 2 mg or 10 μmol/24 h. Orotic acid is generally measured by a colorimetric method but appropriate blanks must be included since falsely raised values can be produced by histidine, septrin etc.[41] Orotic acid may now be measured in plasma and urine by HPLC and raised plasma levels of 40 μmol/l, compared to the normal of less than 0.1 μmol/l, have been found in homozygotes. Orotic acid clearance exceeds the GFR.

The defect may be confirmed by the low to undetectable levels of OPRT and ODC in lysed red cells. It should be noted that OPRT is unstable even in frozen red cells, but ODC is not so unstable. The red cell enzyme levels in heterozygotes overlap the lower end of the normal range so definitive diagnosis of heterozygosity requires both a low enzyme level coupled with a slightly raised urinary excretion of orotic acid. Both enzyme activities and orotic acid excretion may be affected by a variety of factors, such as haematological status, reticulocytosis, iron and pharmacological agents such as 5-azauridine, 5-azaorotic acid, or allopurinol.[40,42] This may confuse the diagnosis. Pharmacological agents have also produced near normal OPRT/ODC levels in enzyme deficient fibroblasts in vitro[40] and a reduction in orotic acid excretion in vivo in hereditary orotic aciduria.[42] These effects have been attributed to stabilisation of the enzyme complex by nucleotide derivatives.

Purine metabolism is normal but uric acid clearance is high in the defect, probably due to the uricosuric effect of orotic acid. Purine enzymes are likewise normal, apart from APRT which is raised.[42] However, this cannot be due to stabilisation by raised PP-ribose-P levels as in HGPRT deficiency, since PP-Ribose-P levels are normal in orotic aciduria.

Treatment

Large doses of oral uridine (150 mg/kg or 0.5 mmol/kg/24 h in three divided doses) will reverse the clinical symptoms and reduce orotic acid excretion to below 1 g or 5 mmol/24 h. Uracil is ineffective.[38] One patient who was treated successfully for 20 years relapsed immediately when compliance was poor, indicating a life long requirement for therapy. Despite the high level of orotic acid and uric acid in the urine, renal function is not impaired, but a high water intake is advisable.

Secondary orotic aciduria

Orotic aciduria secondary to defects involving four of the six enzymes associated with the urea cycle, results from stimulation of de novo pyrimidine biosynthesis following overflow of mitochondrial derived CP into the cytoplasm.[41] The orotic aciduria can equal that in the hereditary disorder, but can be distinguished by the raised blood ammonia levels and, in some cases, by grossly raised levels of uridine and uracil in plasma and urine. The orotic aciduria is considered secondary to PP-ribose-P depletion in consequence of the greatly increased flux through the de novo pathway. Orotic-aciduria secondary to two purine defects associated with immunodeficiency was originally reported but has not been found in subsequent studies. Patients with dietary deficiencies of essential amino acids, Reyes syndrome, hereditary protein intolerance or on parenteral nutrition, can also mimic the degree of orotic aciduria seen in the urea cycle defects.[41]

Hereditary thymine-uraciluria and uraciluria

Biochemical disorder

Pyrimidine metabolism, unlike purine metabolism, normally lacks an identifiable end-product (Fig. 6.2). However, several cases have been reported recently in which the over-excretion of pyrimidine bases was noted. In all but one instance a defect in the enzyme dihydropyrimidine dehydrogenase (di HPyDH: EC 1.3.1.2) was demonstrated.[43] This enzyme normally catalyses the first step in the degradation of the pyrimidine bases, uracil and thymine to β-alanine and β-amino-isobutyric acid respectively (Fig. 6.12).

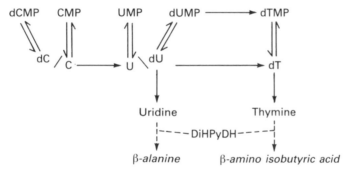

Fig. 6.12 Dihydropyrimidine dehydrogenase (DiHPyDH) is essential for the catabolism of the end-products of pyrimidine metabolism (uracil and thymine) to amino acids. A deficiency of DiHPyDH leads to accumulation of these end-products.

In one case over-excretion of uracil alone was observed (uraciluria). The biochemical defect in this instance is unknown, but decreased salvage of uridine, or increased pyrimidine synthesis resulting from fluctuations in the levels of either the pyrimidine synthetic or urea cycle enzymes was proposed.[43]

Clinical presentation

There is insufficent data to give a clear clinical picture. The first reported case was the third child of healthy parents. The second sibling had died of perinatal asphyxia. Cyanosis and respiratory distress developed a few hours after birth and, later, pneumothorax with hyperbilirubinaemia. Psychomotor development appeared normal until 1 to 1½ years when speech failed to develop and behavioural changes occurred. Intelligence was normal and there were no auditory defects. Similar symptoms with varying degrees of involvement have been reported in some but not all cases. Microcephaly has also been a consistent finding.

The case of uraciluria was the first child of healthy unrelated parents and presented at 4 years with psycho-motor and speech retardation, sparse fine hair, hyperlaxity and hypotonia with microcephaly.[43]

Thymine-uraciluria has also been reported in a case of medulloblastoma which was considered to be related to the specific nature of the tumour.[44]

Inheritance and incidence

There are too few cases to provide information on this.

Diagnosis

These defects may be detected by the finding of high levels of thymine and/or uracil in the urine where they are not normally detectable. DiHPyDH deficiency may be confirmed by demonstrating the enzyme defect in cultured fibroblasts and leucocytes. In the first patient oral loading with uracil or thymine resulted in recovery of more than 70% of the load in urine in the following 24 h and this may also be used to confirm the defect.[43] In the infant with uraciluria, oral loading with uracil excluded diHPyDH deficiency and the absence of abnormal thymine excretion was considered to exclude possible heterozygosity for the defect.[43] Neither orotic acid nor orotidine were elevated generally in either defect. In diHPyDH deficiency normal levels of uric acid and pseudouridine were reported, indicating that tissue breakdown was not enhanced. Periodic bouts of hyperammonaemia of unknown aetiology accompanied by transient orotic aciduria and uridinuria were noted in the patient with uraciluria.

Treatment

There is no established treatment for either disorder.

Pyrimidine-5'-nucleotidase deficiency (McKusick 26612)

Biochemical defect

Pyrimidine-5'-nucleotidase (PyrNT, EC: 3.1.3.5) is the first enzyme of the pyrimidine salvage pathway (Fig. 6.13) and catalyses the specific hydrolysis of pyrimidine-5'-nucleotides. It is a cytosolic enzyme requiring Mg^{2+} for activity, while lead, copper and mercury are markedly inhibitory. PyrNT

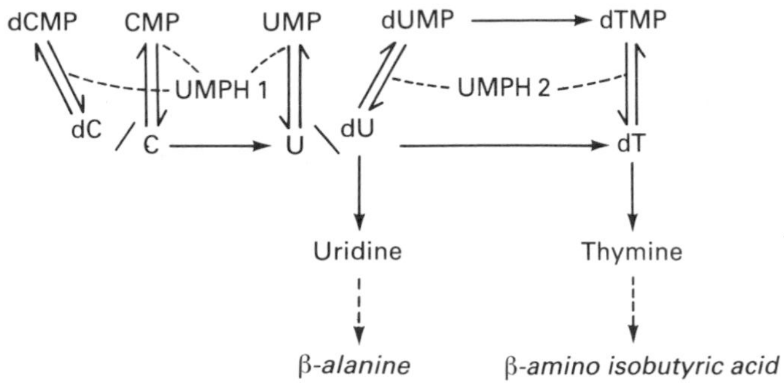

Fig. 6.13 The role of uridine monophosphate hydrolases (UMPH) 1 and 2 in the catabolism of UMP, CMP and dCMP (UMPH1), and dUMP and dTMP (UMPH2).

activity is due, in fact, to two isoenzymes, designated uridine monophosphate hydrolase 1 and 2 (UMPH 1 and 2), which have overlapping substrate specificities and pH optima. UMPH 1 hydrolyses UMP, CMP and dCMP preferentially, whereas UMPH 2 prefers dUMP and TMP as substrates and has a wide pH optimum. UMPH 1 and 2 activities have been demonstrated in a wide range of human tissues, including lymphoblasts, and there is evidence for tissue specificity of isoenzyme composition.[45] The purified enzyme from normal red cells has a pH optimum of 7–7.5 with CMP as substrate. The major part of this activity, 90–95%, resides in UMPH 1, the remainder is due to overlapping specificity of UMPH 2.[45]

Deficiency of UMPH 1[45] results in the accumulation of high levels of pyrimidine nucleotides in the red cells of homozygotes and it was proposed originally that these were derived from RNA degradation in maturing red cells, trapped because of the enzyme defect.[46] Others have shown active uptake of uridine or orotic acid into nucleotides by normal and deficient red cells, suggesting an important role for the red cell in pyrimidine transport and hence an alternative explanation for the raised nucleotide levels.[47] Accumulation of slightly raised levels of UTP and UDP-sugars in lymphoblasts deficient in UMPH 1, has also been noted recently.

Clinical presentation

Homozygotes present with non-spherocytic haemolytic anaemia characterised by marked basophilic stippling in their erythrocytes.[46,47] The age of presentation has varied widely. Other characteristic findings include reticulocytosis, anisocytosis, splenomegaly and sometimes cholelithiasis. Increased levels of indirect bilirubin, increased erythrocyte levels of reduced glutathione, with reduced activity of PP-ribose-P synthetase may also be found. In addition, two recent cases showed intravascular haemolysis, haemoglobulinuria, urinary iron loss and enlarged kidneys. Biopsy showed iron in the epithelium of the proximal tubules.[48] Heterozygotes are clinically and haematologically normal.

Inheritance and incidence

Approximately 35 cases of this autosomal recessive disorder have been reported in both children and adults following the identification of the biochemical basis for the clinical disorder in 1974. Electrophoretic analysis of erythrocytes and lymphoblasts from patients with the disorder have shown a complete deficiency of the major isoenzyme UMPH 1. Normal levels of UMPH 2 have been found, both by assay and electrophoresis. The fact that this isozyme appears unaffected by the genetic deficiency of UMPH 1 suggests it may be determined by an independent genetic locus. Enzyme levels in lysed erythrocytes by conventional assay have shown activity approximately 10% of the normal range of 8–15 nmol/mg Hb/h. Most of the residual activity in affected individuals is undoubtedly attributable to the deoxy-pyrimidine nucleotidase UMPH 2. In some cases the abnormal UMPH 1 has been reported to have different electrophoretic characteristics, pH optima, heat stability and increased K_m.

Diagnosis

The enzyme defect should be suspected in patients with non-spherocytic haemolytic anaemia and may be detected by the method of Valentine et al in lysed red cells, using CMP or UMP as substrate.[46] A preliminary screening test is based on the characteristic U.V. absorption profile at 280 nm and 254 nm for deproteinised extracts of enzyme deficient red cells compared with normal cells. Electrophoretic analysis coupled with staining for the different isozymes is a useful confirmatory test.[45]

HPLC should be used to demonstrate the grossly increased pyrimidine nucleotide levels in the red cells, principally UDP glucose, UDP-N-acetyl glucosamine and CDP choline. In the normal red cell adenine nucleotides comprise over 90% of the total nucleotide pool and, apart from low levels of UDP glucose, pyrimidine nucleotides are undetectable. In PyrNT deficiency the concentration of pyrimidine nucleotides may exceed those of the adenine nucleotides, although the former may vary possibly due to the episodic nature of the disease. It is now established that the level of adenine nucleotides remains normal.

Recent studies using ^{31}P, NMR spectroscopy have shown that the additional pyrimidine triphosphates are Mg^{++} bound and there is a nearly proportional increase in red cell Mg^{++}. The near doubling of the triphosphate pool results in a low intracellular pH, which is thought to explain a low oxygen affinity and altered levels of glycolytic intermediates in the deficient cells, despite a normal 2,3-diphosphoglycerate concentration.[49]

Erythrocyte PP-ribose-P synthetase activity is 30% that for normal cells of comparable age, related to a decrease in enzyme protein. Whether production or degradation is altered is uncertain. Impairment of pentose phosphate shunt activity may contribute to the pathogenesis of the haemolysis and the reduced PP-ribose-P synthetase activity in the defect. Glutathione reductase activity has been reported normal or increased. Unfortunately, neither pyrimidine nor purine levels have been reported in the body fluids in this defect.

Treatment

The disease is relatively benign. Anaemia in the defect has usually been moderate with transfusion rarely necessary. Splenectomy has not proved beneficial.

Acquired pyrimidine-5'-nucleotidase deficiency

Severe lead intoxication is associated with a similar syndrome which may include haemolytic anaemia and marked red cell basophilic stippling. All subjects with lead intoxication have shown substantial reductions in red cell enzyme activity. However, only in severe cases has significant accumulation of red cell pyrimidine nucleotides been demonstrated, associated with anaemia and prominent basophilic stippling. At concentrations of blood lead in excess of 200 μg/100 ml, lead induced deficiency mimics the genetic disorder.

Laboratory diagnosis

All the above defects apart from AMPDA deficiency may be detected by altered levels of metabolites in plasma, urine or red cells. For summary of findings see Table 6.3. In HGPRT deficiency and aberrant PP-R-PS activity, uric acid levels are grossly raised in urine relative to creatinine, as is total purine excretion in PNP deficiency. Xanthine oxidase or PNP deficiency should be suspected in any patient with low to undetectable plasma urate levels on routine screening, and appropriate clinical manifestations.

Xanthine oxidase deficiency may be distinguished from renal hypouricaemia (tubular reabsorption defect) by the absence of uric acid from both plasma and urine, and replacement by xanthine and hypoxanthine. In PNP deficiency, inosine, guanosine and their deoxyanalogues, deoxyinosine and deoxyguanosine replace uric acid in plasma and urine. In ADA deficiency the abnormal metabolite excreted is deoxyadenosine and in APRT deficiency, adenine, 8-hydroxyadenine and 2,8-dihydroxyadenine are found.

The defects can be confirmed by enzyme assay in lysed red cells, cultured lymphoblasts or fibroblasts, except in xanthine oxidase and AMPDA deficiencies where biopsy is essential. In HGPRT, ADA and PNP deficiencies characteristic alterations in red cell nucleotides are also found using high pressure liquid chromatographic (HPLC) techniques. These techniques may also be employed for rapid prenatal diagnosis using fetal blood.[17]

Table 6.3 List of abnormal metabolites which may accumulate (or possible alteration in normal levels) in body fluids and red cells, in the ten different inherited disorders of purine and pyrimidine metabolism which have been identified to date.

	Classic gout	HGPRT⁻	PPRPs↑	APRT⁻	PNP⁻	ADA⁻	XOD⁻	AMPDA⁻	OPRT⁻/ODC⁻	diHPYDH⁻	PyrNT
BLOOD											
RBC											
Enzyme	N	→	↑	→	→	→	No	N	→	→	→
Nucleotide	N	GTP↓	GTP↓	N	dGTP↑	dATP↑↑	N	N	UDPG↑	? ?	UDPS↑↑
PPRP	N	↑	↑	N	↑	N	N	?	N	?	?
Plasma											
Uric acid	N → ↑	↑↑	↑↑	N	Nil	N	Nil	? ?	→ N ←	N ?	? ? ?
Other purine	N	↑↑	↑↑	N	↑↑	N	↑		N	?	
Orotic acid	—	—	—	—	—	—	—	—	—	—	—
URINE											
Uric acid	N → ↑	↑↑	↑↑	N	Nil	N	Nil	?	← N	N	? ? ?
Xanthine	N	N	N	N	Nil	N	↑	?	N	N	
Hypoxanthine	N	↑	↑	N	Nil	N	↑	?	N	N	
8-hydroxyadenine	—	—	—	↑	—	—	—	—	—	—	—
Adenine	—	—	—	↑	—	—	—	—	—	—	—
2,8-dihydroxyadenine	—	—	—	↑	—	—	—	—	—	—	—
I	—	—	—	—	↑↑	—	—	—	—	—	—
G	—	—	—	—	↑↑	—	—	—	—	—	—
dI	—	—	—	—	↑	—	—	—	—	—	—
dG	—	—	—	—	↑	↑	—	—	—	—	—
dA	—	—	—	—	—	↑	—	—	—	—	—
Orotic acid	—	—	—	—	—	—	—	—	↑ ←	N ←	?
Uracil	—	—	—	—	—	—	—	—	—	←	?
Thymine	—	—	—	—	—	—	—	—	—	←	?
Total Purine	N	2–4x↑	2–4x↑	N	4x↑	N	N	?	N	N	?

N Normal
— Not normally detected
? Not known
↓ decreased
↑ increased

In the pyrimidine disorders grossly raised orotic acid levels in urine and plasma are found in OPRT/ODC deficiency. Uracil plus thymine are excreted in diHPyDH deficiency. In UMPH 1 deficiency high levels of pyrimidine nucleotides are found in red cell extracts (Table 6.3).

REFERENCES

1 Simmonds H A, Cameron J S, Dillon M J, Barratt T M, Van Acker K J 1981 'Uric Acid' stones in children: problems of diagnosis and treatment. Fortschritte der Urologie und Nephrologie 16: 52–57
2 Lowry B A, Williams M K, London J M 1962 Enzymatic deficiencies of purine nucleotide synthesis in the human erythrocyte. Journal of Biological Chemistry 245: 3043–3046
3 Webster A D B, Shah T, Peters T J 1984 Lymphocyte ecto 5'-nucleotidase in immunodeficiency and leukaemia. In: De Bruyn C H M M, Simmonds H A, Muller M M (eds) Purine metabolism in man, IVA. Plenum, New York, p 67–72
4 Wyngaarden J B, Kelley W N 1976 Gout and hyperuricaemia. Grune and Stratton, New York
5 Simmonds H A, Cameron J S, Potter C F, Warren D, Gibson T, Farebrother D 1980 Renal failure in young subjects with familial gout. In: Rapado A, Watts R W E, De Bruyn C H M M (eds) Purine metabolism in man, IIIA. Plenum, New York, p 15–21
6 Burke J R, Inglis J A, Craswell P W, Mitchell K R, Emmerson B T 1982 Juvenile nephronophthisis and medullary cystic disease—the same disease (report of a large family with medullary cystic disease associated with gout and epilepsy). Clinical Nephrology 18: 1–8
7 Liberman U A, Samuel R, Halabe A, Sperling O 1981 Juvenile gout and hyperuricosuria due to chronic compensated haemolytic syndrome. Fortschritte der Urologie und Nephrologie 16: 32–35
8 Simmonds H A, Stutchbury J H, Webster D R, Spencer R E, Wooder M, Buckley B M 1984 Pregnancy in xanthinuria: demonstration of foetal uric acid production? Journal of Inherited Metabolic Disease 7: 77–80
9 Harkness R A, Coade S B, Walton K R 1983 Xanthine oxidase deficiency and 'Dalmation' hypouricaemia: incidence and effect of exercise. Journal of Inherited Metabolic Disease 6: 114–120
10 Wilson J M, Daddona P E, Simmonds H A, Van Acker K J, Kelley W N 1982 Human adenine phosphoribosyltransferase: immunochemical quantitation and protein blot analysis of mutant forms of the enzyme. Journal of Biological Chemistry 257: 1508–1515
11 Nyhan W L 1982 Inborn errors of purine metabolism. In: Cockburn F, Gitzelmann R (eds) Inborn errors of metabolism in humans. MTP Press, Lancaster, p 13–37
12 Holmes E W 1978 Regulation of purine biosynthesis de novo. In: Kelley W N, Weiner I M (eds) Uric acid. Springer Verlag, Berlin, p 21–43
13 Emmerson B T, Thompson L 1973 The spectrum of hypoxanthine-guanine phosphoribosyltransferase deficiency. Quarterly Journal of Medicine 166: 423–440
14 Cameron J S, Simmonds H A, Webster D R, Wass V, Sahota A 1984 Problems of diagnosis and in vitro enzyme instability in an adolescent with hypoxanthine-guanine phosphoribosyltransferase deficiency presenting in acute renal failure. In: De Bruyn D H M M, Simmonds H A, Muller M M (eds) Purine metabolism in man, IVA. Plenum Press, New York, p 7–12
15 Wilson J M, Baugher B W, Landa L, Kelley W N 1981 Human hypoxanthine-guanine phosphoribosyltransferase: purification and characterisation of mutant forms of the enzyme. Journal of Biological Chemistry 256: 10306–10312
16 Watts R W E, Spellacy E, Gibbs D A, Allsop J, McKeran R O, Slavin G E 1982 Clinical, post-mortem, biochemical and therapeutic observations on the Lesch-Nyhan syndrome with particular reference to the neurological manifestations. Quarterly Journal of Medicine 201: 43–78
17 Simmonds H A, Rodeck C H, Levinsky R J, Lynch D C, Fairbanks L D, Webster D R 1983 Rapid prenatal diagnosis of adenosine deaminase deficiency and other purine disorders using foetal blood. Bioscience Reports 3: 31–38

18 Nuki G, Astrin K, Brenton D, Cruikshank M, Lever J, Seegmiller J E 1977 Purine and pyrimidine nucleotides in some mutant human lymphoblasts. In: Ciba Foundation Symposium 48—(new series) Purine and pyrimidine metabolism. Elsevier, Amsterdam, p 127–143

19 Simmonds H A, Webster D R, Watson A R, Barratt, T M, Wilson J 1982 Erythrocyte GTP depletion associated with severe muscular hypotonia in three inherited disorders of purine metabolism. Clinical Science 63: 61–66

20 Rassin D K, Lloyd K G, Kelley W N, Fix I 1982 Decreased amino acids in various brain areas of patients with Lesch-Nyhan syndrome. Neuropaediatrics 13: 130–134

21 Elion G B, Benezra F M, Beardmore T D, Kelley W N 1980 Studies with allopurinol in patients with impaired renal function. In: Rapado A, Watts R W E, De Bruyn C H M M (eds) Purine metabolism in man, IIIA. Plenum Press, New York, p 263–267

22 Becker M M 1984 Phosphoribosylpyrophosphate synthetase superactivity: detection, characterisation of underlying defects, and treatment. In: De Bruyn C H M M, Simmonds H A, Muller M M (eds) Purine metabolism in man, IVA. Plenum, New York, p 91–96

23 Losman M J, Hecker S, Woo S, Becker M 1984 Diagnostic evaluation of phosphoribosylpyrophosphate synthetase activities in haemolysates. Journal of Laboratory and Clinical Medicine 103: 932–943

24 Cohen A, Barankiewicz J, Issekutz A, Galfand E W 1984 Purine metabolism in intact cells from a purine nucleoside phosphorylase deficient child. In: De Bruyn C H M M, Simmonds H A, Muller M M (eds) Purine metabolism in man, IVB. Plenum, New York, p 163–166

25 Cohen A, Gudas L J, Ammann A J, Staal G E J, Martin D W 1978 Deoxyguanosine triphosphate as a possible toxic metabolite in the immunodeficiency associated with purine nucleoside phosphorylase deficiency. Journal of Clinical Investigation 61: 1405–1409

26 Carson D A, Kay J, Matsumoto A, Seegmiller J E, Thompson L 1979 Biochemical basis for the enhanced toxicity of deoxynucleosides towards malignant human T-cells. Proceedings of the National Academy of Sciences 76:2430

27 Henderson J F 1983 Mechanisms of toxicity of adenosine, 2'-deoxyadenosine and inhibitors of adenosine deaminase. In: Berne R M, Rall T W, Rubio R (eds) Regulatory function of adenosine. Martinus Nijhoff, The Hague, p 223–234

28 Stoop J W, Zegers B J M, Spaapen L J et al 1984 The effect of deoxycytidine and tetrahydrouridine in purine nucleoside phosphorylase deficiency. In: De Bruyn C H M M, Simmonds H A, Muller M M (eds). Purine metabolism in man, IVA. Plenum, New York, p 61–66

29 Watson A R, Simmonds H A, Webster D R, Layward L, Evans, D I K 1984 Purine nucleoside phosphorylase (PNP) deficiency: a therapeutic challenge. In: De Bruyn C H M M, Simmonds H A, Muller M M (eds) Purine metabolism in man, IVA. Plenum, New York, p 53–59

30 Simmonds H A, Panayi G S, Corrigall V 1978 A role for purine metabolism in the immune response: adenosine deaminase activity and deoxyadenosine catabolism. Lancet 1: 60–63

31 Hirschhorn R 1983 Genetic deficiencies of adenosine deaminase and purine nucleoside phosphorylase: overview, genetic heterogeneity and therapy. In: Wedgewood R J, Rosen F S, Paul N W (eds) Primary immunodeficiency diseases, birth defects, original Article Series. Alan R Liss, New York 19: 73–83

32 Daddona P E, Kelley W M 1978 Human adenosine deaminase binding protein: assay, purification and properties. Journal of Biological Chemistry 253: 4617–4623

33 Matsumoto S S, Ravio K O, Seegmiller J E 1979 Adenine nucleotide degradation during energy depletion in human lymphoblasts: adenosine accumulation and adenylate energy charge correlation. Journal of Biological Chemistry 254: 8956–8962

34 Lowenstein J M 1972 Ammonia production in muscle and other tissues: the purine nucleotide cycle. Physiological Reviews 52: 382–414

35 Fishbein W N 1984 Human myoadenylate deaminase deficiency. In: De Bruyn C H M M, Simmonds H A, Muller M M (eds). Purine metabolism in man, IVA. Plenum, New York, p 77–84

36 Lecky B R F 1983 Failure of D-ribose in myoadenylate deaminase deficiency. Lancet 1:193

37 Jaeken J, Van den Berghe G 1984 An infantile autistic syndrome characterised by the presence of succinylpurines in body fluids. Lancet 2: 1058–1061
38 Becroft D M O, Phillips L I, Simmonds H A 1969 Hereditary oroticaciduria: long-term therapy with uridine and a trial of uracil. Journal of Paediatrics 75: 885–891
39 Jones M E 1980 Pyrimidine nucleotide biosynthesis in mammals: genes, enzymes and regulation of UMP biosynthesis. Annual Reviews of Biochemistry 49: 253–279
40 Krooth R S, Lam G E M, Chen Kian S Y 1974 Oxipurinol and oroticaciduria: efffect on the orotidine-5'-decarboxylase activity in cultured human fibroblasts. Cell 3: 55–57
41 Harris M L, Oberholzer V G 1980 Conditions affecting the colorimetry of orotic acid and orotidine in urine. Clinical Chemistry 26: 473–479
42 Simmonds, H A, Webster D R, Becroft D M O, Potter C F 1980 Purine and pyrimidine metabolism in hereditary oroticaciduria: some unexpected effects of allopurinol. European Journal of Clinical Investigation 10: 333–339
43 Wadman S K, Beemer E A, De Bree P K et al 1984 New defects of pyrimidine metabolism. In: De Bruyn C H M M, Simmonds H A, Muller M M (eds) Purine metabolism in man, IVA. Plenum, New York, p 109–114
44 Berglund G, Greter J, Linsdtedt S, Steen G, Waldenstrom J, Weiss U 1979 Urinary excretion of thymine and uracil in a two year old child with a malignant tumour of the brain. Clinical Chemistry 25: 1325–1328
45 Hopkinson D A, Swallow D M, Turner V S, Aziz I 1984 Evidence for a distinct deoxypyrimidine 5'nucleotidase in human tissues. In: De Bruyn C H M M, Simmonds H A, Muller M M (eds) Purine metabolism in man, IVA. Plenum, New York, p 535–541
46 Valentine W N, Fink K, Paglia D E, Harris S R, Adams S 1974 Hereditary haemolytic anaemia with human erythrocyte pyrimidine-5'-nucleotidase deficiency. Journal of Clinical Investigation 54: 866–879
47 Harley E H, Berman P 1984 Diagnostic and therapeutic approaches in pyrimidine 5'-nucleotidase deficiency. In: De Bruyn C H M M, Simmonds H A, Muller M M (eds) Purine metabolism in man, IVA. Plenum, New York, p 103–108
48 Hanson T W R, Seip M, de Verdier C H, Erickson A 1983 Erythrocyte pyrimidine 5'-nucleotidase deficiency. Scandinavian Journal of Haematology 31: 122–128
49 Swanson M S, Angle C R, Stohs S T, Salhany J M, Elliot R S, Markin R S 1983 ^{31}P NMR study of erythrocytes from a patient with hereditary pyrimidine-5' nucleotidase deficiency. Proceedings of the National Academy of Sciences 80: 169–172

The porphyrias

INTRODUCTION

The porphyrias are a group of disorders of haem biosynthesis in which characteristic clinical features are associated with specific patterns of over-production of haem precursors. The clinical features are of two types: acute attacks of porphyria which are neurological in origin and are always associated with increased excretion of the porphyrin precursors, porphobilinogen (PBG) and 5-aminolaevulinic acid (ALA), and skin lesions which are caused by photosensitization by porphyrins. The six main types of porphyria are classified in Table 7.1. Very occasionally other porphyrias are encountered; a number of these rare variants have been identified in recent years and are described later. In Table 7.1 the porphyrias are divided into two groups according to the concentration of protoporphyrin in erythrocytes. This is a useful practical division and serves to separate those conditions in which detectable accumulation of haem precursors is restricted to the liver, the hepatic porphyrias, from those in which porphyrin concentrations are increased in erythroid and other tissues and which in the past were classified as erythropoietic porphyrias.

HAEM BIOSYNTHESIS

Haem is synthesised in all mammalian cells, although erythroid cells lose this capacity as they mature into erythrocytes. Normal adults produce about 7 μmol of haem/kg body weight each day, of which 80–85% is used for the formation of haemoglobin. Most of the remaining 15–20% is synthesised in the liver. In the rat about 70% of haem produced in the liver is incorporated into microsomal haemoproteins of the cytochrome P-450 series which catalyse the oxidative metabolism of a wide range of endogenous compounds, drugs and other foreign substances. In humans, the amount of haem that is synthesised for this purpose is probably lower because cytochrome P-450 constitutes a smaller proportion of the total haem concentration in hepatocytes.

Table 7.1 The main types of porphyria

Disorder	Clinical presentation	
	Acute porphyria	Photocutaneous
1. Conditions in which erythrocyte free-porphyrin concentration is increased		
a. Congenital erythropoietic porphyria (26370)	−	+
b. Protoporphyria (17700)	−	+
2. Conditions in which erythrocyte free-porphyrin concentration is normal (hepatic porphyrias)		
a. Acute hepatic porphyrias		
(i) Acute intermittent porphyria (17600)	+	−
(ii) Hereditary coproporphyria (12130)	+	+
(iii) Variegate porphyria (17620)	+	+
b. Porphyria cutanea tarda (17610)	−	+

McKusick numbers are shown in parentheses

The pathway of haem biosynthesis

The pathway of haem biosynthesis consists of a series of irreversible reactions which are outlined in Figure 7.1. The formation of the first committed haem precursor, 5-aminolaevulinate, from glycine and succinyl CoA is catalysed by the mitochondrial enzyme, ALA-synthase (EC 2.3.1.37). ALA then enters the cytosol where two molecules condense to form the colourless monopyrrole, porphobilinogen (PBG). Next PBG deaminase (uroporphyrinogen-I-synthase; hydroxymethylbilane synthase; EC 4.3.1.8) catalyses the formation of the symmetrical, linear tetrapyrrole, hydroxymethylbilane from four molecules of PBG. This compound is very unstable and, particularly in the presence of acid, undergoes rapid non-enzymatic cyclisation to the symmetrical porphyrinogen, uroporphyrinogen I. However, in normal physiological circumstances, uroporphyrinogen III synthase catalyses a reaction in which cyclisation occurs with reversal of the order of the side chains on ring D so that the asymmetrical series III isomer, uroporphyrinogen III, is formed. As a consequence, normally less than 1% of hydroxymethylbilane is diverted to the formation of series I porphyrinogens, which cannot be metabolised to haem (Fig. 7.1).

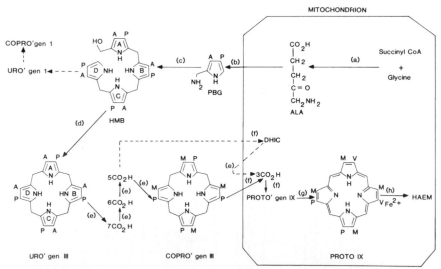

Fig. 7.1 The pathway of haem biosynthesis. Substituents in pyrrole rings, A: CH_2CO_2H; P: $CH_2CH_2CO_2H$; M: CH_3; V: $CH = CH_2$. HMB: hydroxymethylbilane; DHIC: dehydroisocoproporphyrinogen; ALA: 5-aminolevulinic acid; PBG: porphobilinogen; URO'gen: uroporphyrinogen; COPRO'gen: coproporphyrinogen; PROTO'gen: protoporphyrinogen; 3-,5-,6-,7 CO_2H:tri-, penta-, hexa-, heptacarboxylic porphyrinogen. Reactions are catalysed by ALA synthase (a), PBG synthase (b), PBG deaminase (c), uroporphyrinogen III synthase (d), uroporphyrinogen decarboxylase (e), coproporphyrinogen oxidase (f), protoporphyrinogen oxidase (g) and ferrochelatase (h). In normal circumstances, the alternative pathway via DHIC is unlikely to function to any extent; accumulation of $5CO_2H$, as in porphyria cutanea tarda, leads to increased production of DHIC and the isocoproporphyrins derived from it.

In the subsequent series of reactions the side chains of uroporphyrinogen III are progressively modified to form protoporphyrinogen IX. Uroporphyrinogen decarboxylase (EC 4.11.37) catalyses the sequential decarboxylation of the four acetic acid substituents of uroporphyrinogen to produce coproporphyrinogen with the formation of hepta-, hexa- and pentacarboxylic porphyrinogens as intermediates. Coproporphyrinogen III is then converted to protoporphyrinogen IX by coproporphyrinogen oxidase (EC 1.3.3.39). Since this enzyme does not metabolise coproporphyrinogen I, the pathway becomes isomer specific at this stage. Finally, protoporphyrinogen IX undergoes enzymatic aromatization to protoporphyrin IX before ferrochelatase (EC 4.99.1.1) catalyses the insertion of ferrous iron to form protohaem. Like ALA-synthase, the last three enzymes of the pathway are located in the mitochondrion. Although in theory transport of substrates and haem across the inner mitochondrial membrane provides potential regulatory sites for the control of haem metabolism, there is no evidence to suggest that these processes are important in the pathogenesis of the porphyrias.

It is important to appreciate that, apart from protoporphyrin IX, porphyrinogens rather than porphyrins are intermediates of the pathway (Fig. 7.1). These compounds are colourless, unstable hexahydro derivatives of porphyrins that readily autoxidise to porphyrins within tissues, especially when they accumulate in pathological conditions, and during excretion.

Regulation of haem biosynthesis

The pathway of haem biosynthesis is identical in all tissues, but there are major differences between the mechanisms for the regulation of the rate of haem formation in hepatocytes and erythroid cells.

Regulation in liver

The rate of haem synthesis is determined by the activity of the first enzyme of the pathway, 5-aminolaevulinate synthase (ALA synthase). Alterations in the rate of haem synthesis are accompanied by parallel changes in ALA-synthase activity. In hepatocytes, the activity of ALA-synthase appears to be under negative feedback control by haem.[1] Depletion of a regulatory free-haem pool leads to an increase in ALA-synthase activity which can be prevented by administration of haem. Haem acts by depressing the synthesis of ALA-synthase, rather than through direct inhibition of the enzyme. This provides an effective mechanism for the short-term regulation of enzyme activity because the turnover of ALA-synthase in mammalian liver is rapid; the half-life of the enzyme in rat liver being about 70 minutes. Haem blocks the synthesis of ALA-synthase by several mechanisms: by inhibiting both transcription and translation and by preventing the processing of a precursor form of the enzyme for insertion into mitochondria. The relative importance of these different actions remains uncertain.

The induction of ALA-synthase can also be modified by compounds other than haem. Thus, induction is prevented by loading with carbohydrate, while glucocorticoids and possibly other hormones may be required for maximum induction.

A large variety of drugs, chemicals and endogenous compounds, including various steroid metabolites, induce ALA-synthase activity in liver cells.[2,3] Many of these substances decrease the concentration of free haem in the regulatory pool and thus promote synthesis of new enzyme. Most of the drugs that have this action, for example phenobarbitone, induce microsomal cytochromes of the P-450 series and the small accompanying increase in ALA-synthase activity appears to be related to the need to supply the additional haem required for this purpose. Drugs of this type primarily stimulate the synthesis of apocytochrome P-450 which, by combining with available free haem, depletes the regulatory haem pool and leads to secondary induction of ALA-synthase. This mechanism ensures close co-ordination between haem and apoprotein synthesis. In contrast, a small number of drugs and chemicals produce a much more marked increase in ALA-synthase, with massive over-production of porphyrin by the liver and experimental porphyria.[4] Compounds in this group, for example 2-allyl-2-isopropylacetamide and griseofulvin, have two properties: they are lipophilic and stimulate apocytochrome P-450 synthesis, and they deplete haem directly, either by inhibiting haem synthesis or by increasing haem catabolism. Similar enhanced induction of hepatic ALA-synthase occurs when a drug that induces apocytochrome P-450 synthesis is given together with an inhibitor of haem synthesis.

Thus, in the liver, haem synthesis is regulated in a way which enables the supply of haem for microsomal haemoprotein synthesis to change rapidly in response to a wide variety of external stimuli. Impairment of the supply of haem enhances the sensitivity of ALA-synthase to induction by a wide variety of common drugs that are metabolised in the liver by the cytochrome P-450-dependent mono-oxygenase system.

Regulation in erythroid cells

The regulation of haem synthesis in erythroid cells appears to be much less flexible.[2] Alterations in the rate of haem formation largely reflect changes in the number of cells that differentiate to produce haem. ALA-synthase activity increases early in erythroid differentiation and the few factors that stimulate erythroid ALA synthase activity—erythropoietin, hypoxia and some steroid metabolites—may act through promoting differentiation rather than by increasing enzyme activity in individual cells. In reticulocytes, haem inhibits ALA-synthase activity directly. In less differentiated cells, haem may also prevent the induction of ALA-synthase that follows inhibition of haem synthesis, but the mechanism of this action and its relation to differentiation are unclear.

Co-ordination of haem and globin synthesis in erythroid cells is achieved by a mechanism which involves initiation of globin chain synthesis by haem. The efficiency of the process that terminates haem synthesis when the cell is fully haemoglobinised is such that, in mature erythrocytes, haem is in 26 000-fold molar excess of porphyrin, which is present as zinc-protoporphyrin.

Metabolism and excretion of haem precursors

Under normal circumstances, the total daily excretion of haem precursors represents less than 2.5% of the amount of ALA used for haem synthesis. There is little or no alternative metabolism so the quantities excreted indicate the extent of loss of intermediates from the pathway. Table 7.2 shows the reference ranges of haem precursors in urine, faeces, erythrocytes and plasma.

The figures given in Table 7.2 for porphyrins include porphyrinogen, because most methods for the measurement of porphyrins include an oxidation stage to convert porphyrinogens to porphyrins.[5]

ALA and PBG are excreted in the urine while porphyrins and porphyrinogens are excreted in the urine and the bile. Hydrophilic porphyrins with more than four acidic side chains, such as uroporphyrin and heptacarboxylic porphyrin, are preferentially excreted in the urine, while the relatively water-insoluble di- and tricarboxylic porphyrins are restricted to the bile (Table 7.2). Coproporphyrin is excreted by both routes with preferential excretion of the series I isomer in the bile. Impairment of biliary excretion by cholestasis leads to increased urinary excretion of coproporphyrin I. Part of the dicarboxylic 'protoporphyrin' fraction of faeces is formed within the gut, particularly by the action of micro-organisms on haem from the diet and other sources. In addition, protoporphyrin is converted to other dicarboxylic porphyrins by the action of the gut flora.[5]

ENZYME DEFECTS IN THE PORPHYRIAS

Enzyme deficiencies

Each type of porphyria results from a partial deficiency of one of the enzymes of haem biosynthesis. The sites of the primary enzyme defects in each type of porphyria are listed in Table 7.3. All are inherited, with the exception of some abnormalities of uroporphyrinogen decarboxylase (Table 7.3). Studies of the tissue distribution of enzyme defects in the inherited porphyrias indicate that they are present in all cells that synthesise haem, in keeping with biochemical and genetic evidence that each of the enzymes that metabolise ALA to haem is encoded by allelic genes at a single autosomal locus.

Table 7.2 Haem precursors in normal urine, faeces and blood

Sample	PBG (μmol/d)	ALA (μmol/d)	Total porphyrin (nmol/l)	Porphyrin fractions[1] (nmol/d or g dry wt.)			Porphyrins (mean % of total)						
				Copro	Proto	Ether-insoluble	Proto	Copro	Iso-copro	$5CO_2H$	$6CO_2H$	$7Co_2H$	Uro
Urine	0–11	0–46	40–320	40–280	—	0–48[2]	—	76.8 (50–60)	—	2.3	0.8	4.5	15.3
Faeces				0–46	0–220	0–24[3]	72.5	23.5 (5–15)	0.03	1.7	0.6	0.2	1.0
Plasma			0.5–5										
Erythrocytes			90–1690				>90	<10	—	—	—	—	—

See Figure 1 legend for explanation of abbreviations; figures in parentheses indicate % isomer Type III. Units for urinary porphyrin fractions are nmol/d; for faecal fractions nmol/g dry wt.
[1] Determined by solvent partition techniques
[2] Uroporphyrin fraction
[3] X-porphyrin fraction (see text, p. 270)

Table 7.3 Enzyme deficiencies in the porphyrias

Defective enzyme	Activity in porphyria (% normal)	Condition	Inheritance	Chromosomal location of defective gene
1. PBG synthase	1–2	PBG synthase deficiency	AR	9q
2. PBG deaminase (uroporphyrinogen-I-synthase)	47	Acute intermittent	AD	11q
3. Uroporphyrinogen-III-synthase)	a. 16 b. 15	Congenital erythropoietic porphyria Late onset form of a.	AR } AR	Unknown
4. Uroporphyrinogen decarboxylase	a. 41–65 b. 40* c. not measured d. 5–11	Familial PCT Sporadic PCT Toxic PCT Hepatoerythropoietic porphyria	AD Pathogenesis unknown Acquired See text	1 1
5. Coproporphyrinogen oxidase	a. 48–53 b. 2 c. 10	Hereditary coproporphyria Homozygous coproporphyria Harderoporphyria	AD AD See text }	9
6. Protoporphyrinogen oxidase	a. 43–55 b. 14	Variegate porphyria Homozygous variegate porphyria	AD } 	Unknown
7. Ferrochelatase	13–23	Protoporphyria	AD	Unknown

AD, AR: autosomal dominant, autosomal recessive *decreased activity restricted to the liver.

In the autosomal dominant porphyrias, with the exception of protoporphyria, enzyme activities are decreased by approximately 50% in all tissues (Table 7.3). This level is consistent with the idea that the residual enzyme activity in these conditions represents expression of a normal gene which is allelic to a 'silent' mutant gene. In support of this concept, no major differences in the kinetic, physicochemical or immunochemical properties of enzymes from normal and affected individuals have yet been reported. In protoporphyria, the level of enzyme activity (Table 7.3) is lower than would be predicted from the presumed presence of a normal gene allelic to the mutant gene. Furthermore, the residual enzyme appears to be kinetically abnormal. The explanation of these findings is uncertain; although there is some evidence that in vitro measurements of ferrochelatase activity in protoporphyria may not accurately reflect the activity in intact cells.

Nature of mutations

In recent years, progress has been made in understanding the nature of some of the mutations that give rise to porphyrias. In some patients with acute intermittent porphyria, direct evidence for a point mutation in the coding sequence of the gene has been obtained by demonstrating the presence of a catalytically-inactive gene product that cross-reacts with a monospecific antiserum for normal PBG-deaminase. However, this type of mutation is uncommon, most cases of acute intermittent porphyria being cross-reactive material (CRM)-negative. Additional evidence for genetic heterogeneity in acute intermittent porphyria comes from the description of a large Finnish family in which erythrocyte PBG-deaminase activity was found to be normal. The usual mutation in familial porphyria cutanea tarda also appears to be CRM-negative. However, the identification of patients who may be homozygous for the gene for familial porphyria cutanea tarda, and who have less than 10% of the normal concentration of catalytic and immunoreactive uroporphyrinogen decarboxylase (Table 7.3) suggests that the mutation in at least some patients with familial porphyria cutanea tarda does not completely prevent production of active enzyme. Now that DNA probes are available for human PBG-deaminase and uroporphyrinogen decarboxylase genes, rapid progress in defining the nature of these mutations is to be expected.[6] Rare patients that appear to be homozygous for coproporphyrinogen oxidase and protoporphyrinogen oxidase defects have also been described (Table 7.3), and again indicate that gene defects in the corresponding autosomal dominant conditions may lead to a marked suppression, rather than elimination, of enzyme activity.

Two types of porphyria are inherited as autosomal recessive conditions: congenital erythropoietic porphyria and PBG-synthase deficiency (Table 7.3). In both conditions, the residual enzyme activity (Table 7.3) must indicate production of either an enzyme with abnormal kinetic properties or decreased expression of normal enzyme. In PBG-synthase deficiency, a structurally-modified enzyme with impaired catalytic activity is produced. The relationship between this abnormality and the asymptomatic, autosomal dominant PBG-synthase defect described by Bird et al[7] is unknown.

Consequences of enzyme deficiencies

Metabolic consequences

The pattern of haem precursor overproduction that is typical of each type of porphyria reflects accumulation of substrate proximal to the primary enzyme defect. This response to the enzyme deficiency is brought about through operation of the system for negative feed-back control of ALA-synthase by haem. In normal circumstances, the K_m values of the enzymes of the pathway of haem biosynthesis are higher than the concentrations of their substrates (Table 7.4). Thus an increase in substrate production, secondary to increased ALA-synthase activity, will compensate for decreased enzyme activity and restore the rate of haem synthesis to normal. Accumulation of substrate, with its clinical consequences, appears to be the price that is paid for maintaining normal, or near normal, rates of haem synthesis in the porphyrias.

Table 7.4 Enzymes of haem biosynthesis in human liver: activities, K_m values and substrate concentrations
Activities are expressed as nmol ALA or ALA equivalents produced or utilized/hour/mg protein. One mole of porphyrin is equivalent to 8 mole ALA. Mean values or ranges are shown.

	Activity (nmol/hour/mg)	Substrate concentration (nmol/g wet wt.)	Apparent Km (μM)
ALA-synthase	0.22	—	11[3] 2500[4]
PBG-synthase	9.8–15.9	0.04[1]	270
PBG-deaminase	0.15	1.0	6
Uroporphyrinogen decarboxylase	11.0[2]	0.01–0.05[1]	1.5
Coproporphyrinogen oxidase	13.0	0.04–0.11	0.9
Protoporphyrinogen oxidase	—	—	—
Ferrochelatase	16.6	0.13–0.62	1.8[5] 17[6]

1 Rat liver
2 Pentacarboxylate porphyrinogen III as substrate
3 Succinyl-CoA
4 Glycine
5 Protoporphyrin IX
6 Fe^{2+}

These compensatory changes do not occur in all tissues in which there is an enzyme defect. In the hereditary hepatic porphyrias, haem precursor accumulation can be detected in the liver but not in the bone marrow, and the liver appears to be the main source of the increased quantitities of porphyrins and porphyrin precursors that are excreted. Similarly, increased ALA-synthase activity has been detected only in the liver and peripheral blood leucocytes. In spite of the absence of compensatory changes in erythroid cells, anaemia is not a clinical feature of the hepatic porphyrias and haemoglobinisation appears to be unimpaired by the 50% decrease in enzyme activity that is present in these conditions.

The severe enzyme defects that are present in homozygous individuals (Table 7.3) appear to invariably produce accumulation of haem precursors. With the quantitatively less severe defects that are found in the autosomal dominant conditions (Table 7.3), the metabolic consequences vary widely between individuals. Thus similar deficiency of the same enzyme may be associated with marked overproduction of haem precursors in one individual and with no detectable accumulation in another. Much of this variation between individuals seems to be determined by interaction between enzyme defects and acquired factors. In the acute hepatic porphyrias, drugs and steroid hormones are important in this respect while the role of alcoholic liver disease in the development of overt porphyria cutanea tarda is well-established. However, interaction with other genes may also be important. In protoporphyria, clinical expression may involve co-inheritance of a second abnormal allele;[8] but there is as yet no evidence that allelic interactions of this type are important in other porphyrias.

Clinical consequences

The clinical consequences of enzyme deficiencies in the haem biosynthetic pathway are directly related to overproduction of haem precursors. Acute porphyria is always associated with overproduction of PBG and ALA: predominantly PBG in the acute hepatic porphyrias (Table 7.1) and predominantly ALA in the very rare PBG-synthase (EC 4.2.1.24) deficiency (Table 7.3). PBG and ALA excretion are normal in those conditions in which acute attacks never occur (Table 7.1). The relationship between the biochemical and clinical features of acute porphyria is discussed later.

Skin lesions are seen in all porphyrias in which there is over-production of porphyrins, or their unstable porphyrinogen or hydroxymethylbilane precursors. Porphyrins are potent photo-sensitizers so that lesions develop in areas of skin exposed to sunlight. This photodynamic effect of porphyrin requires oxygen and has an action spectrum that resembles the electronic absorption spectrum of porphyrin with a major peak around 400 nm. Irradiation of porphyrin with light at these wavelengths in the presence of oxygen leads to the formation of singlet oxygen, and possibly other oxygen radicals, that are capable of causing local oxidative damage in skin, perhaps through peroxidation of membrane lipids and the release of hydrolytic enzymes from lysosomes. Histological changes include the presence of PAS-staining material in and around sub-papillary capillaries and non-specific deposition of IgG. In some patients with porphyria cutanea tarda or congenital erythropoietic porphyria sclerodermatous plaques may occur in either light-exposed or light-protected areas; a change that may be related to stimulation of collagen formation by uroporphyrin.

Latent porphyria

In all types of autosomal dominant porphyria, individuals who have inherited the enzyme defect but have not developed symptoms (latent porphyrics) are much commoner than those with clinically overt porphyria. Many individuals remain asymptomatic throughout life and in a patient who presents with one of these conditions lack of a family history is common and of no diagnostic significance. Some latent porphyrics may show abnormalities of haem precursor excretion or have increased tissue porphyrin concentrations (subclinical porphyria) but others can only be identified by enzyme measurements. There is no evidence that any biochemical investigation can be used to predict which individuals are most likely to develop symptoms.

THE ACUTE PORPHYRIAS

Acute hepatic porphyrias

The most important clinical feature of the three acute hepatic porphyrias (Table 7.1) is the occurrence of episodic attacks of acute porphyria, which may end fatally. In acute intermittent porphyria (McKusick 17 600) acute attacks are the only clinical manifestation. In hereditary coproporphyria (McKusick 12 130) and variegate porphyria (McKusick 17 620), skin lesions, which are indistinguishable from those of porphyria cutanea tarda, also occur (Table 7.1). Almost all patients with hereditary coproporphyria present with acute porphyria; about a third also have mild skin lesions. In variegate porphyria, the mode of presentation shows some geographical variation. About 60% of South African patients present with skin lesions alone; about 20% have skin lesions and acute porphyria while the remainder have acute attacks only. A similar pattern is found in the United Kingdom but in Finland acute attacks predominate.

The acute hepatic porphyrias occur throughout the world. In Europe the prevalence of acute attacks of porphyria is about 2–3 per 100 000 of the population. Most of these attacks are caused by acute intermittent porphyria, with variegate porphyria accounting for no more than a third and hereditary coproporphyria being uncommon. In South Africa, variegate porphyria provides a classical example of a founder effect with a prevalence as high as 1:250 among the White Afrikaans-speakers of the Eastern Cape. Since most cases of acute intermittent porphyria are latent, the gene frequency may approach 0.5–1 per 10 000.

Clinical features of acute porphyria

The clinical features of acute porphyria show remarkable constancy, whether they are caused by acute intermittent porphyria, variegate porphyria or hereditary coproporphyria.[9] The frequency of acute attacks tends to be lower in hereditary coproporphyria and variegate porphyria than in acute intermittent porphyria.

Acute porphyria is about three times commoner in women than in men, and is most frequent during the third decade in women and the fourth decade in men. Attacks are very uncommon before puberty and do not appear to have been reported before the age of 6. At the other extreme, attacks have occurred for the first time after the age of 80. The main symptoms and signs are listed in Table 7.5. Over 90% of patients present with the sudden onset of severe abdominal pain. Some abdominal tenderness is usually present but is much less than expected from the amount of pain. About 60% of patients develop a predominantly motor peripheral neuropathy, usually after the onset of pain. Convulsions are common and, in a patient with abdominal pain, may provide the first indication of the diagnosis. Presentation with a neuropathy that is neither accompanied nor preceded by pain is very rare. Although mental confusion and other psychiatric disorders are common (Table 7.5), they rarely, with the exception of depression, persist beyond the acute phase. Vomiting may be severe, and is one factor contributing to the hyponatraemia, which is a frequent feature. Another cause is inappropriate secretion of antidiuretic hormone which is one of several hypothalamo-pituitary abnormalities that have been described.[10]

Table 7.5   Acute porphyria: signs and symptoms

Symptoms	% of cases	Signs	% of cases
Abdominal pain	95	Tachycardia	80
Extremity pain/paraesthesia	50	Dark urine	74
Constipation	48	Peripheral motor neuropathy	60
Nausea, vomiting	43	Bulbar involvement	46
Mental changes	40	Mental confusion/hallucinations	40
Back pain	29	Hypertension (diastolic > 90 mm Hg)	36
Chest pain	12	Absent reflexes	29
Diarrhoea	5	Peripheral sensory neuropathy	26
		Postural hypotension	21
		Palpable dilated loops of bowel	21
		Convulsions	20
		Bladder distension	12
		Coma	10

Adapted from Bonkowsky & Schady[12]

Attacks usually subside after several days but they occasionally persist for weeks or even months. The pattern of attacks is variable. Most patients have less than three but they may be multiple or even merge with intermittent exacerbations against a background of chronic pain over many months. Attacks may occur in relation to the menstrual cycle and a few women have regular, disabling premenstrual attacks. About 5% of attacks that are severe enough to require hospitalization end fatally, usually through respiratory paralysis. Weakness, and other neurological sequelae, may remain for years. Persistent hypertension and premature death from chronic renal failure have been reported.

A number of factors are known to precipitate acute porphyria and are implicated in the onset of about 75% of attacks. The list of known precipitants includes more than 100 drugs, hormone preparations, including oral contraceptive preparations, alcohol and low-calorie weight-reducing diets.[3] The development of acute attacks is also facilitated by endogenous steroid hormones. Thus some women suffer cyclical pre-menstrual attacks, and various abnormalities of androgen metabolism, particularly impaired 5-β-hydrogenation of C_{19} and C_{21} metabolites, have been described in symptomatic patients with acute intermittent porphyria.

Biochemical features and pathogenesis of acute porphyria

Attacks of acute hepatic porphyria are accompanied by a number of characteristic biochemical changes. There is a marked increase in urinary PBG and, to a lesser extent, ALA excretion with increased activity of ALA-synthase in the liver. Formation of cytochrome P-450 in the liver is impaired. These changes are similar to those produced in laboratory animals by the combination of inhibition of haem synthesis and induction of apocytochrome P-450. Many of the drugs and other compounds that provoke attacks of acute hepatic porphyria are known to induce both cytochrome P-450 and ALA-synthase. It appears that in the acute hepatic porphyrias, the increased demand for haem imposed by these drugs cannot be met because enzyme defects are present that either directly or indirectly limit haem synthesis at the level of PBG-deaminase.[11]

All the clinical features of acute porphyria, including the abdominal pain, are neurological in origin, the main histological lesion being axonal degeneration with secondary demyelination. The relationship between the biochemical and neurological abnormalities is unexplained. Of several theories that have been proposed,[12] a direct neurotoxic effect of ALA seems to be supported by the most evidence. ALA can cross the blood brain barrier and is known to have various neuropharmacological actions, while manoeuvres that depress ALA production may be effective therapeutically. In addition, other conditions in which there is excessive formation of ALA, but not PBG, for example PBG-synthase deficiency, hereditary tyrosinaemia (tyrosinosis) and lead poisoning are associated with identical or similar neurological syndromes. Nevertheless, little is known about haem metabolism in nervous tissue and the possibility that the enzyme deficiency, which is presumably present in this tissue, has a direct effect within neurones cannot be discounted. It is also unclear whether the mental disturbances arise in the same way as the neuropathy. Haem is a major determinant of tryptophan pyrrolase activity in the liver and disordered tryptophan metabolism has been implicated in the pathogenesis of affective disorders.

Diagnosis of the acute hepatic porphyrias

The diagnosis of an acute attack of acute intermittent porphyria, variegate porphyria or hereditary coproporphyria is established by demonstrating a coincidental increase in urinary PBG excretion (Table 7.6). Virtually all patients with abdominal pain caused by porphyria excrete sufficient PBG to give a positive result with the simple Watson-Schwartz screening test, or one of its modifications, which detect PBG by the red colour given with Ehrlich's reagent (p-dimethylaminobenzaldehyde in acid).[13] However, false-positive results may occur and it is essential that all positive tests are confirmed by a specific, quantitative test. In all three conditions PBG excretion is higher during acute attacks than during remission. In both variegate porphyria and hereditary coproporphyria, PBG excretion may fall very rapidly after the onset of symptoms and usually returns to normal in remission. Return to normal is less common in acute intermittent porphyria, but may occur. The diagnosis of acute porphyria cannot be excluded, therefore, particularly when patients present late in the attack, unless PBG and faecal porphyrin excretion are both shown to be normal. In this situation it is important to quantify PBG because the Watson-Schwartz screening test does not detect small, but diagnostic, increases in PBG concentration. Urine containing large amounts of PBG is normal in colour, but darkens to reddish-brown on standing due to the polymerisation of PBG to porphyrins and the brown pigment, porphobilin. These changes may occur before micturition, especially if the urine is acid.

Acute intermittent porphyria, variegate porphyria and hereditary coproporphyria are differentiated by measuring faecal porphyrin concentrations (Table 7.6).[5,14] In acute intermittent porphyria, faecal porphyrin concentrations are usually normal. Occasional small increases are probably caused by constipation. In both hereditary coproporphyria and variegate porphyria, there is a marked increase in total faecal porphyrin excretion. This increase is caused by coproporphyrin III in hereditary coproporphyria while in variegate porphyria the faeces contain increased concentrations of protoporphyrin IX, coproporphyrin III and a mixture of hydrophilic dicarboxylic porphyrin-conjugates of uncertain origin, which have been called peptide-porphyrins or porphyrin-X (Table 7.6; Fig. 7.2).

Latent acute intermittent porphyria is best detected by measuring PBG-

Table 7.6 Laboratory diagnosis of acute hepatic porphyrias and PBG-synthase deficiency

CONDITION	Increased concentration of:			
	Urine	Faeces	Erythrocytes	Plasma
AIP (acute attack)	PBG>ALA Porphyrin (mainly due to polymerisation of PBG to uroporphyrin)	N (very occasionally slight increase)	N	PBG ±uroporphyrin (615 nm)
HC (acute attack)	As for AIP Coproporphyrin III	Coproporphyrin III	N	Coproporphyrin III (615 nm)
VP (acute attack)	As for HC	Coproporphyrin III Protoporphyrin (Proto>copro) Porphyrin-X	N	Unidentified porphyrin (626 nm)
VP (cutaneous phase)	±PBG (often normal) Coproporphyrin III (occasionally normal)	As above	N	As above
PBG-synthase deficiency	ALA>PBG Coproporphyrin III	N	Zinc-protoporphyrin	

N = no increase in concentration of PBG, ALA or porphyrin. Figures in parentheses give approximate positions of fluorescence emission maxima in aqueous solution at neutral pH. AIP, acute intermittent porphyria.; HC, hereditary coproporphyria; VP, variegate porphyria.

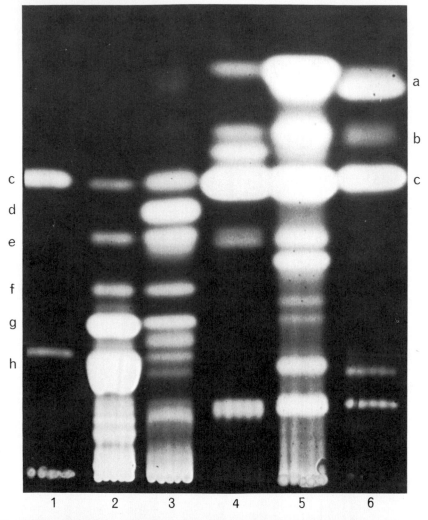

Fig. 7.2 Porphyrin excretion patterns. Thin-layer chromatogram of the methyl ester derivatives of porphyrins from urine and faeces. Tracks show porphyrins from normal urine (1); porphyria cutanea tarda urine (2); porphyria cutanea tarda faeces (3); hereditary coproporphyria faeces (4); variegate porphyria faeces (5); and normal faeces (6). a, protoporphyrin and other dicarboxylic porphyrins; b, tricarboxylic porphyrin; c, coproporphyrin; d, isocoproporphyrin; e–g, penta-, hexa- and heptacarboxylic porphyrin; h, uroporphyrin. The silica gel plate was developed with toluene:ethylacetate:ethanol (80:15:3, by vol.) and photographed in u.v. light.

deaminase in erythrocytes. This test has the advantage over urinary PBG measurement of being able to detect latent acute intermittent porphyria before puberty, when PBG excretion is normal, and in the 70% of adult gene carriers who have normal excretion. Because there is some overlap between the ranges of PBG-deaminase activities in normal subjects and patients with acute intermittent porphyria, this test either alone or in combination with measurement of urinary PBG only identifies about 75% of individuals with latent acute intermittent porphyria. But when it is combined with pedigree analysis, so that use can be made of the clear-cut gene dosage effects that operate within families, or with measurement of leucocyte ALA-synthase activity,[15] only about 5% of putative gene carriers remain unassigned. Because PBG-deaminase activity falls rapidly as erythrocytes mature, the activity of unfractionated haemolysates is influenced by changes in the age distribution of circulating erythrocytes. Thus this test cannot be used to detect latent acute intermittent porphyria before the age of four months and may be difficult to interpret in patients with haematological disorders. Prenatal diagnosis of acute intermittent porphyria is practicable but is rarely indicated.

Latent variegate porphyria and hereditary coproporphyria are most simply detected by measurement of faecal porphyrin concentrations; urinary PBG and porphyrin excretion are usually normal (Table 7.6). However, in both conditions, faecal porphyrin excretion is normal before puberty and in at least 20% of adult carriers of the genes. Identification of latent porphyria in putative gene carriers in these categories, or when faecal analyses are equivocal, requires measurement of the appropriate mitochondrial enzyme in lymphocytes or fibroblasts: coproporphyrinogen oxidase for hereditary coproporphyria and protoporphyrinogen oxidase for variegate porphyria (Table 7.3).

Management of the acute hepatic porphyrias

In spite of recent improvements, there is still no reliable therapy for acute porphyria.[9] In addition to the general supportive measures, precipitants should be removed and a high carbohydrate intake started as soon as possible. If these measures fail, intravenous haematin may be useful.[3,16] Both carbohydrate loading and haematin decrease PBG and ALA production, presumably by repressing the induction of ALA synthase in the liver; but their effect on the clinical progression of the attack is less predictable.

Prevention of the acute attack remains of paramount importance. The relatives of all patients who present with acute porphyria should be investigated so that those identified as latent porphyrics can be given appropriate advice, particularly about the need to avoid known precipitants.[3,9] Cyclical premenstrual attacks may be prevented by LH-RH inhibitors.[17]

Homozygous variants of the acute hepatic porphyrias

Very rarely patients are encountered who have inherited coproporphyrinogen oxidase or protoporphyrinogen oxidase defects from both parents (Table 7.3). These conditions are distinguished from hereditary coproporphyria and variegate porphyria by the appearance of skin lesions in early childhood. They are otherwise clinically heterogeneous. Short stature has been reported in some patients with homozygous coproporphyria[18] and in homozygous variegate porphyria[19] while a neurological syndrome of mental retardation, ocular nystagmus and fits is present in some cases of homozygous variegate porphyria.[20] Porphyrin excretion patterns resemble those of their single gene counterparts, except in one form of homozygous coproporphyria where the mutation alters the kinetics of the enzyme so that a tricarboxylic porphyrinogen intermediate of the reaction, harderoporphyrinogen, accumulates.[21]

PBG-synthase deficiency (McKusick 12527)

This condition has been described in three individuals in two unrelated families (Table 7.3).[22] All three patients presented in their teens with attacks of abdominal pain and polyneuropathy closely resembling those seen in the acute hepatic porphyrias. These attacks were accompanied by a marked increase in the urinary excretion of ALA and coproporphyrin III with only a minimal increase in PBG excretion. Two other conditions are known in which there is severe inhibition of PBG-synthase: lead poisoning and hereditary tyrosinaemia (tyrosinosis). In lead poisoning, the pattern of haem precursor over-production is very similar to that found in PBG-synthase deficiency but the two conditions can be distinguished by measuring the blood lead concentration and by family studies. In hereditary tyrosinaemia (p. 199), where PBG-synthase is specifically inhibited by the abnormal metabolite, succinylacetone, increased excretion of ALA is unaccompanied by any abnormality of porphyrin metabolism. These differences have not been explained.

PORPHYRIA CUTANEA TARDA AND RELATED SYNDROMES

Porphyria cutanea tarda is the commonest type of porphyria in Europe and N. America. Unlike other types of porphyria it is not a distinct entity with a well-defined pattern of inheritance but an aetiologically diverse group of conditions that share the same primary enzyme defect: decreased activity of uroporphyrinogen decarboxylase in the liver (Table 7.3). All types of porphyria cutanea tarda, and the rarer allied conditions that also result from uroporphyrinogen decarboxylase deficiency (Table 7.3), have certain characteristics in common. Their sole clinical features are cutaneous and, although their severity may vary, the skin lesions that result from porphyrin accumulation are indistinguishable from those in congenital erythropoietic porphyria, variegate porphyria, and hereditary coproporphyria. Acute attacks of porphyria do not occur and patients do not react adversely to barbiturates and the other lipophilic compounds that precipitate acute porphyria. All have a similar pattern of over-production of haem precursors which is characteristic of uroporphyrinogen decarboxylase deficiency. Uroporphyrin and other acetic acid substituted porphyrins derived from the substrate and intermediates of the uroporphyrinogen decarboxylase reaction (Fig. 7.1), are excreted in excess and accumulate in the liver. Typically, the urine contains large amounts of uroporphyrin and heptacarboxylic porphyrin, while isocoproporphyrin and heptacarboxylic porphyrin predominate in faeces (Fig. 7.2). Uroporphyrin is mainly the Type I isomer; heptacarboxylic porphyrin is almost entirely Type III. PBG excretion is always normal.

Porphyria cutanea tarda (McKusick 17610)

Classification

Porphyria cutanea tarda can be divided into two types by measuring uroporphyrinogen decarboxylase in erythrocytes. In one type, familial porphyria cutanea tarda, uroporphyrinogen decarboxylase activity is decreased to about 50% of normal in erythrocytes and all other tissues that have been investigated. This defect is inherited as an autosomal dominant characteristic, and is frequently latent so that patients with familial porphyria cutanea tarda may not have a family history of overt porphyria.

In the other type of porphyria cutanea tarda, erythrocyte uroporphyrinogen decarboxylase activity is normal. Most patients in this group have the sporadic form of porphyria cutanea tarda, but it also includes a toxic form of porphyria cutanea tarda which results from exposure to polyhalogenated aromatic hydrocarbons, notably hexachlorobenzene and 2,3,7,8-tetrachlorodibenzo-p-dioxin. In addition, there are very rare families in which porphyria cutanea tarda affects more than one individual yet erythrocyte uroporphyrinogen decarboxylase activity is normal. The relative frequency of the sporadic (or Type I) and autosomal dominant (or Type II) forms of porphyria cutanea tarda, which account for almost all patients with this condition, has not been established; although the sporadic form appears to be commoner in most countries.

Clinical features

Porphyria cutanea tarda usually presents during the fourth to sixth decades and is commoner in men. The familial type tends to occur at a younger age. Onset before the age of 20 is a strong indicator of the familial type but otherwise, in the absence of a family history, the familial and sporadic types cannot be distinguished clinically. The commonest clinical feature is increased fragility of the skin with superficial erosions, most characteristically on the backs of the hands, following trivial trauma. The next most frequent symptom, and the usual reason for seeking medical advice, is the appearance of subepidermal vesicles and bullae. These break to form erosions which heal slowly and often leave atrophic scars. Milia are common in areas which suffer repeated trauma. Other common features are hypertrichosis, pigmentation and scleroderma-like lesions.

Most adults with porphyria cutanea tarda have some associated condition, usually affecting the liver.[23] The commonest is alcoholic liver disease, but porphyria cutanea tarda has been reported in many other types of liver disease, including chronic active hepatitis, infective hepatitis, haemochromatosis and various granulomatous conditions. Liver disease is usually mild and only revealed by investigation, although in some series as many as 30% of patients have been reported to have cirrhosis. Only a minority present with liver disease and are then found to have porphyria cutanea tarda. After alcohol, the most important aetiological factor is oestrogen therapy. In recent years, the widespread use of oestrogens in oral contraceptive and other preparations has led to an increased prevalence of porphyria cutanea tarda in women. Even in this group the liver may be histologically abnormal with some peripheral inflammation and focal hepatocellular necrosis. Porphyria cutanea tarda is also associated with systemic lupus erythromatosus and occurs with increased frequency in patients undergoing long-term haemodialysis. About 15% of patients have diabetes mellitus. Hepatoma may develop in long-standing cases of porphyria cutanea tarda, and there is some evidence that the incidence of this complication is greater than in other types of long-standing liver disease. In general, the prognosis of porphyria cutanea tarda is largely related to the severity of the underlying liver disease.

Many patients with porphyria cutanea tarda show some evidence of iron overload. About 85% of those undergoing liver biopsy have some degree of hepatic siderosis with stainable iron in parenchymal cells. Siderosis is usually no more than moderate; deposition of iron to the extent seen in haemochromatosis is unusual. Total body iron stores are slightly to moderately increased in about three-quarters of European patients. However, although porphyria cutanea tarda has been recorded in association with idiopathic haemochromatosis and other iron storage disorders, it is a very rare complication of these conditions and experimental iron overload in animals does not decrease uroporphyrinogen decarboxylase activity.

Subclinical porphyria cutanea tarda appears to be more frequent than the overt condition. Surveys of patients with chronic liver disease and of chronic alcoholics have shown that abnormalities of porphyrin metabolism of the type found in patients with porphyria cutanea tarda who have gone into clinical remission may be present in 10–20%. Although some of these patients undoubtedly have subclinical porphyria cutanea tarda, there is no direct evidence that the abnormalities in the majority, particularly those in which coproporphyrin excretion predominates, are related to porphyria cutanea tarda.

Laboratory diagnosis of porphyria cutanea tarda

Porphyria cutanea tarda and other uroporphyrinogen decarboxylase defects can be distinguished from all other types of porphyria by demonstrating the characteristic pattern of porphyrin excretion in urine and faeces, and by showing that erythrocyte porphyrin concentration is normal (Table 7.7; Fig. 7.2).[5] Omission of faecal porphyrin analysis may lead to mis-diagnosis since some patients with variegate porphyria have a urinary porphyrin excretion pattern that is indistinguishable from porphyria cutanea tarda. Urinary, faecal and plasma porphyrin concentrations decrease during remission, eventually returning to normal. The abnormal porphyrin excretion pattern persists after total urinary and faecal porphyrin concentrations have become normal, until in prolonged remission the pattern also eventually becomes normal. The liver contains high concentrations of uroporphyrin and heptacarboxylic porphyrin. Needle biopsy samples show bright red fluorescence due to porphyrin when viewed in long-wave ultraviolet light, and hepatocytes contain needle-like inclusions, resembling uroporphyrin crystals, which appear to be a specific feature of porphyria cutanea tarda.

A small number of patients with a condition that is clinically indistinguishable from porphyria cutanea tarda have been shown to have porphyrin-producing hepatic tumours.[24]

Treatment

Porphyria cutanea tarda is the only form of porphyria for which specific and effective treatments exist.[25] The treatment of choice is reduction of total body iron stores to the verge of iron-deficiency by repeated venesection.[26] This manoeuvre is invariably followed by remission which may be prolonged for many years or even permanent. Treatment with low-dose chloroquine is as effective for producing clinical remission but relapse may be more frequent and the theoretical possibility of exacerbating the underlying liver cell damage has not been entirely excluded.[27] Neither treatment is dependent on withdrawal of aetiological agents, such as alcohol and oestrogens, although this should be encouraged and may in itself lead to prolonged remission.

Pathogenesis of porphyria cutanea tarda

The occurrence of porphyria cutanea tarda as an uncommon complication of such common disorders as alcoholic liver disease led to the suggestion that such patients are in some way predisposed to the development of porphyria cutanea tarda. The current view is that an abnormality of uroporphyrinogen decarboxylase in the liver is the predisposing factor and that precipitating agents such as iron, alcohol, oestrogens and, possibly, liver cell damage interact with this enzyme defect to increase the over-production of substrate and thus produce clinically overt porphyria. The mechanism of this interaction is obscure; although for iron, the agent which has been most investigated, a number of theories have been proposed.[23]

The identification of the autosomal dominant form of porphyria cutanea tarda indicated that the predisposition of this group of patients is inherited. Whether the same is true for the sporadic form remains controversial. At present there is little clinical or biochemical evidence to suggest that the majority of these patients have an inherited disorder. However the possibility that they have inherited an enzyme variant that is susceptible to inactivation by toxic processes that operate only in the liver has not been excluded.

Other uroporphyrinogen decarboxylase defects

Hepatoerythropoietic porphyria (McKusick 17610)

11 cases of hepatoerythropoietic porphyria have been reported since its first description in 1969. The condition presents in early childhood with skin lesions similar to those of porphyria cutanea tarda.[28] In older children and adults, the persistence of severe skin lesions with associated infection, scarring and atrophy may lead to photomutilation. Porphyrin is deposited in bone, and the teeth may show red fluorescence in ultra-violet light although they do not become as visibly discoloured by porphyrin as in congenital erythropoietic porphyria. Liver disease is absent or minimal; and patients may survive to the age of 60 or more.

The porphyrin excretion pattern is variable but in general closely resembles that of porphyria cutanea tarda. However, in hepatoerythropoietic porphyria, the concentration of zinc-protoporphyrin and, to a lesser extent, free protoporphyrin is moderately increased in erythrocytes. Erythrocyte uroporphyrinogen decarboxylase activity is decreased to less than 10% of normal (Table 7.3) and a similarly severe enzyme defect appears to be present in nucleated cells. The mutation appears to be CRM-negative in most cases and family studies suggest that these patients may be homozygous for the gene for familial porphyria cutanea tarda. However one family with hepatoerythropoietic porphyria has been found to be CRM-positive.

Uroporphyrinogen decarboxylase deficiency and dyserythropoiesis

A patient with severe photomutilation, a porphyria cutanea tarda-like pattern of porphyrin excretion, an inherited 50% reduction of erythrocyte uroporphyrinogen decarboxylase activity, minimal increase in liver proporphyrin concentration and dyserythropoietic anaemia has been described by Kushner et al.[29]

OTHER CUTANEOUS PORPHYRIAS

Congenital erythropoietic porphyria (McKusick 26370)

Clinical features

Less than 100 cases of congenital erythropoietic porphyria CEP have been reported since it was first described in 1874. Most patients present in early infancy either with severe skin lesions of the type seen in porphyria cutanea tarda or because red urine, due to the presence of large amounts of porphyrin, is noted before the onset of skin symptoms. Photosensitisation is severe and frequently leads to gross photomutilation. Erythrodontia, a brown discoloration of the teeth due to deposition of porphyrin, is common. Haemolytic anaemia, probably caused by the action of light on porphyrin-containing erythrocytes in superficial capillaries, is a frequent complication. Its severity varies greatly both with time in individual patients and from patient to patient; in many patients it contributes to the poor prognosis with few patients surviving beyond the age of 40. A mild, late-onset, type of congenital erythropoietic porphyria, which presents during adult life and is clinically indistinguishable from porphyria cutanea tarda, has been described.[30]

Biochemical features and laboratory diagnosis

Defiency of uroporphyrinogen III synthase is the primary inherited enzyme defect in congenital erythropoietic porphyria. Activity is decreased to the same extent in the classical and late-onset forms (Table 7.3). The low activity of uroporphyrinogen III synthase leads to massive over-production of uroporphyrinogen I which is presumably formed by non-enzymatic cyclisation of accumulated hydroxymethylbilane (Fig. 7.1). Uroporphyrinogen I is decarboxylated to coproporphyrinogen I but cannot be metabolised further. The main site of overproduction is the bone marrow. Erythroid cells contain large amounts of porphyrinogens, and porphyrins derived from them by oxidation, and thus show characteristic red autofluorescence in ultraviolet light. Formation of haem from uroporphyrinogen III is not decreased, and in many patients may be considerably increased due to the presence of haemolytic anaemia.

The diagnosis of congenital erythropoietic porphyria is established by analysis of the isomer type of the excreted porphyrins and by measurement of porphyrins in erythrocytes (Table 7.7).

Management

The treatment of congenital erythropoietic porphyria is aimed at preventing exposure to sunlight and at controlling the haemolytic anaemia.[25,30] However, such measures do no more than ameliorate the condition. The

Table 7.7 Laboratory diagnosis of the cutaneous porphyrias

| CONDITION | Urine | Increased concentration of: | | |
		Faeces	Erythrocytes	Plasma
PCT	Uroporphyrin (30% III), 7CO$_2$H (>90% III) (uro>7 CO$_2$H) with smaller amounts of 6-, 5-CO$_2$H and copro	Isocoproporphyrin, 7CO$_2$H with smaller amounts of copro, 6-,5- CO$_2$H and uro	N	Uroporphyrin (615 nm)
CEP	Uroporphyrin (>80% I) Coproporphyrin (>80% I) (Uro>copro)	Coproporphyrin I	Uroporphyrin I Coproporphyrin I ±Zinc-protoporphyrin	Uroporphyrin I (615 nm)
PP	N	Protoporphyrin IX in about 40% of patients	Protoporphyrin IX (Proto>>Zn-proto)	Protoporphyrin IX (634 nm)

PCT, porphyria cutanea tarda; CEP, congenital erythropoietic porphyria; PP, protoporphyria. Other abbreviations as for Figure 1 and Table 6.

severe photomutilation, restricted life-style, and relatively poor prognosis, make congenital erythropoietic porphyria probably the only porphyria in which prevention by termination following prenatal diagnosis should be considered for all families. Measurements of uroporphyrinogen III synthase in cultured amnion cells and of uroporphyrin I in amniotic fluid can be used for this purpose.[30]

Protoporphyria (McKusick 17700)

In most countries, protoporphyria (erythropoietic protoporphyria) is less common than porphyria cutanea tarda. Many individuals who inherit the gene for protoporphyria show no abnormality other than decreased ferrochelatase activity, and the risk of a gene carrier developing symptoms has been estimated as less than 10%.[8]

Clinical features

In contrast to all other cutaneous porphyrias, the dominant feature of protoporphyria is photosensitivity.[31] Onset usually occurs during early childhood but may be delayed until adult life. Exposure to sunlight provokes burning, itching or painful sensations in the skin which are accompanied by slight oedema and reddening. Vesicle formation is uncommon. Repeated episodes of oedema and erythema may lead to some thickening and lichenification, particularly over the bridge of the nose and the backs of the hands. Skin fragility, hypertrichosis and pigmentation do not occur. Patients may be very pale due to many years of assiduous avoidance of sunlight.

   Some patients have a mild hypochromic, microcytic anaemia, and there is an increased incidence of cholelithiasis with the formation of stones that contain protoporphyrin IX. However, the most important complication is liver disease. Minor abnormalities of biochemical liver function tests and deposits of protoporphyrin in the liver are common; but a small minority of patients develop cirrhosis and hepatic failure which is rapidly fatal. Of 17 such cases that have been reported, most have died within a few months of developing jaundice.[32]

Biochemical features and laboratory diagnosis

Protoporphyria is characterised biochemically by an increased concentration of free protoporphyrin IX in erythrocytes. Erythrocyte protoporphyrin concentrations may also be increased in lead poisoning, in iron deficiency and in some anaemias.[33] However in these conditions, as in normal subjects, virtually all the protoporphyrin is present as its zinc-chelate, whereas in protoporphyria free, uncomplexed protoporphyrin predominates. In addition, plasma protoporphyrin concentrations are increased in protoporphyria but not in the other conditions. Urinary porphyrin excretion is normal but faecal protoporphyrin concentrations are increased in about 40% of patients (Table 7.7).

Identification of the major site of protoporphyrin production in this condition has been controversial. In most patients, erythroid cells appear to be the main source of excess protoporphyrin. Porphyrin accumulates during the later stages of erythroid maturation but as circulating erythrocytes mature some leaks into the plasma to be excreted by the liver into the bile. However production of protoporphyrin by the liver may also be increased. Most of this probably enters the bile, although some plasma porphyrin may be of hepatic origin. The source of the protoporphyrin that accumulates in the liver as crystalline deposits, and which may cause liver cell damage leading to hepatic failure, is unclear.

Management

The treatment of photosensitivity in protoporphyria has been described by Bickers.[25] Administration of sufficient β-carotene, or related carotenoids, to produce photoprotective pigmentation of the skin is effective in many patients. The management and prevention of liver disease has been less successful. At present, there is no reliable method for predicting which patients are likely to develop this complication. Patients with abnormal liver function tests, or very high red cell and plasma protoporphyrin concentrations, should undergo liver biopsy. Cholestyramine has been used to interrupt the enterohepatic circulation of protoporphyrin, and thus lessen accumulation in the liver, and may reverse early hepatic damage in some patients. This and other approaches to treatment are discussed by Bloomer.[34]

Erythropoietic coproporphyria

Two patients with the clinical features of protoporphyria but with an excess of coproporphyrin in their erythrocytes have been described.[35]

REFERENCES

1 Granick S, Sinclair P, Sassa S, Groeninger G 1975 Effects by heme, insulin and serum albumin on heme protein synthesis in chick embryo liver cells cultured in a chemically defined medium, and a spectrofluorometric assay for porphyrin composition. Journal of Biological Chemistry 250: 9212–9225
2 Ibrahim N G, Friedland M L, Levere R D 1983 Heme metabolism in erythroid and hepatic cells. Progress in Haematology 13: 75–130
3 Moore M R, Disler P B 1983 Drug-induction of the acute porphyrias. Advances in Drug Reactions and Acute Poisons Review 2: 149–189
4 Smith A G, De Matteis F 1980 Drugs and the hepatic porphyrias. Clinics in Haematology 9: 399–425
5 Elder G H 1980 The porphyrias: Clinical chemistry, diagnosis and methodology. Clinics in Haematology 9: 371–398
6 Romeo P-H, Raich N, Dubart A et al 1986 Molecular cloning and tissue specific expression analysis of human porphobilinogen deaminase and uroporphrinogen

decarboxylase. In: Nordmann Y (ed) Porphyrins and Porphyrias. Colloques INSERM/John Libbey Eurotext Ltd, Paris, p 25–34

7 Bird T D, Hamernyik P, Butter J Y, Labbe R F 1979 Inherited deficiency of delta-aminolaevulinic acid dehydratase. American Journal of Human Genetics 31: 662–668

8 Went L N, Klasen E C 1984 Genetic aspects of erythropoietic protoporphyria. Annals of Human Genetics 48: 105–117

9 Brodie M J, Goldberg A 1980 Acute hepatic porphyrias. Clinics in Haematology 9: 253–272

10 Brodie M J, Graham D J M, Goldberg A et al 1978 Thyroid function in acute intermittent porphyria: a neurogenic cause of hyperthyroidism. Hormone and Metabolic Research 10: 327–331

11 Elder G H, Evans J O, Thomas N et al 1976 The primary enzyme defect in hereditary coproporphyria. Lancet 2: 1217–1219

12 Bonkowsky H L, Schady W 1982 Neurologic manifestations of acute porphyria. Seminars in Liver Disease 2: 108–124

13 Pierach C A, Cardinal R, Bossenmaier, J, Watson C J 1977 Comparison of the Hoesch and the Watson-Schwartz tests for urinary porphobilinogen. Clinical Chemistry 23: 1666–1668

14 Moore M R 1982 Laboratory investigation of disturbances of porphyrin metabolism. Broadsheet 109, Association of Clinical Pathologists, London

15 McColl K E L, Moore M R, Thompson G G, Goldberg A 1982 Screening for latent acute intermittent porphyria: the value of measuring both leucocyte δ-aminolaevulinic acid synthase and erythrocyte uroporphyrinogen-I-synthase activities. Journal of Medical Genetics 19: 271–276

16 Pierach C A 1982 Hematin therapy for the porphyric attack. Seminars in Liver Disease 2: 125–131

17 Anderson K E, Spitz I M, Sassa S, Wayne Bardin C, Kappas A 1984 Prevention of cyclical attacks of acute intermittent porphyria with a long-acting agonist of luteinizing hormone-releasing factor. New England Journal of Medicine 311: 643–645

18 Grandchamp B, Deyback J C, Grelier M, Verneuil H de, Nordmann Y 1980 Studies of porphyrin synthesis in fibroblasts of patients with congenital erythropoietic porphyria and one patient with homozygous coproporphyria. Biochimica et Biophysica Acta 629: 577–586

19 Murphy G, Hawk J L M, Magnus I A et al 1986 Homozygous variegate porphyria: two similar cases in unrelated families. Journal of the Royal Society of Medicine 79: 361–362

20 Korda C V, Deybach J C, Martasek et al 1984 Homozygous variegate porphyria. Lancet 1:851

21 Nordmann Y, Grandchamp B, Verneuil H de, Phung L, Cartigny B, Fontaine G 1983 Harderoporphyria: a variant hereditary coproporphyria. Journal of Clinical Investigation 72: 1139–49

22 Doss M, von Tiepermann R, Schneider J, Schmid H 1979 New type of hepatic porphyria with porphobilinogen synthase defect and intermittent acute clinical manifestations. Klinische Wochenschrift 57: 1123–1127

23 Pimstone N R 1982 Porphyria cutanea tarda. Seminars in Liver Disease 2: 132–142

24 Grossman M E, Bickers D R 1978 Porphyria cutanea tarda, a rare cutaneous manifestation of hepatic tumours. Cutis 21: 782–784

25 Bickers D R 1981 Treatment of the porphyrias: mechanisms of action. Journal of Investigative Dermatology 77: 197–113

26 Ramsay C A, Magnus I A, Turnbull A, Baker H 1974 The treatment of porphyria cutanea tarda by venesection. Quarterly Journal of Medicine 43: 1–24

27 Cainelli T, Di Padova C, Marchesi et al 1983 Hydroxychloroquine versus phlebotomy in the treatment of porphyria cutanea tarda. British Journal of Dermatology 108: 593–600

28 Lim H W, Poh-Fitzpatrick M B 1984 Hepatoerythropoietic porphyria: a variant of childhood-onset porphyria cutanea tarda. Journal of American Academy of Dermatology 11: 1103–1111

29 Kushner J P, Barbuto A J, Lee G R 1976 An inherited enzymic defect in porphyria cutanea tarda. Decreased uroporphyrinogen decarboxylase activity. Journal of Clinical Investigation 58: 1089–1097

30 Nordmann Y, Deybach J C 1982 Congenital erythropoietic porphyria. Seminars in Liver Disease 2: 154–163

31 De Leo V, Poh-Fitzpatrick M, Matthews-Roth M, Harber L C 1976 Erythropoietic protoporphyria. 10 years experience. American Journal of Medicine 60: 8–22.
32 Romslo I, Gadenholt H G, Hovding G 1982 Erythropoietic protoporphyria terminating in liver failure. Archives of Dermatology 118: 668–671
33 McColl K E L, Goldberg A 1980 Abnormal porphyrin metabolism in disease other than porphyria. Clinics in Haematology 9: 427–444
34 Bloomer J R 1982 Protoporphyria. Seminars in Liver Disease 2: 143–153
35 Heilmeyer L, Clotten R 1964 Die kongenitale erythropoietische Coproporphyrie. Deutsche Medicine Wochenschrift 89: 649–655

Collagen disorders

INTRODUCTION

The collagens are the most ubiquitous proteins in the animal kingdom. They constitute the major structural component of all connective tissues in such diverse organs as skin, bone, tendon, ligaments, cornea, cartilage, gut, lung and blood vessels. The physical and mechanical properties of such tissues are dependent upon the formation and precise organization of large supramolecular structures and their interaction with other matrix components such as elastin, proteoglycans and glycoproteins. There is also substantial evidence[1] that collagen plays a major role in fetal development. It is not surprising therefore that a large number of clinical syndromes with a wide spectrum of symptoms are known or suspected of being caused by molecular abnormalities of collagen. These include the osteochondrodysplasias, Marfan's syndrome, the Ehlers-Danlos syndrome, pseudoxanthoma elasticum and cutis laxa among others.

THE COLLAGEN FAMILY

Once collagen was defined as a protein that contained two unusual amino acids, hydroxyproline and hydroxylysine, a high content of glycine (one third of total residues) and demonstrated a particular X-ray diffraction pattern indicative of a coiled-coil triple-helical structure. At the time only one protein was known to meet these criteria and this was the major component of skin and bone. In 1969 the first suggestion of molecular diversity came with the discovery that cartilage contained a distinct collagen species[2] and then a third molecular species was identified in fetal skin and other tissues.[3,4] Now the number of proteins identified in this family has expanded to 10 types (Table 8.1) with some evidence for even further heterogeneity. These 10 proteins contain the products of some 20 different structural genes. All the proteins are comprised of 'collagenous' and 'non-collagenous' domains, the relative proportions of which vary with the collagen type and help to determine the type of supramolecular organization of the molecules. The 'collagen' domains contain a high proportion of

Table 8.1   Collagen types, structure, characteristics and localization

Type	Chain composition	Characteristics	Tissue localization
I	$\alpha1(I)_2\alpha2(I)$	subunit MW, 95 kd. low hylys, 1/3 gly.	skin, bone, tendon, lung, ligament, blood vessel walls etc.
I (trimer)	$\alpha1(I)_3$	subunit MW, 95 kd. low hylys	embryonic tendons, skin, membranous bones
II	$\alpha1(II)_3$	subunit MW, 95 kd. medium hylys	hyaline cartilage, intervertebral disc, vitreous humour
III	$\alpha1(III)_3$	subunit MW, 95 kd. S-S bonds within helix	blood vessels, skin, lung, gut, etc.
IV	? $\alpha1(IV)_2\alpha2(IV)$	subunit MW, 140 kd. extensively S-S bonded high hylys, <1/3 glycine	basement membranes
V	$\alpha1(V)_2\alpha2(V)$ $\alpha1(V)_3$ $\alpha1(V)\alpha2(V)\alpha3(V)$	subunit MW, 95 kd. high hylys	pericellular, skin, periostium, blood vessel walls, placental membranes
VI	$\alpha1(VI)\alpha2(VI)\alpha3(VI)$	subunit MW, 140 kd. S-S bonded aggregates combined collagenous/non-collagenous domains	skin, blood vessel intima, placenta
VII	$\alpha1(VII)_3$	subunit MW, 170 kd. extended triple helix	foetal membranes, skin anchoring fibrils?
VIII	? EC1, EC2	subunits 177 kd, 125 kd interrupted collagenous domains	endothelial cells and other cell types
IX	$\alpha1(IX)\alpha2(IX)\alpha3(IX)$	S-S bonded 3 interrupted collagen domains	hyaline cartilage
X	? $\alpha1(X)_3$	subunit MW, 59 kd.	hypertrophic region of hyaline cartilage
$1\alpha,2\alpha,3\alpha$	?	95 kd MW. High hylys 1α, 2α similar to $1\alpha(V)$ and $\alpha2(V)$ 3α similar to $\alpha1(II)$	hyaline cartilage

imino acids and glycine is commonly one third of the total residues. They also contain the distinctive amino acids hydroxyproline and hydroxylysine. The primary structure is a repetitive gly-X-Y-sequence where X is often proline and Y often hydroxyproline but can be any amino acid. In the native molecules three polypeptide chains in a polyproline-like helix coil about each other giving a triple-helical coiled-coil structure rather like a three stranded rope which is responsible for the characteristic X-ray diffraction pattern (Fig. 8.1). For a detailed description of this structure see Ref. 5. When the three component chains of the molecule are identical it is called a homopolymer, when they are genetically distinct it is referred to as a heteropolymer. The molecules of Types I, II and III collagen aggregate in vivo and in vitro to form fibrils and are called the interstitial collagens. Type IV collagen appears to produce a complex 'chicken-wire'

A. TYPICAL SEQUENCE

GLY - X - Y - GLY - PRO - Y - GLY - X - HYP - GLY - PRO - HYP

B. MINOR HELIX

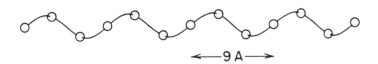

←—9 A—→

C. MAJOR (TRIPLE) HELIX

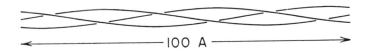

←————————— 100 A —————————→

D. MOLECULE

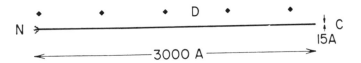

E. FIBRIL

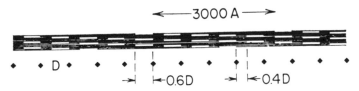

Fig. 8.1 The molecular structure of a typical interstitial collagen. A.—The repetitive triplet sequence of amino acid residues. B.—The minor helix conformation adopted by each polypeptide chain. C.—The major helix conformation adopted by the trimeric molecule. D.—The overall dimensions of the complete molecule. D represents 234 residue spacings. E.—The aggregation of individual molecules to form fibrils. Each molecule is staggered by 1D with respect to its neighbour. 0.6D and 0.4D represent 'hole zones' and 'overlap-zones' respectively which give rise to the banded appearance of collagen fibres in the electron microscope.

mesh structure in vivo (Fig. 8.2). The supramolecular structures adopted by the other collagens in vivo has yet to be established with certainty (Fig. 8.2). Some of them appear to be restricted to the pericellular environment.

Cross-linking sites: (1) 7-S collagen domain
                        (2) Non-collagenous domain

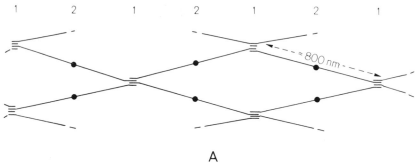

A

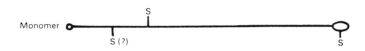

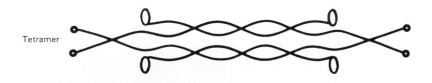

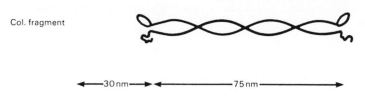

B

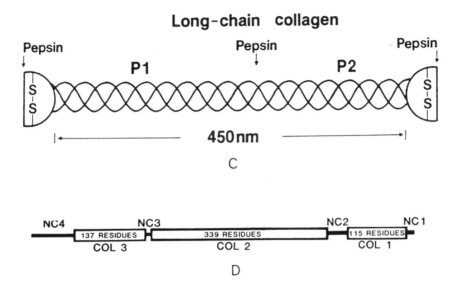

Long-chain collagen

Pepsin   Pepsin   Pepsin

P1   P2

|←   450 nm   →|

C

NC4   NC3   NC2   NC1

137 RESIDUES   339 RESIDUES   115 RESIDUES

COL 3   COL 2   COL 1

D

Fig. 8.2 Proposed molecular structures of some minority collagens. (A) the 'chicken-wire' structure of Type IV collagen (reproduced from Ref. 6). The molecules are arranged so that four like-termini are intermolecularly crosslinked in the 7-S domain (1) and two adjacent complexes are linked by interaction of the non-collagenous domains (2) at the opposite end. (B) structures of type VI collagen (reproduced from Ref. 9). The molecule consists of a triple helical domain flanked by two globular domains. In the electron microscope evidence is seen for associations of these molecules into overlapping dimers and tetramers as shown. (C) structure of type VII collagen (reproduced from Ref. 13). The molecule has an extended triple helical region, which is sensitive to pepsin, flanked by non-helical domains at N- and C-termini. (D) structure of type IX collagen (reproduced from Ref. 15) derived from protein chemistry, electron microscopy and DNA sequence analysis. The protein consists of three separate 'collagenous' domains.

Here only a brief description of the structure and distribution of individual collagens is given as a background to the description of the various molecular defects.

Type I collagen

Type I collagen is the archetypal collagen, it is the most abundant form in the body, constituting greater than 95% of the organic matrix of bone and tendon and 80% of adult skin. It is a major constituent of the cornea, ligaments, sclerae, heart valves, and the annulus fibrosus of the intervertebral disc and a significant component of blood vessel walls, the lung parenchyma, gut, joint capsule and foetal membranes, it is in fact found in virtually all connective tissue matrices.

  The basic molecule is a heteropolymer with two identical polypeptide chains designated $\alpha 1(I)$ and a third, homologous but genetically distinct, $\alpha 2(I)$ chain. Each chain contains 1050 residues with 330 residues of glycine and approximately 100 residues each of proline and hydroxyproline. The presence of hydroxyproline is critical since the formation of additional interchain hydrogen bonds through the hydroxyl group enhances the stability of the triple helix giving it a denaturation temperature a few degrees above ambient body temperatures. Nearly 95% of the residues are contained in the gly-X-Y triplet sequence of the triple-helical domain but at both N- and C-termini are short amino acid sequences, called telopeptides, that cannot adopt the triple-helical conformation. Although only 15–20 residues long, the telopeptides play a critical role in maintaining the integrity of the tissue as they contain the sites for intermolecular crosslink formation (see below). The complete molecule which has a rod-like structure some 300 nm long and 1.5 nm in diameter aggregates into fibrils (20–200 nm in diameter) such that all molecules point in the same direction and overlap the adjacent molecule by approximately one quarter of its length (1D if the molecular length is represented by 4.4D, Fig. 8.1). Between consecutive molecules in the fibril is a small gap of 0.6D units which can be filled with electron dense stains giving rise to the characteristic banding pattern seen in the electron microscope (Fig. 8.1).

The different physical properties of the major Type I collagen containing tissues such as skin, bone, tendon and cornea are derived in part by its interaction with other matrix components but also by an exquisite regulation of fibril organization and size. For example, in tendon the fibrils aggregate in large fibre bundles which run parallel to the direction of stress and produce a tissue that has the tensile strength of an equivalent steel wire. In skin the fibres are oriented more or less randomly allowing for some flexibility yet providing strength in every direction. In the cornea however the transparency of the tissue is achieved by having sheets of parallel fibres with a strictly controlled, uniformly small diameter arranged with the fibre orientation in each sheet almost perpendicular to that above and below.

Some tissues from embryonic sources contain minute amounts of a homopolymer containing only $\alpha1(I)$ chains. Molecules of this composition have also been identified in cultures of certain cell types, particularly amniotic fluid cells and transformed cells. The molecular structure of this molecule appears to be the same as the normal Type I molecule. Its function is unknown.

Type II collagen

Type II collagen is a homopolymer of $\alpha1(II)$ chains which are the same size as and homologous to $\alpha1(I)$ and $\alpha2(I)$ but they are genetically distinct. Type II thus has a similar molecular structure to Type I collagen. The $\alpha1(II)$ chains have a similar content of glycine, proline and hydroxyproline to $\alpha1(I)$ and $\alpha2(I)$ but a somewhat higher content of hydroxylysine, most of which is glycosylated (see below). Type II is found only in hyaline cartilages, intervertebral discs (associated with Type I collagen) and the vitreous humour of the eye. The molecules form small fibrils which physically entrap the giant proteoglycan complexes and the associated water in a complex network. This allows the cartilage to withstand large compressive forces.

Sequencing and other biochemical data have indicated that isolated α1(II) chains are heterogeneous, so more than one Type II collagen molecule may exist.

Type III collagen

Type III collagen was first identified as a significant component of foetal skin, blood vessel walls and leiomyomas.[3,4] It is a homopolymer of α1(III) chains each containing 1000 residues with the same molecular structure as Types I and II collagen. It is distinguished from these by the presence of interchain disulphide bonds within the helical domain of the molecule. This serves as a convenient marker in the analysis of pathological conditions described below. Type III collagen has a similar tissue distribution to Type I collagen but it does not occur in bone and forms only a very minor component of tendon where it is restricted to the endotendineum. In some tissues such as blood vessel walls and fetal skin it constitutes the major collagenous component.

The relative abundance of Type III collagen shows some interesting developmental changes, particularly in the skin. Fetal skin contains as much as 50% Type III collagen but after parturition this level slowly declines to the adult levels of 10–15% during the first decade.[4] Type III collagen production is stimulated in adult skin during wound healing so that early scar tissue contains high levels of Type III collagen. This level usually returns to normal as the wound retracts and matures but in hypertrophic scars, for some unknown reason, the Type III collagen remains artificially high even after scar maturation. These observations suggest that Type III collagen plays a role in the early development of connective tissues but it is no longer considered to be an 'embryonic protein'.

Type IV collagen

Type IV collagen is the collagen of basement membranes, it does not form fibres like Types I, II and III. The molecule consists of three collagen chains with an apparent molecular weight of 140 kilodaltons forming a triple helix which is 390 nm long. It is somewhat flexible due to interruptions in the gly-X-Y triplet sequence and the inclusion of a short non-collagenous sequence. At one end of the helix is a globular protein sequence of about 25 kilodaltons. The molecule is inter- and intramolecularly crosslinked by disulphide bonds and other covalent crosslinks. The current concept of its supramolecular structure.[6] (shown in Fig. 8.2) envisages 4 triple helices being tightly crosslinked between like ends (the 7-S domain) and each globular domain crosslinking with the globular domain of an adjacent molecule, forming a complex 'chicken wire' network.

Two distinct collagen chains α1(IV) and α2(IV) have been isolated from Type IV collagen preparations and it is thought they form a hetero-polymer but this has not been determined unequivocally. Type IV collagen chains are distinguished from those of other collagens by their lower content of glycine and high content of hydroxylysine and cysteine.

Type V collagen

Type V collagen was originally identified in proteolytic extracts of fetal membranes, it is thought to be a heteropolymer of two α1(V) [originally known as αB] and one α2(V) [originally αA] chains[7] although occasionally the stoichiometry of α1(V) and α2(V) and the presence of a third chain (α3(V)) suggests that other structures may exist. The α chains are approximately 1000 residues long giving the molecule similar overall dimensions to the interstitial collagens. Unlike the latter proteins it will not readily precipitate as fibrils in vitro although in cell cultures the Type V appears as filamentous pericellular fibrils. Type V is not intramolecularly disulphide bonded but has a relatively high content of hydroxylysine. The protein is a minor component of many tissues including skin, bone, liver, tendon, gingiva and muscle but its major source is fetal membranes.

Type VI collagen

Type VI collagen was first identified in peptic extracts of aortic intima and placenta as a high molecular weight disulphide-bonded aggregate containing three non-identical chains with molecular weights 40–55 kilodaltons. More recent studies using non-degradative procedures have shown that these polypeptides represent the triple-helical domain of a complex structure with subunit molecular weight 110–145 kilodaltons having globular domains at both ends of the triple helix.[8,9] Polymeric forms of this collagen containing dimers and tetramers linked end-to-end through the globular domains probably reflect the supramolecular organization within the tissue (Fig. 8.2). Immunofluorescence studies have shown Type VI is the product of fibroblasts and smooth muscle cells and is found in virtually all interstitial connective tissues particularly the skin, the aortic media, cartilage perichondrium (but not the cartilage itself) and the corneal stroma but it is absent from basement membranes.[8] Recently Type VI collagen has been identified with a previously characterized transformation-sensitive cell surface glycoprotein GP140[10] and with a microfibrillar glycoprotein.[11,12]

Type VII collagen

Type VII collagen is a homopolymer containing α chains with a molecular weight of approximately 170 kilodaltons giving a triple-helical domain about

1.5 times the length of the interstitial collagens. This triple helix is susceptible to prolonged proteolysis indicative of interruptions in the gly-X-Y
triplet sequence. The molecule is internally disulphide bonded (Fig. 8.2).
The fibril structure in vivo has not been ascertained but fibrils generated
in vitro contain head to head dimers. The appearance of these fibrils, the
isolation from epithelial basement membrane rich tissues and some immuno-
localization studies have suggested that Type VII collagen may be a major
component of the anchoring filaments and anchoring fibrils associated with
such membranes.[13]

Type VIII collagen

Type VIII collagen (EC collagen) was originally identified as a product of
endothelial cell cultures. It is a homopolymer with a subunit molecular
weight of 177 kilodaltons. The triple helix is not continuous and mild
proteolytic digestion produces at least three 'collagenous' domains.[14]

Type IX collagen

Several low molecular weight collagenous peptides have recently been
isolated from proteolytic digests of cartilage matrices from the chick, pig
and cow. Although there appears to be some species differences in the
proteinase susceptibility these molecules all seem to derive from a similar
parent molecule now called Type IX collagen. This is a disulphide bonded
molecule containing three distinct polypeptide chains. The molecule
consists of three triple-helical domains containing 137, 339 and 115 residues
separated by short non-collagenous sequences. There are additional short
non-collagenous sequences at both N- and C-terminals[15] (Fig. 8.2). The
structure and function of this collagen in tissues is not yet clear, rotary
shadowing electron micrographs suggest it is quite flexible and it has been
localized to the pericellular region of the cartilage by immunofluorescence.
However one recent study has identified Type IX collagen with a small
chondroitin sulphate proteoglycan (Lt) from chick sternum which has a
more widespread distribution within the cartilage matrix.[16] This hybrid
collagen/proteoglycan molecule may play a significant role in the collagen-
proteoglycan interaction in the cartilage.

Type X collagen

Type X collagen is another short chain collagen identified in cartilagenous
tissues and chondrocyte cultures. It is a non-disulphide bonded trimer of
polypeptide chains with a molecular weight of 59 kilodaltons, of this 45
kilodaltons are involved in the typical collagenous triple helix the remainder
forms a globular 'knob' at the end of the triple helix.[17] The supramolecular
structure adopted by this molecule in vivo is not known although molecules

do have a tendency to associate via their globular domains in vitro.[17] Immunofluorescence has shown that this collagen accumulates around the hypertrophic chondrocytes in the diaphysis of the cartilage.

Unclassified collagens

Cartilage is also the source of three other collagenous chains designated 1α, 2α and 3α. Each has a molecular weight of 100 kilodaltons (~1000 amino acid residues) and resembles the interstitial or Type V collagens. Peptide mapping of 3α has shown a remarkable similarity to $\alpha1(II)$ chains and 3α may represent an overmodified form. However, whilst 1α and 2α bear a close resemblance to the chains of Type V collagen, similar peptide mapping experiments have shown that they are genetically distinct.[18] The molecular structure of these proteins remains unclear.

THE BIOSYNTHESIS OF COLLAGENS

The biosynthesis of the major collagens has been well established[19] and the following description refers primarily to the interstitial collagens, Types I, II and III. However, all available evidence suggests that other collagens follow a similar pathway although details may vary slightly.

Briefly the steps in the biosynthesis of collagens are:

1. Gene selection, transcription
2. Processing to mature mRNA
3. Translation of mRNA to yield preproαchain
4. Cleavage of signal peptide
5. Lysyl and prolyl hydroxylation, hydroxylysyl glycosylation (glucose and galactose), mannose oligosaccharide addition to C-propeptide
6. Molecular assembly, disulphide bond formation in C-propeptide, triple helix formation
7. Secretion of procollagen
8. Cleavage of amino-terminal and carboxy-terminal propeptides
9. Fibril formation
10. Oxidation of specific lysines and hydroxylysines, covalent crosslink formation
11. Maturation of crosslinks

The interstitial collagens, like many other proteins destined for export, are initially synthesized as a precursor form. The secreted protein is some 50% larger than the mature molecule found in tissues. The increased size

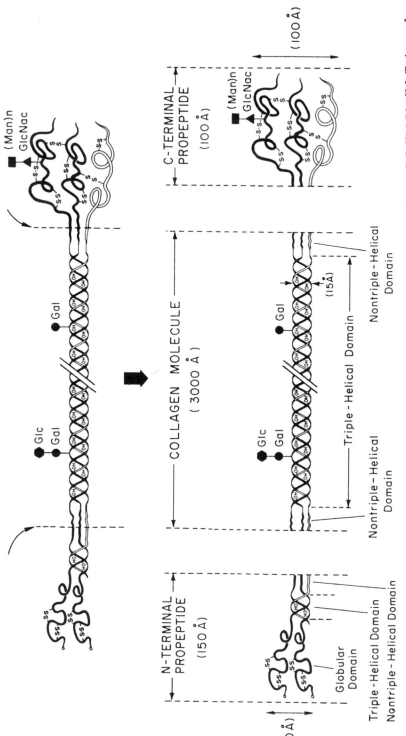

Fig. 8.3 A schematic representation of the Type I procollagen molecule and its various domains (reproduced from Prockop D J, Kivirikko K I, Tuderman L, Guzman N A 1979 New England Journal of Medicine 301: 16). This is the typical procollagen structure for the interstitial collagens.

is accounted for by additional peptide sequences (called the pro-peptides) at both the N- and C-terminals of the α chain. Thus the initial translation product for the pro α chain is a polypeptide with a molecular weight of 150 kilodaltons comprising a transient hydrophobic leader sequence at the N-terminus to facilitate transfer into the lumen of the rough endoplasmic reticulum followed by the N-propeptide which itself has three discrete domains, a globular domain, a short collagenous domain containing Gly-X-Y sequences and a short non-helical domain (which includes the telopeptide) leading to the major collagenous domain of the α chain itself. At the C-terminus of the pro α chain is a propeptide containing 300 amino acid residues with a typical globular amino acid sequence (Fig. 8.3). Comparative DNA sequencing has shown that the C-propeptide sequence is highly conserved between different collagen chains implying a major role for this domain in molecular assembly.[20] It appears that this region directs the assembly of the three chains, stabilizes the trimer by interchain disulphide bonds and initiates triple helix formation. The N-propeptides also contain cysteine residues, in Type I collagen disulphide bonding is purely intra-chain but in Type III collagen interchain disulphide bonds are formed.

The initial translation product undergoes several post-ribosomal modifications. Certain lysine and proline residues are hydroxylated to produce hydroxylysine and hydroxyproline. This is accomplished by two distinct enzymes, lysyl hydroxylase and prolyl hydroxylase, respectively, each of which requires ferrous iron, α-ketoglutarate, molecular oxygen and a reducing agent, such as ascorbic acid, as cofactors. Some hydroxylysine residues are further modified by the sequential addition of galactose and glucose moieties to the side chain hydroxyl group by specific glycosyl trans-ferase enzymes. The degree of post-translational modification of lysines varies from collagen type to collagen type, from tissue to tissue for a given collagen type and with age, embryonic tissues being more hydroxylated than adult. Other sugar residues—particularly mannose—are added as asparagine-linked oligosaccharide to the C-terminal propeptide. The post-translational modifications continue only whilst the chains are not in a triple-helical conformation. As the three chains come together via the C-terminal propeptides and triple helix formation propogates toward the N-terminus, hydroxylation ceases. The level of hydroxylation of the proline residues is the critical factor in helix formation, the thermal stability of the triple helix is directly proportional to the number of hydroxyprolines because of the formation of additional hydrogen bonds through the hydroxyl group, unhydroxylated collagen is unstable at body temperature.

The completed triple-helical precursor molecule, procollagen, is secreted via the golgi and microtubules into the extracellular space. Recently it has become apparent that a significant proportion (10–30%) of all newly synthesized collagen never leaves the cell but is degraded intracellularly. The precise role of this process is not clear, it seems to serve as a quality control mechanism since incorporation of destabilizing amino acid

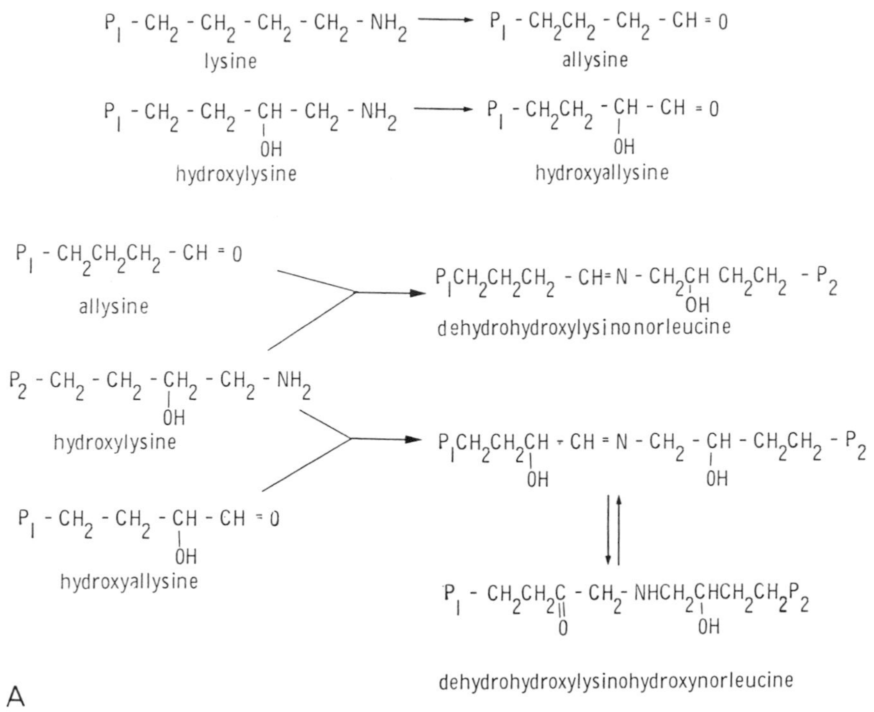

$$P_I - CH_2 - CH_2 - CH_2 - CH_2 - NH_2 \longrightarrow P_I - CH_2CH_2 - CH_2 - CH = O$$

lysine   allysine

$$P_I - CH_2 - CH_2 - \underset{\underset{OH}{|}}{CH} - CH_2 - NH_2 \longrightarrow P_I - CH_2CH_2 - \underset{\underset{OH}{|}}{CH} - CH = O$$

hydroxylysine   hydroxyallysine

$$P_I - CH_2CH_2CH_2 - CH = O$$

allysine

$$P_I CH_2CH_2CH_2 - CH = N - CH_2\underset{\underset{OH}{|}}{CH} CH_2CH_2 - P_2$$

dehydrohydroxylysinonorleucine

$$P_2 - CH_2 - CH_2 - \underset{\underset{OH}{|}}{CH} - CH_2 - NH_2$$

hydroxylysine

$$P_I CH_2CH_2\underset{\underset{OH}{|}}{CH} - CH = N - CH_2 - \underset{\underset{OH}{|}}{CH} - CH_2CH_2 - P_2$$

$$P_I - CH_2 - CH_2 - \underset{\underset{OH}{|}}{CH} - CH = O$$

hydroxyallysine

$$P_I - CH_2CH_2\underset{\underset{O}{||}}{C} - CH_2 - NHCH_2\underset{\underset{OH}{|}}{CHCH_2}CH_2P_2$$

dehydrohydroxylysinohydroxynorleucine

A

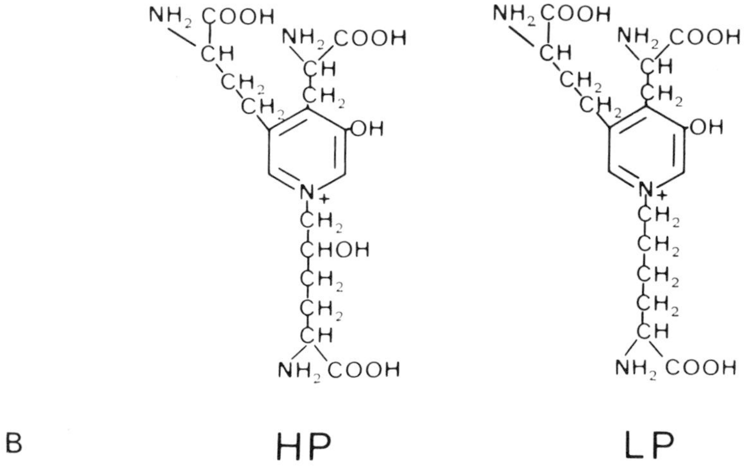

B   HP   LP

Fig. 8.4 Covalent intermolecular crosslinking of collagen: (A) The formation of bifunctional crosslinks. Peptidyl lysine or hydroxylysine residues are enzymically oxidised to allysine or hydroxyallysine by lysyl oxidase. An allysine and hydroxylysine react to form dehydrohydroxylysinonorleucine, whilst an hydroxylallysine and hydroxylysine react to produce dehydrohydroxylysinohydroxynorleucine. This is stabilized by an Amadori-type rearrangement, existing mostly as the keto-form. (B) structures of the pyridinolines, HP = hydroxypyridinoline, LP = pyridinoline. They differ by being derived from an hydroxylysine or lysine respectively.

analogues into the protein cause an increase in intracellular degradation. Similar increases are also seen in some diseases (see below).

Prior to incorporation of the molecule into a fibril the N- and C-terminal propeptides are removed by separate enzymes which cleave all three chains simultaneously. The collagen molecules thus produced can self-assemble into the quarter stagger arrangement in the fibril. The fibril is then stabilized by the formation of unique intermolecular crosslinks. Crosslinking is initiated by the oxidative deamination of the ε-amino group of specific lysine or hydroxylysine residues in the N- and C-terminal telopeptides by a copper requiring enzyme called lysyl oxidase. This produces a terminal aldehyde (allysine) which can then react with the ε-amino group of specific hydroxylysines within the helix of an adjacent molecule, or molecules, by a Schiff-base condensation (Fig. 8.4). These crosslinks, which can be identified by reduction with ^{3}H-borohydride, are only intermediate products and disappear as the tissue matures forming more complex structures which have not been identified. One complex crosslinking component called pyridinoline (Fig. 8.4) has been postulated as the mature crosslink in certain tissues because it can be derived by further condensation of the Schiff-base intermediates. The critical importance of crosslinking to the mechanical integrity of connective tissues is demonstrated by a drug-induced disease called lathyrism. Here a compound, β-aminopropionitrile, derived from the seeds of the sweet pea Lathyrus odoratus irreversibly inhibits the lysyl oxidase responsible for the oxidative deamination. The outcome is a marked decrease in the tensile strength of the connective tissues causing extreme skin friability, skeletal deformities and a blood vessel weakness which leads to aneurisms and rupture.

The biosynthesis described here applies to a typical interstitial collagen, many of the steps must apply to all collagens. One possible distinction for the non-interstitial collagens is that the extracellular processing of the procollagen form may not proceed to the same extent and the precursor form itself may be incorporated directly into the matrix.

THE COLLAGEN GENES AND MESSENGER RNA

The structural genes for the proα-chains of the interstitial collagens (Types I, II & III) have been cloned and characterized (Table 8.2). The structure of the α2(I) gene has been reviewed in great detail[21] and this gene serves as the model for the interstitial collagen genes (Fig. 8.5). It is large, 38 kb, and complex with the coding sequences separated into more than 50 exons. The exons coding for the amino acid residues of the central triple-helical domain consist of only 54 base pairs or low order multiples thereof. This represents 6 Gly-X-Y triplets and although a few exons have more or less bases they always code for a whole number of triplets; splice sites are never found within the Gly-X-Y sequence. It has been postulated that the

THE CHICK a-2 (type I) COLLAGEN GENE

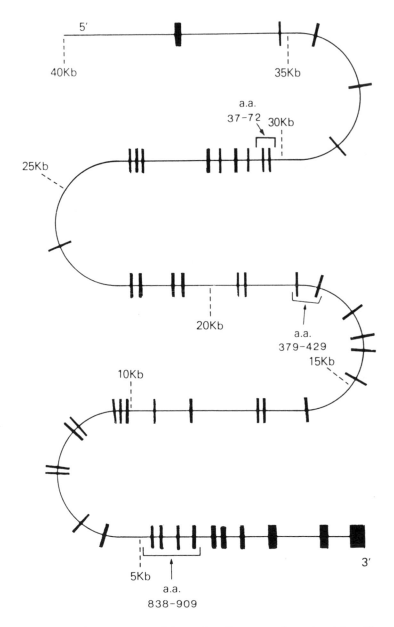

Fig. 8.5 The intron/exon structure of the α2(I) collagen gene (reproduced from Yamada Y, Avvedimento E, Mudrys M, Ohkulso H, Vogeli G, Irani M, Pastan I, de Crombrugghe B 1984 Cell 22: 887–892). The genes for all interstitial collagen chains have a similar organization of introns and exons.

Table 8.2   The collagen genes, characteristics and location

Gene	Size	Introns	Exon size	Chromosomal location
α1(I)	18 000bp	>50	54bp	17q 21.31–22.05
α2(I)	38 000bp	>50	54bp	7q 21.3–22.1
α1(II)	38 000bp	>50	54bp	12
α1(III)	38 000bp	>50	54bp	2q 24.3–>q 31
α1(IV)	?	?	?	13
α2(V)	?	?	?	2q 24.3–>q 31
α1(IX)	?	multiple	variable 33–1100bp	?
α2(IX)	?	multiple	variable 33–1100bp	?

multiple 54 base pair exon structure may have arisen by duplication of a primordial gene of this size or by insertion of non-coding sequences into the gene to discourage crossovers that might arise from the high degree of homology of the different collagens. This exon/intron structure has been highly conserved among different pro α-chains. Virtually the same number and size of exons are found in the α1(II) and α1(III) genes which are 38–40 kb long and the α1(I) gene which is only 18 kb long, the difference in size being accounted for by changes in the length of the various introns.

Quantitative and clinical data suggest that there is only a single copy of each collagen gene in the haploid genome. Despite their apparent structural conservation the various collagen genes are spread throughout the chromosomes. The α1(I) gene is found on chromosome 17 (q21.31–22.05) and the α2(I) gene is on 7 (q21.3–22.1) while the α1(II) gene is on chromosome 12, the α1(III) and α2(V) are on chromosome 2 and the gene for the α1(IV) chain is on chromosome 13. Transcription of these genes gives rise to multiple forms of mRNA for each protein due to the recognition of more than one polyadenylation site at the 3' end of the message. It is not certain if this performs any particular function.

The genes for two of the polypeptides of Type IX collagen do not conform to the 54 base pair exon pattern. Indeed of the 11 exons in genomic clones for α1(IX) and α2(IX) sequenced recently only one contained 54 bp; the others ranged in size from 33 to 1100 bp implying that the non-interstitial collagens represent a separate class of collagen genes derived from a different precursor.[22]

MOLECULAR ABNORMALITIES OF COLLAGEN SYNTHESIS

Inherited diseases of connective tissues in which molecular abnormalities of collagen are suspected (Table 8.3) reflect the widespread distribution of these proteins. They present with a range of clinical findings from brittle bones to weak blood vessels, from loose skin to lax joints. For technical reasons molecular abnormalities have been demonstrated in only collagen

Table 8.3 Inherited diseases thought to involve collagen abnormalities

Disease	Inheritance
Osteogenesis Imperfecta	AD, AR, Sporadic
Ehlers-Danlos Syndrome	AD, AR, XLR
Marfan Syndrome	AD
Cutis Laxa	AD, AR, XLR
Menkes Syndrome	XLR
Progeria	?AR
Epidermolysis Bullosa	AR, AD
Werner's Syndrome	?AR

Types I and III. These proteins have been well characterized, the skin provides a readily accessible tissue source but, most significantly, they are major products of fibroblasts in culture. It is the ability to manipulate such cell cultures to study collagen biosynthesis, the development of improved methods of analysing the proteins they produce and the advent of recombinant DNA technology that has led to significant advances in our understanding of the molecular pathology of these diseases in recent years.

Osteogenesis imperfecta

The most obvious clinical manifestation of osteogenesis imperfecta (OI) is that the bones are poorly calcified and exceedingly fragile causing multiple fractures. It is however a generalized disorder and abnormalities of skin, teeth, heart valves and vasculature are all observed in certain cases.[23] Clinically it is a heterogeneous disorder with severity ranging from a mild disease with relatively few fractures and no major skeletal deformity through progressive deformity to intrauterine or perinatal death (Fig. 8.6). Both autosomal dominant and recessive inheritance are known. The disease has been separated into four major groups based on clinical criteria[24] (Table 8.4) but there is further heterogeneity within each group and many patients cannot be classified.

The tissues affected in this syndrome contain predominantly Type I collagen implying that this protein or its interactions with other matrix components are faulty. All available biochemical data support this premise.

Type II OI

Osteogenesis imperfecta Type II is the lethal form of the disease, it is heterogeneous but many affected individuals have broad crumpled bones some have beaded ribs on X-ray whilst some have long, thin bones. The major breakthrough in the characterisation of this disease was made in 1975 when Pentinnen et al[25] showed that cultured skin fibroblasts

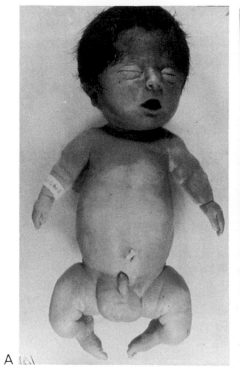
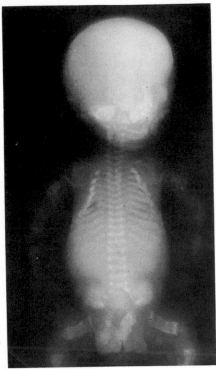

A

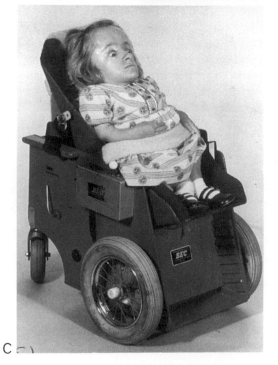

C

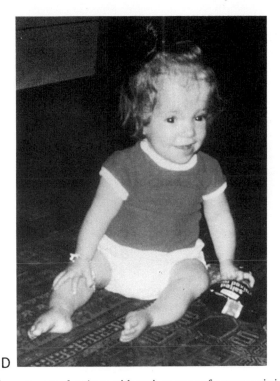

D

Fig. 8.6 Clinical appearance of patients with various types of osteogenesis imperfecta.
(A) broad boned lethal Type IIA OI (B) radiologic features of Type IIA OI
(C) progressively deforming Type III OI (D) mild dominant Type I OI
Photographs by courtesy of Dr. F. M. Pope, Clinical Research Centre, Harrow.

from a particularly severely affected individual synthesized abnormal ratios of Type I and III collagens indicative of reduced Type I. It is now known that cells from this patient synthesize two forms of proα1(I) chain, one of normal length and one missing some 80 amino acid residues from the triple helical domain (Fig. 8.7A). The shortened chains can be incorporated into a trimeric Type I protein with either a normal or abnormal proα1(I) chain but the molecules produced are thermally unstable, poorly secreted and degraded intracellularly.[26,27] The amount of functional Type I collagen produced is thus only one quarter of normal levels (Fig. 8.7B). This destruction of normal protein chains by association with the abnormal protein has been termed 'protein suicide' by one laboratory.[27] Analysis of the DNA revealed a deletion from the affected allele of some 500 base pairs which resulted in the loss of three complete exons coding for the amino acid sequence around the junction of α1(I)CB8 and α1(I)CB3 (Fig. 8.7C).

Fibroblasts from another lethal OI patient synthesized only shortened proα2(I) chains in reduced amounts. It was estimated that between 15 and 20 residues were missing from the C-terminal half of the helical region. The

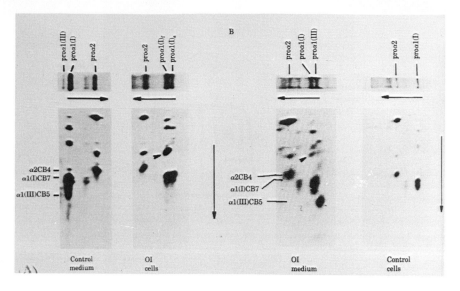

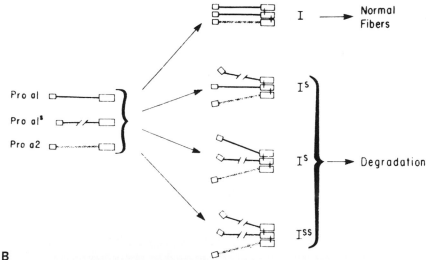

B

Fig. 8.7 (A) Gel electrophoretograms showing the synthesis of shortened proα1(I) chains in a Type II OI patient (reproduced from Ref. 26). Whole chains are first separated by electrophoresis in a low concentration acrylamide gel (shown horizontally at the top of the figure with arrows marking the direction of migration of the proteins). In the OI cells the proα1(I) band appears as a doublet of proα1(I)f and proα1(I)s. After separation in the first dimension the proteins are digested with cyanogen bromide *in situ* and re-electrophoresed at right angles in a higher concentration gel. The proteins from the OI cells show an additional spot (marked with arrowhead) and a distortion of other spots derived from the proα1(I) doublet. This can also be seen to a lesser extent in the proteins from the OI medium but not in those from control cells or medium. (B) 'suicide protein' hypothesis of the effect of the deletion in this Type II OI patient (reproduced from Ref. 27). All trimeric molecules containing a shortened proα1(I) chain cannot be secreted from the cells and are destined for intracellular degradation. (C) order of the cyanogen bromide peptides in the α chains of the major interstitial collagens. In this Type II OI patient the deletion removes the methionine at the junction of α1(I) CB8 and α1(I) CB3.

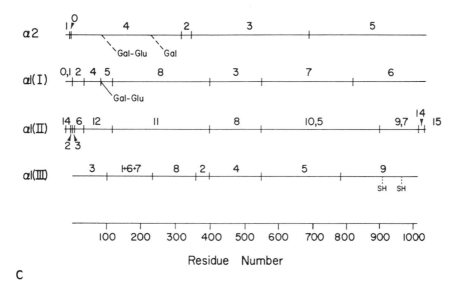

C

Table 8.4 Classification and characteristics of osteogenesis imperfecta after Sillence

Type	Inheritance	Clinical Features
I	Autosomal dominant	A. bone fragility, blue sclerae, deafness, late onset of fractures, normal teeth B. as A but with dentinogenesis imperfecta C. as B but with few fractures
II	Autosomal recessive sporadic	extremely severe osseous fragility, stillborn or death in neonatal period A. broad crumpled long bones and beaded ribs B. broad crumpled long bones, no beading of ribs C. thin, fractured, long bones, thin beaded ribs D. as A but includes microcephaly and cataracts E. as A but bones more hypoplastic
III	Autosomal recessive	Moderate to severe osseous fragility, normal sclerae (blue in infancy), ± severe deformity of long bones and spine. Non-lethal in newborn, progressively deforming.
IV	Autosomal dominant	Osseous fragility with normal sclerae (blue in infancy) ± severe deformity of long bones and spine A. without dentinogenesis imperfecta B. with dentinogenesis imperfecta

α1(I) chains associated with the mutant α2(I) chains migrated more slowly on SDS-polyacrylamide gels indicating excessive post-translational modification of lysine residues. When cells from the parents were examined neither produced the shortened proα2(I) chain but the father did show reduced synthesis of α2(I) chains. It was concluded that the child was a compound heterozygote with a new mutation causing the shortened α2(I) chain and a silent α2(I) allele inherited from the father.

Major deletions are not the only cause of lethal disease, one recent study has implied that point mutations at critical sites in the α chains can also be lethal. In this case two forms of α1(I) chain were observed. One was normal, the other contained a cysteine residue within the helical domain (cysteine does not usually occur in this region of the Type I molecule). When two mutant chains were incorporated into the same molecule disulphide bonded dimers were formed. Cyanogen bromide peptide mapping localized the mutation to the C-terminal peptide α1(I)CB6 (Fig. 8.7C). Molecules containing one or more mutant chains were poorly secreted, were overhydroxylated along the entire chain and were thermodynamically unstable (denaturation temperature 38°C compared to 41°C in normals). These observations were explained by a single base change causing a glycine → cysteine substitution in the Gly-X-Y sequence. The effect of the cysteine substitution in this patient is very different to another cysteine substitution in a patient with a dominant form of OI (see below).

Excessive post-ribosomal modification of lysine residues is a common feature of Type II OI but the extent seems quite variable (see Fig. 8.8 for some patients studied in our laboratory). An explanation for these observations has recently been suggested by Bonadio and Byers.[28] They postulate that most cases of Type II OI are not the result of large deletions from the genome but are caused by point mutations or small deletions which affect the stability of the triple helix. They propose that the mutant collagen chains initiate triple helix formation from the C-terminal propeptide as normal but the mutation causes an energy barrier to further propagation of the helix. Until this barrier is surmounted the chains amino-terminal to the mutation remain substrates for the hydroxylases and become overhydroxylated. The site of the mutation can thus be mapped by determining the point of onset of overhydroxylation. Three types of patient were identified, those with mutations in α1(I)CB6 which have a denaturation temperature (Tm) of 36–37°C, those with mutations in the carboxy-terminal half of α1(I)CB7 having a Tm of 38–39°C and those with mutations in the amino-terminal half of α1(I)CB7 with a Tm of 39–40°C (Fig. 8.9).

There have been a few reports of other collagens as well as Type I being overhydroxylated. In one child which died at 3 months the Type I and Type III collagen chains isolated from skin were all overhydroxylated and in another the Type II collagen of the cartilage was also excessively modified.

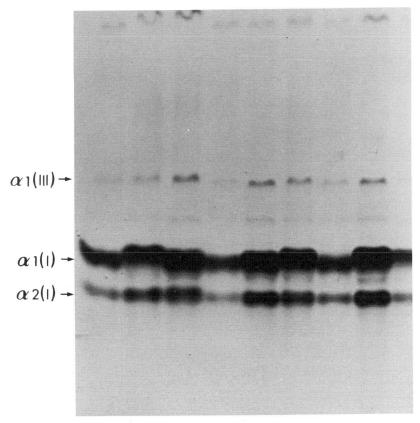

$\alpha 1(\text{III}) \rightarrow$

$\alpha 1(\text{I}) \rightarrow$

$\alpha 2(\text{I}) \rightarrow$

Fig. 8.8 Gel electrophoretogram of α chains from several patients with Type II OI. It can be seen that the migration of the α1(I) chain is slower in the patients (tracks 2,3,5,6,8 and 9) than the normal α1(I) (tracks 1,4 and 7) and also that the retardation is different for individual patients. The slow migration is attributed to overhydroxylation of the molecules prior to secretion.

The clinical data on Type II OI is insufficient to determine whether it is inherited as an autosomal recessive or sporadic new mutation. With the exception of the patient with shortened α2(I) chains all cases of broad-boned lethal OI characterized biochemically have demonstrated both normal and abnormal products. Whenever parents were also examined no protein abnormality was found. This would suggest that this form of the disease results from a new dominant mutation.

Type III OI (McKusick 25942)

Type III osteogenesis imperfecta is a severe, progressively deforming disease (Fig. 8.6). Skin fibroblasts from one patient secreted a Type I

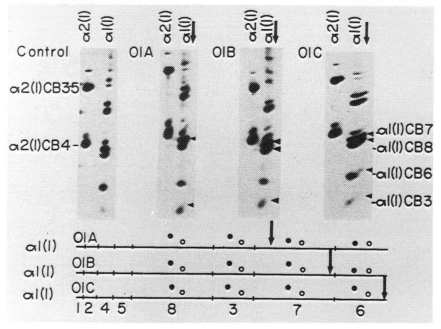

Fig. 8.9 Two dimensional electrophoretic maps of collagens produced by patients with Type II OI (reproduced from Ref. 28). The α chains have been separated horizontally as in Fig. 7(A), cyanogen bromide digested in situ and electrophoresed vertically. Three categories of patient are identified (OIA, OIB and OIC) where either two, three or four cyanogen bromide peptides of the α1(I) chain are distorted due to overhydroxylation (arrowheads). The lower part of the figure gives a schematic representation of the α1(I) chain in each category of patient. The circles represent the relative migration of the normal (open circles) and abnormal (closed circles) peptides and the arrows indicate possible sites for the mutation in each category which could give rise to this pattern.

procollagen that precipitated into the cell layer. The decreased solubility of the protein was caused by excessive mannosylation of the C-terminal propeptide, probably as a result of an amino acid substitution in this domain.

A second patient produced a Type I collagen containing only α1(I) chains (Fig. 8.10). Although a functional α2(I) mRNA was isolatable from skin fibroblasts only small amounts of pro α2(I) chain were synthesized and none of them were incorporated into a trimeric molecule. Further analysis of the α2(I) mRNA by S1-nuclease protection experiments and finally cloning and sequencing of the defective α2(I) gene revealed a 4 base pair deletion causing a frame shift mutation of the last 33 residues of the C-terminal propeptide.[29] As a result this C-propeptide could not interact with the C-propeptides of the α1(I) chains to initiate triple-helix formation, a third α1(I) chain was recruited instead producing α1(I)-trimer molecules (Fig. 8.10B). The child was homozygous for this defect, both parents, who produced half normal levels of $\alpha 1(I)$ chains, showed no clinical signs of osteogenesis imperfecta but both were considered prematurely osteoporotic.

Osteogenesis imperfecta Types I and IV (Mckusick 16620 and 16622)

Osteogenesis imperfecta Types I and IV are the less severe, dominantly inherited forms of the disease. In some families the disease is associated with dentinogenesis imperfecta but in others it is not (Table 8.4).

There have been several reports that tissues and skin fibroblast cultures from these patients show a higher proportion of Type III collagen than controls but for others this observation has been variable. For most of these patients the molecular defect is unknown. In one group of patients the abnormal ratio of Type III/Type I collagen was associated with a reduced production of Type I collagen. The Type I collagen secreted by the cells contained $\alpha 1(I)$ and $\alpha 2(I)$ chains in the required 2:1 ratio but within the cells the pro $\alpha 1(I)$:pro $\alpha 2(I)$ ratio was close to 1:1. This implies that only half the normal amount of $\alpha 1(I)$ chain was being synthesized and that one $\alpha(I)$ allele was 'silent'. In similar patients we have found reduced levels of cytoplasmic mRNA for $\alpha 1(I)$ implying either defective transcription or faulty processing of the nuclear transcript.

Not all Type I OI patients show depressed synthesis of Type I collagen. One child with a very mild disease produced normal proportions of Types I and III collagens but the Type I collagen contained two forms of $\alpha 1(I)$ chain. One was normal, the other contained cysteine, so as in the lethal OI case, disulphide bonded dimers were formed when there were two mutant chains in a molecule (Fig. 8.11). The cysteine has been mapped to $\alpha 1(I)$ CB6 (Fig. 8.7C). The contrast in the pathological consequences of the two cysteine substitutions can be explained by the effect the mutation has on the molecule. Whereas the mutation in the Type II OI patient resulted in molecules which were poorly secreted, overhydroxylated, thermally unstable and degraded intracellularly in the Type I OI patient the mutant molecules were thermally stable, hydroxylated normally and secreted normally. Thus the mutation did not affect the net collagen production. At present there is no direct evidence, but it is likely that in the mildly affected patient the substitution has occurred in the X or Y position of the Gly-X-Y triplet.

A change in the Type I:Type III collagen ratio does not necessarily reflect an abnormality in the $\alpha 1(I)$ chain. In one patient with Type IV OI two forms of $\alpha 2(I)$ chain were observed. One $\alpha 2(I)$ chain seemed to be missing some 18–20 amino acids (one exon?) from the $\alpha 2(I)$CB4 peptide. Incorporation of the shortened $\alpha 2(I)$ chains into a molecule destabilized the triple helix. The findings in this patient may be contrasted with those reported for the lethal OI where shortened $\alpha 2(I)$ chains were the only species produced.

Thus, although the classification of Sillence et al[24] has facilitated the

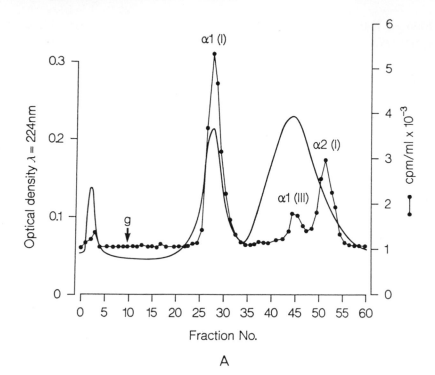

A

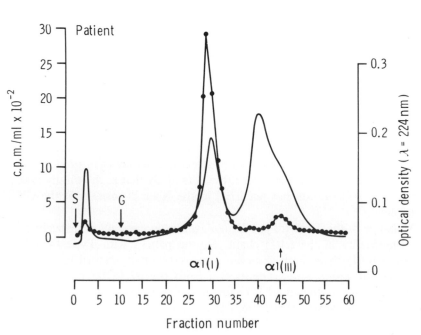

B

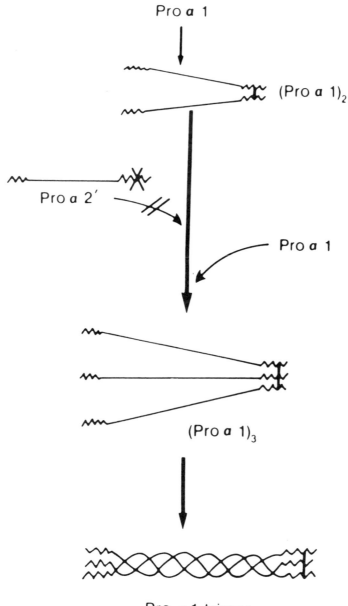

C   Pro *a* 1 trimer

Fig. 8.10 Characterization of an α2(I) deficiency in an OI Type III patient.
(A) carboxymethyl cellulose separation of collagen chains produced by normal fibroblasts.
(B) a similar separation of the collagen chains produced by this particular patient with Type
III OI. Note the complete absence of α2(I) chains. (C) schematic representation of the
effect of the mutation in this Type III OI patient (reproduced from Deak S B, Nicholls A,
Pope F M, Prockop D J 1983 Journal of Biological Chemistry 258: 15192-15197). The
mutation in the C-terminal propeptide of the proα2(I) chain prevents its incorporation into
a trimeric molecule so a third proα1(I) chain is recruited.

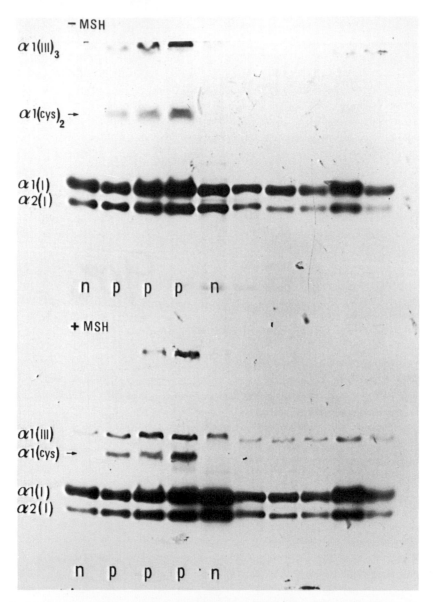

Fig. 8.11 Gel electrophoretogram of the collagens produced by a Type I OI patient with a cysteine substitution in the α1(II) chain (reproduced from Nicholls A C, Pope F M, Craig D 1984 British Medical Journal 288: 112–113). The upper part of the figure shows the proteins electrophoresed without mercaptoethanol reduction (−MSH). The mutant runs as a dimer α1(cys)$_2$. The lower part of the figure shows the same samples after mercaptoethanol reduction (+MSH) where α1(III) and α1(cys) run as monomers (both α1(III) and α(cys) migrate behind α1(I) although they are the same size because reduction is carried out in the gel after an initial period of electrophoresis to allow resolution of the different chains).

clinical description of osteogenesis imperfecta there is considerable biochemical heterogeneity within each type. Whilst all biochemical studies to date have implicated abnormalities in Type I collagen, the mutations are not restricted to one subunit chain in this disease. The number of patients for whom the molecular defect has been identified is still small but some trends appear to be emerging. For example, Type IIA OI, the most severe form, seems to result from point mutations (probably in the glycine codon), small deletions or rarely from large deletions that destabilize the triple helix, probably inherited as new dominant mutations. The milder Type I OI patients might separate into two distinct groups, those who produce a reduced amount of normal Type I collagen due to an effectively 'silent' allele (i.e. regulatory, transcription or transcript processing defect) and those producing normal amounts of Type I collagen containing the product of one abnormal allele where the mutation (probably in an X or Y residue) has only minimal effect on the stability of the molecule. Many of the latter mutations would remain 'silent' to available analytical techniques.

The Ehlers-Danlos Syndrome

The Ehlers-Danlos Syndrome is perhaps more heterogeneous than osteogenesis imperfecta. All patients are characterized by a velvety soft, fragile skin and a tendency to form tissue paper scars, hypermobile joints and hernias. The variability of these tendencies plus the association with specific clinical signs have allowed the separation of 10 distinct types although, as with osteogenesis imperfecta, further heterogeneity within types is obvious (Table 8.5). In only a few of these types has a biochemical basis been identified and only those forms will be considered in any detail.

Ehlers-Danlos Syndrome Type IV (McKusick 13005)

Type IV EDS is a catastrophic form of the disease. The patients have remarkably thin skin showing a prominent venous network and a prematurely aged appearance of the hands and feet but the major problem is a disastrous tendency for major blood vessels to rupture. All the patients investigated so far have shown a defect in Type III collagen in cell culture or tissue. The disease is clinically and biochemically heterogeneous. Clinically both autosomal recessive and dominant forms have been described. The initial biochemical results showed a lack of Type III collagen in both tissues and cell culture[30] and were supported by immunofluorescence studies showing an absence of this collagen from the cells. Later studies have shown that most patients produce Type III procollagen in reduced amounts. In some cases the cell is unable to secrete the Type III collagen synthesized (Fig. 8.12) this may be analogous to the delayed secretion of Type I collagen in lethal OI. In one patient Type III collagen production

Table 8.5   Classification and features of the Ehlers-Danlos Syndrome

Type	Genetics	Features
EDS I (Gravis)	Autosomal dominant	Severe joint hypermobility, skin hyperextensibility and tissue fragility, skeletal abnormalities
EDS II (Mitis)	Autosomal dominant	Mild-moderate joint laxity, skin hyperextensibility and tissue fragility
EDS III (Benign Hypermobile)	Autosomal dominant	Generalized severe joint hypermobility without skeletal deformity, mild tissue fragility, skin hyperextensibility
EDS IV (Ecchymotic)	Autosomal recessive Autosomal dominant	Severe bruising, low skin hyperextensibility, frequent rupture of large arteries or bowel
EDS V	X-linked recessive	Marked skin hyperextensibility, variable fragility, minimal joint hypermobility, frequent skeletal deformities
EDS VI (Ocular type)	Autosomal recessive	Marked joint hypermobility, mild skin hyperextensibility, severe scoliosis, frequent ocular rupture and retinal detachment
EDS VII (Arthrochalasis multiplex congenita)	Autosomal recessive	Short stature, severe joint laxity with multiple congenital dislocations, moderate skin hyperextensibility and bruising
EDS VIII (Periodontosis type)	Autosomal recessive	Mild-moderate joint laxity, severe skin fragility, severe periodontitis with early tooth loss
EDS IX (X-linked skeletal)	X-linked recessive	Widening and bowing of multiple long bones at site of tendon and ligament insertion
EDS X	?Autosomal dominant	Severe scoliosis, severe hernias, mild joint hypermobility, periodontitis, aortic rupture

by cultured fibroblasts seemed normal but tissues were grossly Type III deficient. Some of the Type III secreted by the cells ran more slowly than normal on polyacrylamide gels and was unusually susceptible to proteolytic enzymes. The slow migrating $\alpha 1(III)$ chain appeared to have an insertion of some 18–20 amino acid residues in the helical region of the molecule. Type III collagen molecules containing mutant chains were not incorporated into fibres.

It can be seen from these few studies that the molecular pathology of

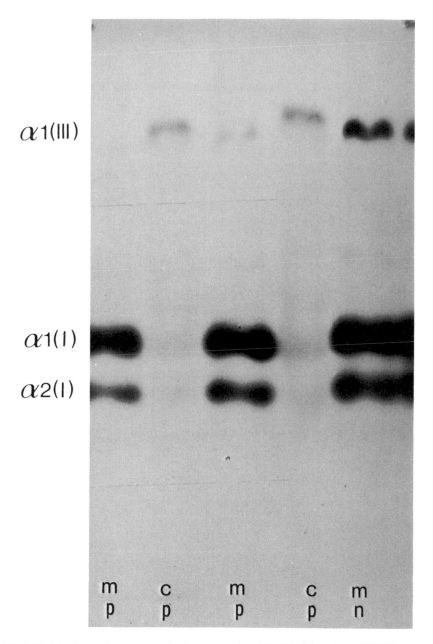

Fig. 8.12 Gel electrophoretogram of collagens produced by fibroblasts from EDS IV patients. Note that the medium (m) from the patients (p) shows virtually no α1(III) chains compared to the control (n). The patient's cells (c) however show significant amounts of Type III collagen accumulating intracellularly.

Type III collagen in EDS IV may be as complex as that of Type I collagen in osteogenesis imperfecta. Unfortunately progress in understanding the biochemical basis of EDS IV has been slower than that for osteogenesis imperfecta because fibroblasts make much smaller quantities of Type III collagen than Type I collagen. It is to be hoped that the application of recombinant DNA technology will facilitate these studies in the future.

Ehlers-Danlos Syndrome Type V (McKusick 30520)

Type V EDS is an X-linked form of the disease where the biochemistry remains unclear. It was initially reported as a deficiency of the crosslinking enzyme lysyl oxidase. However studies of other patients with this form of the disease have revealed normal crosslinking and crosslinking enzyme.

Ehlers-Danlos Syndrome Type VI (McKusick 22540)

EDS VI was the first inherited connective tissue disease to have the biochemical abnormality identified. The disease is typified by marked hyperextensibility of the skin and joint laxity accompanied by severe scoliosis. Analysis of tissues showed a marked diminution of the hydroxylysine content[31] which had a serious effect on the intermolecular crosslinking. The low level of hydroxylysine was caused by a deficiency in the enzyme lysyl hydroxylase. Two forms of enzyme abnormality have been identified. In one the enzyme has an altered affinity for the ascorbate cofactor and a lower thermal stability, in the other normal enzyme is produced in reduced amounts. An interesting observation in these patients was that the degree of underhydroxylation varied with the tissue. In most cases the skin had virtually no hydroxylysine, the tendon and bones were less severely affected but the cartilage was totally unaffected. Each collagen type in a tissue is affected in a similar manner except, possibly, Type IV collagen. The differential effects on tissues and collagen types suggests the existence of tissue or collagen specific isoenzymes of lysyl hydroxylase, but none have yet been identified.

In one family there was a curious discrepancy between the level of lysyl hydroxylation and enzyme activity. While the degree of lysyl hydroxylation in the skin was only moderately depressed the enzyme activity measured in skin fibroblast cultures was only 10–15% of controls.

Ehlers-Danlos Syndrome Type VII (McKusick 22541)

Patients with EDS VII show extreme joint laxity, bilateral hip dislocation and short stature. Skin and tendon from these patients contain appreciable amounts of incompletely processed procollagen. This was originally attributed to a defect in the peptidase which cleaves the N-terminal propeptide.

A subsequent re-examination of one patient has indicated that a structural mutation near the propeptide cleavage site in one of the $\alpha2(I)$ alleles makes it resistant to the enzyme. This observation suggests that this was a new dominant form and that EDS VII may be clinically and biochemically heterogeneous.

In humans the effects of this disease on the ultrastructure of the collagenous tissues is relatively mild but there is a variety in cattle and sheep called dermatosporaxis where skin fragility is extreme. In these animals there is a total absence of N-propeptidase activity leading to an accumulation of collagen molecules with persistent N-propeptides (pN-collagen) in the skin. This has a dramatic effect on fibril formation (Fig. 8.13) and on the intermolecular crosslinking.

Other Ehlers-Danlos Syndromes

The biochemical lesions in the remaining forms of the Ehlers-Danlos Syndrome have not been identified although there is ultrastructural evidence for abnormalities in collagen fibrillogenesis in many of them.

The Marfan Syndrome (McKusick 154700)

This syndrome like the others is a heterogeneous group of diseases which share the common features of skeletal, cardiovascular and ocular abnormalities. The typical Marfan is tall with long arms, hands and feet (arachnodactyly), pectus deformities of the chest, scoliosis, cardiac valve deficiency, myopia and lens dislocation. The disease is life threatening as dilatation of the aortic root and aortic aneurisms are common and can rupture catastrophically.

Some clinical features of this syndrome are similar to those in lathyrism the disease induced by β-aminopropionitrile. This reagent irreversibly inhibits the enzyme lysyl oxidase and prevents intermolecular crosslinking of collagens. Initial biochemical investigations of the Marfan syndrome showed an increased extractability of collagen compatible with a crosslinking defect but no specific abnormality was identified. More recent evidence has suggested that the crosslinking defect may be secondary to a structural abnormality of the collagen. The amounts of identifiable crosslinks were reduced in skin and aorta of patients but the aldehyde precursor was present, indicating normal lysyl oxidase activity. In one study the aorta of a patient contained reduced amounts of Type I collagen but skin fibroblasts from the same individual produced normal amounts of Type I collagen. This could be explained by a structural mutation of the $\alpha1(I)$ or $\alpha2(I)$ chains that did not inhibit synthesis or secretion but would not allow incorporation of the molecule into a fibre. Analysis of aortic tissue and skin fibroblasts from another patient resolved two forms of the $\alpha2(I)$ chain. One

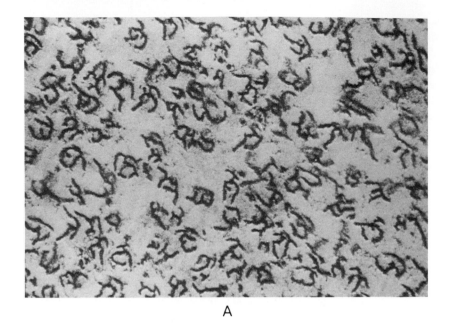

A

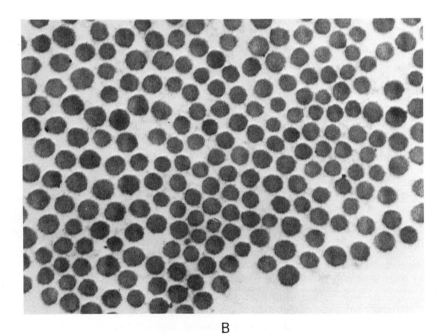

B

Fig. 8.13 Electron micrograph of the collagen fibrils in the skin of a dermatosporactic calf (A). Note the disorganization of the fibrils compared to those of normal skin (B). Photographs courtesy of Dr. P. Fryer, Clinical Research Centre, Harrow.

was normal but the other contained an additional 20–25 residues in the helical domain. The increased length of the mutant molecule seems to have caused a misalignment of crosslinking sites because tissue collagen was highly extractable. Cloning and sequencing of the α2(I) genes in this patient have revealed a 38 bp insertion. Strangely this insertion did not occur within a normal exon nor did it interfere with normal splice sites, so it is debatable whether this is the causal mutation.

Cutis laxa

Cutis laxa is yet another clinically and genetically heterogeneous group of disorders. It can be autosomal dominant (McKusick 12370 and 12380), autosomal recessive (McKusick 21910 and 21920) or X-linked recessive (McKusick 30415). The most obvious clinical feature is lax skin but hernias, emphysema with associated heart disease, gastrointestinal and genitourinary diverticulae are also seen. The recessive form is often fatal in infancy but the X-linked and dominantly inherited forms are less severe.

The affected boys in one family presenting with the X-linked form of the disease were found to have a lower activity of the enzyme lysyl oxidase and reduced immunoreactive protein. Collagen crosslink precursors and reducible crosslinks were decreased and tissue collagen extractability was increased. The serum levels of copper and ceruplasmin were below normal in these patients and since lysyl oxidase is a copper requiring enzyme the low activity may be secondary to the abnormal copper metabolism.

A similar disease is associated with the X-linked *Mottled* locus in mice. All males have a reduced life expectancy, some die in utero, the others— e.g. the Blotchy—die early, frequently as a result of blood vessel rupture. Tissue solubility and crosslink analysis revealed a reduced level of intermolecular crosslinking associated with a decreased lysyl oxidase activity. However serum copper levels were again abnormally low in these animals so the observed affect on enzyme activity may be a secondary phenomenon.

In a male patient with indeterminate inheritance of cutis laxa an over production of a protein with a molecular weight of 140 kilodaltons was identified in skin fibroblasts. This protein was chemically and immunologically related to GP140 and Type VI collagen (see above) suggesting that some forms of this disease may be due to abnormalities of this recently characterized protein.

Epidermolysis bullosa

Epidermolysis bullosa is a group of genetic diseases characterized by the formation of blisters following minimal trauma of the skin. The different types are distinguished by the site of cleavage within the skin. In some forms cleavage occurs along the basement membrane at the dermal/epidermal junction. Some studies on the most severe type, recessive dystrophic epidermolysis bullosa (McKusick 22660), observed an increase in collagenase (a proteolytic enzyme which specifically cleaves interstitial collagen molecules within the triple-helical region) both as enzyme activity and immunoreactive protein. There was evidence that this was a mutant enzyme.

More recent studies have implicated an abnormality of the basement membrane itself or the basement membrane/dermal junction. A specific basement membrane component was absent in the recessive dystrophic epidermolysis bullosa and reduced in the dominant form (McKusick 13170). This component, detected by a monoclonal antibody, was not identified although several types of collagen (including Type IV) were excluded. Other investigators demonstrated an absence or abnormality of anchoring fibrils in this disease. Since it has been suggested that Type VII collagen is a major component of anchoring fibrils this may perhaps be the defective molecule.

Miscellaneous diseases

Convincing evidence of the critical importance of collagen in normal embryonic development has been provided by recent studies of an artificially induced embryonic lethal mutation in mice. When early mouse embryos were infected with murine leukaemia retrovirus, viral DNA became stably integrated into the genome and mutant strains were bred from animals carrying the insertion. One mutant strain, Mov-13, was a recessive embryonic lethal, with homozygous embryos dying on the 13th day of gestation. In Mov-13 a single copy of the viral DNA had been integrated into the first intron of the $\alpha 1(I)$ collagen gene. The insertion altered the surrounding chromatin structure and blocked transcription of the $\alpha 1(I)$ mRNA hence no Type I collagen was produced. In normal embryos Type I collagen mRNA accumulation and protein synthesis was first detected on day 12. Post-mortems showed that homozygous Mov-13 embryos died from rupture of major blood vessels. Curiously heterozygous embryos, capable of producing only half-normal amounts of $\alpha 1(I)$ mRNA, appeared to suffer no ill-effects. This is contrary to our experience with the human condition where half-normal synthesis of Type I collagen results in Type I osteogenesis imperfecta.

CONCLUSION

Abnormalities in one or other of the collagen proteins or their biosynthesis are the cause of a large number of inherited diseases of connective tissues. So far only a few cases involving mutations in the major interstitial collagens, Types I and III, have been precisely characterized but they have provided a fascinating insight into the structure-function relationships of various domains of the collagen molecule or of a particular collagen type. The mutant map for the Type I collagen molecule is shown in Figure 8.14. One interesting feature is the way mutations in different parts of the molecule are expressed in such different phenotypes as the brittle bones of OI, the lax joints of EDS VII or the fragile blood vessels of the Marfan Syndrome and Mov-13 mouse. The types of abnormality that have been identified suggest that, as in the thalassemias and haemoglobinopathies, the range of mutations in the collagen genes will include major or minor deletions of the gene, RNA transcription or processing defects and a host of single base changes giving amino acid substitutions. Further abnormalities need to be characterized by protein chemistry and recombinant DNA techniques to allow the development of a biochemical classification of this remarkably heterogeneous group of diseases for the benefit of the clinical geneticist and patient.

Direct biochemical investigations of individual patients or families may be too complex and time consuming to provide a viable means of prenatal diagnosis especially as collagen types and post-translational modification vary during fetal development. An alternative approach to identifying the abnormal gene without needing to know the specific biochemical defect is to demonstrate linkage of the disease with a DNA variation known as a restriction fragment length polymorphism (RFLP). RFLPs arise because the natural variation of DNA sequences within the population sometimes causes changes in sites susceptible to a particular restriction endonuclease. Thus if a restriction site is created or destroyed in or around the gene of interest, enzyme digests of total DNA will give fragments differing in size

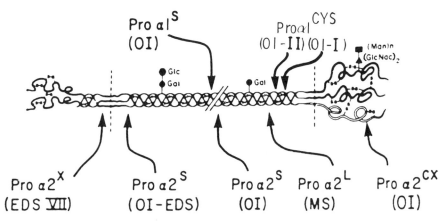

Fig. 8.14 The Type I procollagen molecule showing sites of mutations mapped to date. OI = osteogenesis imperfecta, MS = Marfan Syndrome, EDS = Ehlers-Danlos Syndrome (modified from Prockop D J, Kivirikko K I 1984 New England Journal of Medicine 311: 376–386).

from the norm when hybridized with a radioactive probe complementary to that gene (Fig. 8.15). If one or more polymorphisms for a gene can be shown to segregate with the disease in a particular family then it is highly probable that a mutation in the polymorphic gene is the cause of the disease in that family. Unfortunately restriction fragment length polymorphisms are quite rare in the collagen genes studied to date (Table 8.6). No restriction enzyme generating a RFLP has been found for the $\alpha1(I)$ gene. Only five polymorphisms have been identified for the $\alpha2(I)$ gene, two (Eco RI and Rsa I) have been used to show linkage to dominant OI in some families (Fig. 8.15) and one (MspI) has excluded defects in the $\alpha2(I)$ gene in other kindreds.[32,33] If such an approach can be developed for the collagen genes it will greatly facilitate prenatal diagnosis as fetal genotyping can be performed during the first trimester of pregnancy, but it does require quite extensive family studies. Perhaps a combination of biochemistry and molecular biology will provide the ideal approach.

Table 8.6 Restriction fragment length polymorphisms (RFLP) assocciated with collagen genes

| Gene | Enzyme | RFLP sizes (kb) | |
		+/+	−/−
$\alpha1(I)$	None		
$\alpha2(I)$	MspI	0.5, 1.6	2.1
	Eco RI (i)	3.5, 10.5	14.0
	Eco RI (ii)	2.8, 1.5	4.3
	Rsa I	7.0, 7.0	14.0
	Bgl II	0.7, 2.2	2.9
$\alpha1(II)$	Hind III	7.0, 7.0	14.0
	Pvu II	1.7, 1.6	3.3
$\alpha1(III)$	Ava II	1.7, 4.5	6.2

Whatever the approach there is still a lot to be done. A large number of diseases have not had the molecular pathology identified. Some of these may involve the more recently discovered collagens so further characterization of these minority proteins is required. So too is the isolation and identification of the genes for the remaining collagen chains and an expansion in the range of DNA probes available for the more common collagens. This is a very active area of research and hopefully in a few years time it will be possible to describe the molecular abnormalities of the collagen family more completely.

Fig. 8.15 (A) Southern blot analysis of genomic DNA cut with the restriction enzyme Eco RI and probed with an $\alpha2(I)$ gene clone showing a polymorphic variation giving rise to 14 kb or 10.5 kb fragments. (B) Pedigree showing segregation of this Eco RI $\alpha2(I)$ gene polymorphism (+) with the disease in a family with type I OI. Reproduced from Tsipouras P, Myers J C, Ramirez F, Prockop D J 1983 Journal of Clinical Investigation 72: 1262–1267).

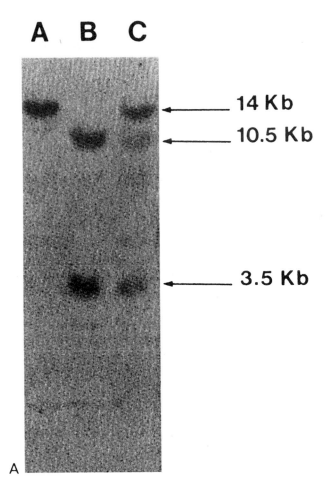

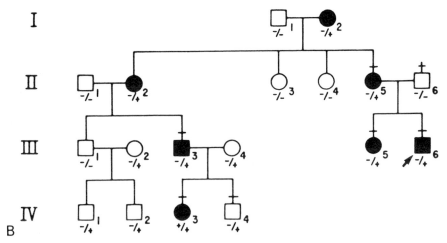

REFERENCES

1 Hay E D 1984 In: Trelsted R L ed. Role of the extracellular matrix in development, Alan R Liss, New York, p 1–31
2 Miller E J, Matukas V J 1969 Chick cartilage collagen: A new type of α1 chain not present in bone or skin of the species. Proceedings of the National Academy of Sciences USA 64: 1264–1268
3 Chung E, Miller E J 1974 Collagen polymorphism: characterization of molecules with the chain composition [α1(III)]₃ in human tissues. Science 183 1200–1201
4 Epstein E H 1974 [α1(III)]₃ Human skin collagen: release by pepsin and preponderance in foetal life. Journal of Biological Chemistry 249: 3225–3231
5 Traub W, Piez K A 1971 The chemistry and structure of collagen. Advances in Protein Chemistry 25: 243–352
6 Timpl R, Wiedemann H, Van Delden V, Furthmayr H, Kühn K 1981 A network model for the organization of Type IV collagen molecules in basement membranes. European Journal of Biochemistry 120: 203–211
7 Burgeson R E, El Adli F A, Kaitila I I, Hollister D W 1976 Foetal membrane collagens: identification of two new collagen α chains. Proceedings of the National Academy of Sciences USA 73: 2579–2583
8 Von Der Mark H, Aumailley M, Wick G, Fleischmajer R, Timpl R 1984 Immunochemistry, genuine size and tissue localization of collagen VI. European Journal of Biochemistry 142: 493–502
9 Furthmayr H, Wiedemann H, Timpl R, Odermatt E, Engel J 1983 Electron microscopical approach to a structural model of intima collagen. Biochemical Journal 211: 303–311
10 Heller-Harrison R, Carter W G 1984 Pepsin Type VI collagen is a degradation product of GP140. Journal of Biological Chemistry 259: 6858–6864
11 Knight K R, Ayad S, Shuttleworth C A, Grant M E 1984 A collagenous glycoprotein found in dissociative extracts of foetal bovine nuchal ligament: evidence for a relationship with Type VI collagen. Biochemical Journal 220: 395–403
12 Jander R, Troyer D, Rauterberg J 1984 A collagen-like glycoprotein of the extracellular matrix is the undegraded form of Type VI collagen. Biochemistry 23: 3675–3681
13 Bentz H, Morris N P, Murray L W, Sakai L Y, Hollister D W, Burgeson R E 1983 Isolation and partial characterization of a new human collagen with an extended triple-helical structural domain. Proceedings of the National Academy of Sciences USA 80: 3168–3172
14 Sage H, Trüeb B, Bornstein P 1983 Biosynthetic and structural properties of endothelial cell Type VIII collagen. Journal of Biological Chemistry 258: 3391–3401
15 Van der Rest M, Mayne R, Ninomiya Y, Seidah N G, Chretien M, Olsen B R 1985 The structure of the Type IX collagen. Journal of Biological Chemistry 260: 220–225
16 Vaugh L, Winterhalter K H, Bruckner P 1985 Proteoglycan Lt from chicken embryo sternum identified as Type IX collagen. Journal of Biological Chemistry 260: 4758–4763
17 Schmid T M, Mayne R, Bruns R R, Linsenmayer T F 1984 Molecular structure of short chain (SC) cartilage collagen by electron microscopy. Journal of Ultrastructural Research 86: 186–191
18 Burgeson R E, Hebda P A, Morris N P, Hollister D W 1982 Human cartilage collagens: comparison of cartilage collagens with human type collagen. Journal of Biological Chemistry 257: 7852–7856
19 Fessler J H, Fessler L I 1978 Biosynthesis of procollagen. Annual Reviews of Biochemistry 47: 129–162
20 Yamada Y, Kühn K, de Crombrugghe B 1983 A conserved nucleotide sequence coding for a segment of the C-propeptide is found at the same location in different collagen genes. Nucleic Acids Research 11: 2733–2744
21 Boedtker H, Fuller F, Tate V 1983 The structure of collagen genes. International Review of Connective Tissue 10: 1–63
22 Lozano G, Ninomiya Y, Thompson H, Olsen B R 1985 A distinct class of vertebrate collagen genes encodes chicken Type IX collagen polypeptides. Proceedings of the National Academy of Sciences USA 82: 4050–4054
23 McKusick V A 1972 Heritable disorders of connective tissue, 4th ed. CV Mosby, St. Louis

24 Sillence D O, Senn A, Danks D M 1979 Genetic heterogeneity in osteogenesis imperfecta. Journal of Medical Genetics 16: 101–116

25 Penttinen R P, Lichtenstein J R, Martin G R, McKusick V A 1975 Abnormal collagen metabolism in cultured cells in osteogenesis imperfecta. Proceedings of the National Academy of Sciences USA 72: 586–589

26 Barsh G S, Byers P H, 1981 Reduced secretion of structurally abnormal Type I procollagen in a form of osteogenesis imperfecta. Proceedings of the National Academy of Science USA 78: 5142–5146

27 Williams C J, Prockop D J 1983 Synthesis and processing of a Type I procollagen containing shortened proα1(I) chains by fibroblasts from a patient with osteogenesis imperfecta. Journal of Biological Chemistry 258: 5915–5921

28 Bonadio J, Byers P H 1985 Subtle structural alterations in the chains of Type I procollagen produce osteogenesis imperfecta Type II. Nature 316: 363–366

29 Pihlajaniemi T, Dickson L A, Pope F M, Korhonen V R, Nicholls A, Prockop D J, Myers J C 1984 Osteogenesis imperfecta: cloning of a proα2(I) collagen gene with a frame shift mutation. Journal of Biological Chemistry 259: 12941–12944

30 Pope F M, Martin G R, Lichtenstein J R, Penttinen R, Gerson B, Rowe D W, McKusick V A 1975 Patients with Ehlers-Danlos Syndrome Type IV lack Type III collagen. Proceedings of the National Academy of Science USA 72: 1314–1316

31 Pinnell S R, Krane S M, Kenzora J E, Glimcher M J 1972 A heritable disorder of connective tissue. Hydroxylysine deficient collagen disease. New England Journal of Medicine 286: 1013–1020

32 Tsipouras P, Myers J C, Ramirez F, Prockop D J 1983 Restriction fragment length polymorphism associated with the proα2(I) gene of human Type I procollagen. Application to a family with an autosomal dominant form of osteogenesis imperfecta. Journal of Clinical Investigation 72: 1262–1267

33 Grobler-Rabie A F, Wallis G, Brebuer D K, Beighton P, Bester A J and Matthew C G 1985 Detection of a high frequency Rsa I polymorphism in the human proα2(I) collagen gene which is linked to an autosomal dominant form of osteogenesis imperfecta. EMBO Journal 4: 1745–1748

Inherited disorders of steroid biosynthesis

INTRODUCTION

The inherited diseases of steroid hormone biosynthesis constitute a large and important group of the inherited metabolic disorders. Biosynthesis of steroid hormones takes place in the adrenal cortex, gonads and placenta: other tissues are involved, however, in both the production of some active steroid metabolites, e.g. dihydrotestosterone from testosterone in the skin, and in the biochemical inactivation, degradation and excretion of the steroids. Inherited disorders of both steroid synthesis and peripheral metabolism have been described.

Physiologically, steroid hormones are divided into three groups, with glucocorticoid, mineralocorticoid or sex hormone activity, each with specific actions, control, etc., though this distinction is by no means absolute. Inherited diseases resulting in impaired steroid biosynthesis are caused by the absence or altered properties of one of the enzymes in the biosynthetic pathways. As a result there is an accumulation of precursor molecules and often increased activity in alternative pathways of steroid metabolism. The biological activity of the precursor molecules, the increased synthesis of other steroids and the antagonism that can occur between different steroids produce a complex situation in which, for example, a primary defect in the synthesis of cortisol can present clinically as a disturbance of sexual differentiation.

A complete understanding of the clinical and pathological aspects of inborn errors of steroid biosynthesis requires a comprehensive knowledge of the anatomy, biochemistry and physiology of steroid hormone metabolism in fetal and postnatal life and also of the process of sexual differentiation. Because steroid hormones are involved in the sexual development of the fetus disorders of steroid synthesis frequently give rise to abnormal sexual development. Detailed reviews have been published elsewhere;[1,2,3,4,5] for the purposes of this chapter only an essential outline will be given. Emphasis will be given to the adrenal cortex since this gland is involved in the synthesis of all three types of steroid and is the major organ involved in inherited disorders of steroid biosynthesis.

THE ADRENAL CORTEX

The adrenal cortex develops from mesodermal tissue beginning in the sixth week of life. By the twentieth week there are two distinct zones; an inner fetal zone which constitutes the bulk of the gland and a thin subcapsular zone of small lipid containing cells termed the adult zone. The adult zone increases in size throughout the remainder of pregnancy and constitutes about 20% of the gland at birth. Postnatally the fetal cortex rapidly degenerates. The steroid biosynthetic activity of the fetal adrenal varies throughout pregnancy but one important function is as an integral part of the fetoplacental unit in the synthesis of oestriol (see later).

During the immediate post natal period there are considerable structural and biochemical changes. The adrenal develops the classical three zones, the glomerulosa, fasciculata and reticularis. In the infant the glomerulosa is a continuous subcapsular band but in the adult it is usually broken up into discrete islets. The glomerulosa is the site of synthesis of aldosterone while the glucocorticoid and adrenal sex steroid hormones are synthesized in the fasciculata and the reticularis.

The blood supply to the adrenal is complex: three separate arteries join to form a subcapsular plexus from which a few twigs go direct to the adrenal medulla. Capillaries pass downwards through the fasciculata into a capillary network in the reticularis which drains in turn into a single central adrenal vein. It has been suggested that this vascular arrangement has some function in controlling steroid biosynthesis and, in particular, the synthesis of androgens in the reticularis.[6,7]

STEROID STRUCTURE

All naturally occurring steroids are based on a 4 ring structure, the cyclopentanoperhydrophenanthrene nucleus (Fig. 9.1) and its derivatives, of which the largest is cholestane. The numbering of the carbon atoms of the steroid nucleus is particularly important since the enzymes of steroid metabolism are in part identified by these numbers e.g. 21-hydroxylase. Hydroxyl

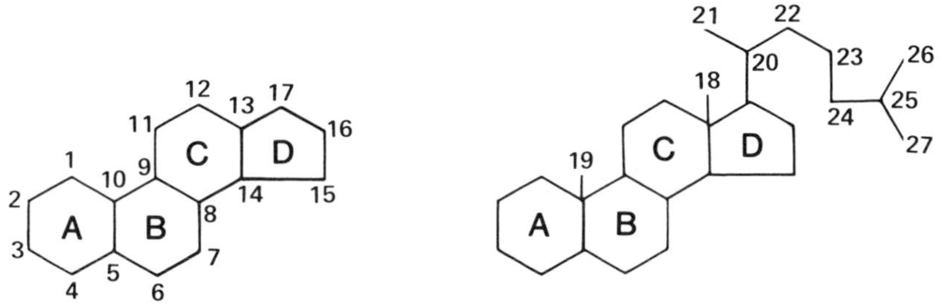

Cyclopentanoperhydrophenanthrene   Cholestane

Fig. 9.1 The steroid nucleus, showing numbering of the carbon atoms.

or other substituents can be orientated towards the reader (α) or away (β). Isomers can occur which radically alter the three dimensional structure of the steroids and therefore their biological activity.

Steroid nomenclature (IUPAC)[8] is complicated and is based on the various parent nuclei, cholestane (C27), pregnane (C21), androstane (C19) and oestrane (C18). For general purposes the standard IUPAC names are abbreviated. Systematic and abbreviated names of the most important steroids are listed in Table 9.1

Table 9.1 Steroid nomenclature

Common name	IUPAC Nomenclature
Cholesterol	cholest-5-en-3β-ol
Pregnenolone	3β-hydroxypregn-5-en-20-one
Progesterone	pregn-4-ene-3,20-dione
17-hydroxypregnenolone	3β,17α-dihydroxypregn-5-en-20-one
17-hydroxyprogesterone	17α-hydroxypregn-4-ene-3,20-dione
11-deoxycortisol	17α,21-dihydroxypregn-4-ene-3,20-dione
11-deoxycorticosterone (DOC)	21-hydroxypregn-4-ene-3,20-dione
Corticosterone	11β,21-dihydroxypregn-4-ene-3,20-dione
Cortisol	11β,17,21-trihydroxypregn-4-ene-3,20-dione
18-hydroxycorticosterone	11β, 18,21-trihydroxypregn-4-ene-3,20-dione
Aldosterone	11β,21-dihydroxy-18-al-pregn-4-ene-3,20-dione
Dehydroepiandrosterone (DHA)	3β-hydroxyandrost-5-en-17-one
Androstenedione	androst-4-ene-3,17 dione
Testosterone	17β-hydroxyandrost-4-en-3-one
Dihydrotestosterone (DHT)	17β-hydroxy-5α-androstan-3-one
Oestrone	3-hydroxyoestra-1,3,5(10)-trien-17-one
Oestradiol	oestra-1,3,5(10)-triene-3,17-βdiol

STEROID HORMONE BIOSYNTHESIS

A generalised pathway of the synthesis of steroid hormones is shown in Fig. 9.2. Not all cells synthesising steroids will have all the enzyme activities of this pathway thus limiting the individual steroids they can produce, e.g. the zona glomerulosa lacks 17-hydroxylase and cannot synthesize cortisol, while the zona fasciculata and reticularis lack the enzyme which catalyses the final step in the synthesis of aldosterone. A deficiency of a specific enzyme in the steroid biosynthetic pathway will manifest itself in all tissues possessing that enzyme. However, there is increasing evidence for the existence of isoenzymes in different or even the same organs, each with a specificity for one particular group of steroids e.g. 11β-hydroxylase, 3β-hydroxysteroid dehydrogenase (3β-HSD) and possibly 21-hydroxylase. The existence of such isoenzymes is one possible explanation for the clinical heterogeneity of many of the disorders of steroid biosynthesis.

The classical pathways shown in Figure 9.2 are of course idealised and

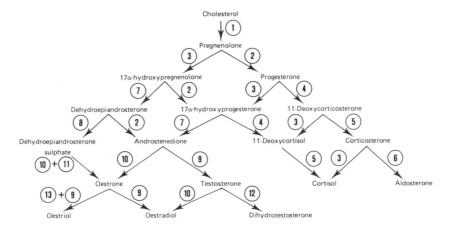

Fig. 9.2 An integrated summary of the synthesis of glucocorticoid, mineralocorticoid and sex steroid hormones. The enzymes catalysing each step are: 1–20,22-desmolase (complex); 2–3β-hydroxysteroid dehydrogenase; 3–17α-hydroxylase; 4–21-hydroxylase; 5–11β-hydroxylase; 6-corticosterone methyl oxidase; (18-hydroxylase and 18-dehydrogenase); 7–17, 20-desmolase; 8–steroid sulphotransferase; 9–17β-hydroxysteroid dehydrogenase; 10-aromatase; 11-steroid sulphatase; 12–5α-reductase; 13–16α-hydroxylase.

there exist alternative enzymes and possible routes for the biosynthesis of individual steroids. The role of these other pathways is unclear in the normal human and their activity is usually very low. Activity of the alternative metabolic pathways can be considerably increased in pathological conditions and this accounts for many of the unusual steroids produced in the inborn errors of steroid metabolism.

Steroids are synthesised from cholesterol which is usually exogenous; alternatively cholesterol can be synthesized 'de novo' from acetate. Cholesterol is converted to pregnenolone by the enzyme 20,22-desmolase (probably a complex of enzymes) with the loss of a 6-carbon side chain. The action of various hydroxylases, dehydrogenases (reductases), 17, 20 desmolase and A-ring aromatase converts pregnenolone to the active steroid hormones. Many of the enzymes in the steroid biosynthetic pathway are cytochromes P-450.[3]

The synthesis of cortisol can proceed along two pathways. In the $\triangle^4$-pathway pregnenolone is first converted to progesterone by the action of 3β-HSD and then to 17α-hydroxyprogesterone (17OHP). In the alternate $\triangle^5$-pathway the steps are reversed with 17α-hydroxypregnenolone being formed first and then being converted to 17OHP. The $\triangle^5$-pathway possibly predominates in humans. Further hydroxylation at positions 21 and 11 produce cortisol.

Aldosterone synthesis, which occurs exclusively in the zona glomerulosa, proceeds along the $\triangle^4$-pathway to progesterone and 11-deoxycorticosterone; the hydroxylation at position 21 prevents any action of 17-hydroxylase. Following 11-hydroxylation the C18 methyl group is converted to an aldehyde in a two step procedure. The first step is 18-hydroxylation to form 18-hydroxycorticosterone; the second step is possibly a dehydrogenase, or alternatively a second hydroxylation and spontaneous or enzymatic dehydration. Only the second step is exclusive to the zona glomerulosa,[9] 18-hydroxycorticosterone can be produced in the zona reticularis and fasciculata.

The major pathway of androgen biosynthesis is via the $\triangle^4$-pathway to 17α-hydroxypregnenolone which is converted to dehydroepiandrosterone (DHA) by 17,20-desmolase (C21 → C19). Testosterone is produced from DHA by the action of 3β-HSD and 17α-hydroxysteroid dehydrogenase. Conversion of testosterone to dihydrotestosterone (DHT) occurs in the testis and also peripherally, the latter accounting for a substantial percentage of circulating DHT in the adult male. The conversion of testosterone to DHT is essential for androgenic activity in certain tissues.

Oestrogen synthesis has a unique step in which the A ring is aromatised and the C19 carbon is lost (C19 → C18). The reaction requires molecular oxygen, NADPH and three sequential hydroxylations, the first two being on the C19 methyl group and the third at C2. Androstenedione and testosterone are converted to oestrone and oestradiol respectively.

Control of steroid biosynthesis

The main regulator of adrenal glucocorticoid and sex hormone biosynthesis is ACTH which acts early in the biosynthetic pathway at the conversion of cholesterol to pregnenolone. A separate adrenal androgen stimulating hormone has been postulated but there is little evidence to support this hypothesis.[6] ACTH can be detected in the fetus by the twelfth week of life and plays a critical role in the development of the adrenal cortex. The regulation of ACTH release is complex and the principal points are shown in Figure 9.3. Secretion of ACTH shows a circadian rhythm with high levels of ACTH (and cortisol) secretion during the early morning which then falls gradually throughout the day. Circadian rhythm is established within the first few weeks and months after birth.[10] ACTH secretion is in turn controlled by the release of corticotrophin releasing factor (CRF) produced in the hypothalamus. CRF release is influenced by many different factors of which stress is a component and which will overide circadian rhythm and other inhibitors of ACTH release.

It has been proposed that the mass of the individual adrenal zones and in particular their width is involved in the control of steroid biosynthesis.[7] This control mechanism relies on the vascular arrangement of the adrenal which can allow the establishment of a metabolic gradient, particularly of steroids, and on the fact that the adrenal cell is pluripotential. Evidence from the study of adrenal cell division and death, and from cell culture

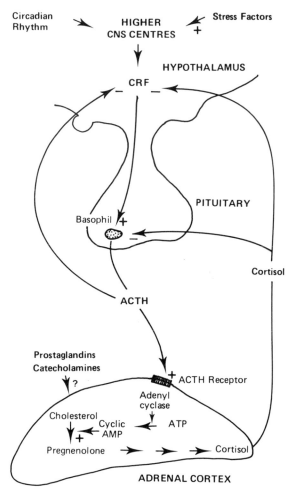

Fig. 9.3 Diagrammatic representation of the major control mechanisms of cortisol biosynthesis.

experiments, suggests that cells produced in the zona glomerulosa migrate as they age through the fasciculata to the reticularis. During this migration they will synthesise in turn mineralocorticoid, glucocorticoid and adrenal androgen, depending on the influence of the immediate environment. There is also a possibility that the adrenal medulla and the adrenergic nervous system may play a role in the control of steroid biosynthesis.[11]

Cortisol has a classical feedback role on ACTH release; an increase in plasma cortisol concentration will rapidly cause a fall in ACTH secretion. In those inborn errors of steroid metabolism which reduce cortisol synthesis, this feedback control mechanism is activated, ACTH secretion is increased and its secretion becomes continuous. This gives rise to glandular hyperplasia and to increased synthesis of cortisol precursors and other metabolites. The glandular hyperplasia occurs in utero and patients with these disorders have congenital adrenal hyperplasia (CAH) but not all steroid biosynthetic defects give rise to CAH. The signs and symptoms of patients with CAH are produced by the lack of cortisol and by other steroid metabolites which can affect sexual differentiation in utero if they are androgenic. Maternal ACTH will not cross the placenta but maternal corticosteroid will do so, though in insufficient quantity to effectively reduce ACTH secretion in fetuses with CAH.

The three major factors involved in the control of aldosterone secretion are sodium, potassium and the renin-angiotensin system (Fig. 9.4). The role of ACTH remains controversial in normals, but it is probably of minor importance, while cathecholamines, prostaglandins and serotonin may also regulate aldosterone secretion. ACTH may have a more important role in aldosterone regulation in patients with the salt losing types of CAH.[12] The

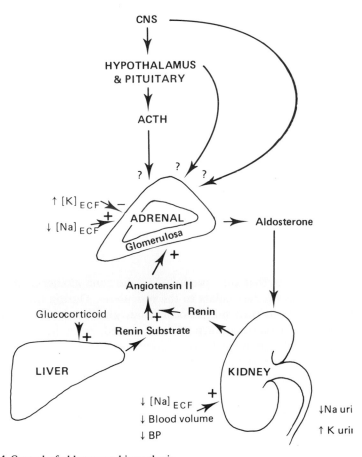

Fig. 9.4 Control of aldosterone biosynthesis.

relationship between aldosterone and the renin-angiotensin system is a negative feedback loop; a fall in aldosterone giving rise to sodium loss and hence
a release of renin from the kidney and production of angiotensin II which
directly stimulates the cells of the zona glomerulosa to synthesise aldosterone. This feedback mechanism is very sensitive and disorders of steroid
biosynthesis which give rise to a loss of body sodium will be accompanied
by high renin levels.

THE FETO-PLACENTAL UNIT (Fig. 9.5)

In the pregnant state the oestrogens, oestrone, oestradiol and particularly
oestriol, are produced in large quantities; the pathway of oestriol synthesis
is different than in the adult adrenal or ovary. The fetus is deficient in 3β-
HSD and thus cannot convert pregnenolone to progesterone. The placenta
can carry out this conversion and supply progesterone to the fetal adrenal
which can metabolise it to DHA-sulphate. This in turn is returned to the
placenta where a sulphatase enzyme is present together with the enzymes
to convert DHA to oestrone and oestriol. The fetal liver is capable of
converting the DHA-sulphate to 16α-hydroxy-DHA-sulphate which can be
further metabolised in the placenta to oestriol. The contribution of maternal
adrenal gland to the feto-placental unit is not clear but DHA-sulphate from
the mother can also be metabolised in the placenta.

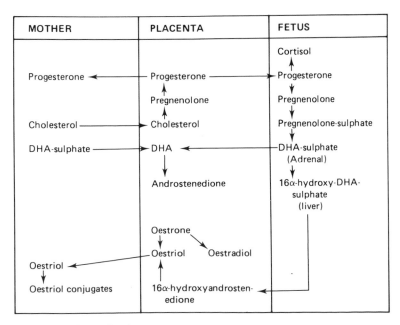

Fig. 9.5 The feto-placental unit

CATABOLISM AND EXCRETION OF STEROIDS

Steroids are catabolised mainly in the liver but additional metabolism of steroids can occur in other tissues.[13] There is some evidence that the adrenal gland itself may also be involved in the catabolism of some steroids, particularly oestrogens. The products of catabolism are excreted in the urine; some products of androgen and oestrogen catabolism are excreted in the bile and undergo enterohepatic circulation the significance of which is not known.

A number of steps are involved in steroid catabolism, these include reduction, oxidation, hydroxylation, side chain cleavage and conjugation usually to form glucuronides or sulphates. A large number of steroid metabolites are produced from one steroid hormone; the major metabolites of cortisol are shown in Table 9.2. Separation of these metabolites by chemical means is difficult and time consuming and they have been measured by techniques which measure groups of steroids with a particular chemical structure. More specific analysis with chromatographic techniques have essentially replaced measurement of oxo-, oxogenic and 17-hydroxy steroids in urine in the investigation of disorders of steroid biosynthesis, particularly as the chromatographic techniques allow identification of unusual steroids (see later).

Table 9.2   Major metabolites of cortisol in urine[15]

Metabolite	Average excretion (%)	
Cortisol	1.7	
Cortisone	1.7	
Tetrahydrocortisol	17.0	
Allotetrahydrocortisol	9.0	C21
Tetrahydrocortisone	27.5	
20 β-cortol	9.8	
20 α-cortolone	11.3	
20 β-cortolone	10.3	
11-oxoaetiocholanolone	3.1	
11 β-hydroxyaetiocholanolone	3.9	C19
11 β-hydroxyandrosterone	1.0	
Others	3.7	

NORMAL SEXUAL DEVELOPMENT IN UTERO (Fig. 9.6)

The differentiation of the primitive gonad is controlled by the presence of H-Y antigen a protein of between 16 500 and 18 000 daltons. The structural gene for H-Y antigen is on the Y chromosome; in its presence the fetal gonad develops into a testis and in its absence an ovary will develop. There is a considerable body of evidence that a controlling gene for H-Y synthesis is sited on the X chromosome.[14] Gonadal sex is irreversible by the eighth

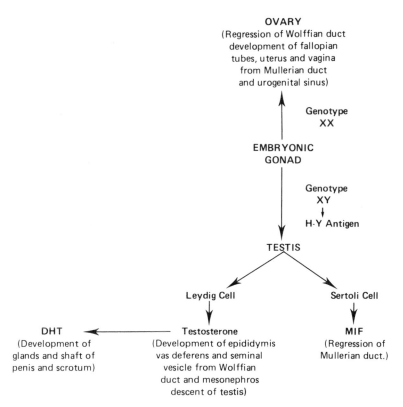

Fig. 9.6 The development and differentiation of the gonad and internal and external genitalia. MIF, Mullerian duct inhibiting factor; DHT, dihydrotestosterone.

week of pregnancy when the primitive gonads are capable of secreting sex hormones.

The internal genitalia are derived from the Mullerian and Wolffian ducts. This time critical process depends entirely on the presence of testosterone and the glycoprotein hormone Mullerian duct inhibiting factor (MIF) produced by the Leydig and Sertoli cells of the testis respectively. In the male fetus MIF causes degeneration of Mullerian structures and subsequently the Wolffian duct develops into the epididymis, vas deferens, seminal vesicles and ejaculating ducts under the influence of testosterone. This action of testosterone does not require its conversion to DHT. Female development occurs in the absence of MIF and testosterone. The major part of the Wolffian duct degenerates while the Mullerian structures become the fallopian tubes, uterus and upper part of the vagina.

The external genitalia develop from the genital tubercle, urethral fold and labioscrotal swelling. In the male these become the glans and shaft of the penis, urethra and scrotum. The process depends on testosterone but in this case conversion to DHT by 5α-reductase is essential for androgen action.

The DHT binds to a cytosolic receptor and is then transferred to the nucleus where it regulates the action of specific genes. The androgen cytosol receptors are X-linked.

The description of sexual differentiation given here is very simplified; the stages in development are complex and often time critical. The process can easily be disturbed by decreased or excessive production of androgenic steroids in utero, disorders of the peripheral metabolism of testosterone or absence of MIF.

LABORATORY INVESTIGATION OF INHERITED DISORDERS OF STEROID BIOSYNTHESIS

A deficiency of activity of any particular enzyme in the steroid pathway leads to a reduction in the formation of the end product of that pathway, accumulation of intermediates and increasing activity in the alternative pathways of metabolism of the precursors. The investigation of inherited disorders of steroid synthesis requires the measurement of the steroid hormones and/or their precursors and metabolites in urine and blood or both.[15] Response to therapy can also be monitored by the measurement of steroids in these same body fluids and also in saliva. Assay of specific enzymes is confined to the situation where tissue is readily available e.g. measurement of 5α-reductase or placental sulphatase in skin biopsy. Many of these assays are demanding technically and are best carried out in specialist laboratories.

Much of the early diagnosis and monitoring of inherited disorders of steroid biosynthesis relied on urine assays of steroid metabolites, especially the oxosteroids, 17-hydroxycorticosteroids and pregnanetriol as chemical techniques to measure specific steroids in blood were not generally available and lacked specificity. Analysis of steroids in urine has been considerably improved by the application of gas and liquid chromatography; the former can be coupled when required to mass spectroscopy.

Collection of urine is a non-invasive technique, potentially highly useful in paediatric practice but with a number of problems which limit its usefulness. Despite its seeming simplicity, 24 hour urine collections are frequently incorrectly performed even in hospital. Collections are particularly difficult in neonates when they may be complicated by the existence of abnormal genitalia. Episodic secretion, e.g. circadian rhythms, are masked by 24 hour urine collection and random collections may be misleading, depending on whether they include or exclude periods of excessive steroid excretion. Urine measurements in the first few days of life are further complicated by the major changes in adrenal function that are occurring at this time, which results in a highly variable pattern of steroid excretion and can give rise to both false positive and negative diagnoses. Urine spot tests such as the 11-oxygenation index, which rely on the ratio of different types of steroids, have not proved universally successful in overcoming this problem. Other factors which can influence measurements of steroids in urine include hepatic and renal function and drugs.

With the advent of ligand binding methods, i.e. competitive protein binding, and later radioimmunoassay which has now almost superseded it, the analysis of specific steroids in plasma, urine and other body fluids was brought within the capacity of many more laboratories. These assays lead to improvements in the understanding of the pathophysiology of disorders of steroid metabolism and in diagnosis and monitoring of therapy. However, production of antibodies with high specificity to steroid molecules is difficult; cross reaction with closely related precursors may cause significant errors and misdiagnoses. Furthermore, even with specific assays, problems arise in the neonatal period as patients with identical disorders can show considerable variations in plasma steroid concentrations and these can also change markedly in the first few weeks of life.[16] High concentrations of 17OHP have been found in sick premature infants without adrenal disease; these concentrations were comparable to those found in patients with 21-hydroxylase deficiency.

Dynamic tests of adrenal or gonadal function are sometimes helpful in establishing the diagnosis. ACTH stimulation is useful if the patient has already been treated with cortisol for urgent reasons and an HCG stimulation test can assist in the investigation of abnormalities of androgen synthesis and metabolism. Other investigations that may be required to clarify the diagnosis include chromosome analysis and radiology of the urogenital tract.

A summary of the patterns of steroids and their metabolites found in the plasma and urine of patients with inborn errors of steroid biosynthesis is given in Table 9.3.

CLINICAL PRESENTATION

Inherited disorders of steroid metabolism can present in a variety of different ways (Table 9.4) The majority of cases are diagnosed in the neonatal period, early infancy or at puberty but an increasing number of patients, particularly with 21-hydroxylase deficiency, are being diagnosed in adult life during investigation of female hirsutism or on the basis of HLA typing in affected families (see later). Occasional patients remain undiagnosed until very late in life. With increasing sophistication of diagnostic methods more patients are being described with presentations differing from the classical descriptions of these defects.

The signs and symptoms of the different disorders reflect both the reduction in the activity of the normal steroid hormones and the biological activity of the accumulated precursors and other steroids. These latter steroids are present in large quantities in those disorders in which a lack of cortisol production causes an increased release of ACTH due to absence of feedback inhibition. Thus the presentation of a defect late in the pathway

Table 9.3 ACTH, renin, steroid hormones and their metabolites in plasma and urine in the individual disorders of steroid biosynthesis

Deficient enzyme	Increased in urine	Decreased in urine	Increased in plasma	Decreased in plasma
20, 22-desmolase		Oxosteroids (Absent) Oxogenic/Steroids (Absent) Pregnanetriol	ACTH Renin	Cortisol Aldosterone Testosterone
3β- hydroxysteroid dehydrogenase	Oxosteroids Pregnenetriol		ACTH Renin 17α-hydroxypregnenolone Pregnenolone DHA	Steroids Aldosterone
17α-hydroxylase	Pregnenediol Pregnanetriol	Oxosteroids(±)	ACTH(±) Progesterone 11-deoxycorticosterone Corticosterone Pregnenolone	Renin 17-hydroxyprogesterone Cortisol Testosterone Aldosterone
21-hydroxylase	Oxosteroids Pregnanetriol Pregnanetriolone 17-hydroxypregnanolone		ACTH Renin 17α-hydroxyprogesterone 21-deoxycortisol DHA Androstenedione Testosterone	Renin(±)

Table 9.3 ACTH, renin, steroid hormones and their metabolites in plasma and urine in the individual disorders of steroid biosynthesis (*contd*)

Deficient enzyme	Increased in urine	Decreased in urine	Increased in plasma	Decreased in plasma
11β-hydroxylase	Oxosteroids Tetrahydro-11-deoxycortisol Tetrahydro-11-deoxycorticosterone		ACTH Renin 11-deoxycortisol 11-deoxycorticosterone Androstenedione Testosterone	
Corticosterone methyl oxidase Type I	Corticosterone metabolites	Tetrahydroaldosterone	Renin	Aldosterone
Corticosterone methyl oxidase Type II	Corticosterone metabolites Tetrahydro-11-dehydro-18-hydroxycortico-sterone	Tetrahydroaldosterone	Renin	Aldosterone
17, 20-desmolase	Pregnanetriol Pregnanetriolone			
17β-hydroxysteroid dehydrogenase	Oxosteroid (±)		Androstenedione	Testosterone(±) (increased Androstenedione: Testosterone ratio) DHT(±)
5α-reductase	Testosterone(±)		Testosterone(±)	Dihydrotestosterone

Table 9.4 Main clinical presentation of inherited disorders of steroid biosynthesis at different ages

Age	Clinical presentation
Prenatal	Elevated or reduced concentrations of specific steroids in amniotic fluid
Neonatal	Ambiguous genitalia Hyponatraemia with renal salt loss Failure to thrive and associated symptoms
Infancy	Hypertension Hyponatraemia
Childhood and Adolescence	Virilisation Hirsutism Precocious puberty Delayed puberty Primary amenorrhoea Gynaecomastia Tall stature
Adulthood	Hirsutism Menstrual disturbances Infertility Family history HLA typing

of cortisol synthesis e.g. 21-hydroxylase can present primarily as a disorder of sexual differentiation due to excess androgen production during fetal development and the signs and symptoms of cortisol deficiency can be minimal or absent. It follows that the definitive diagnosis of the type of steroid biosynthetic defect is dependent on the results of laboratory investigations.

Two presentations in the neonatal period produce particularly urgent diagnostic problems; these are salt loss with hyponatraemia and ambiguous genitalia. The differential diagnosis for both are summarised in the lists below; for each there are a large number of other aetiologies which are not disorders of steroid biosynthesis.

Hyponatraemia in the neonate and in early infancy:
1. Inadequate intake of sodium
   a. Low sodium milk
   b. Intravenous therapy
2. Increased water intake
   Intravenous therapy
3. Increased net sodium loss
   a. Gastrointestinal
      (i) Diarrhoea
      (ii) Fistulae
   b. Renal
      (i) Anatomical kidney abnormalities

   (ii) Obstructive uropathy
   (ii) Renal tubular disorders
   (iv) Pseudohypoaldosteronism
  c. Mineralocorticoid underactivity
   (i) Congenital adrenal hypoplasia
   (ii) 21-hydroxylase deficiency
   (iii) 11β-hydroxylase deficiency
   (iv) 3β-hydroxysteroid dehydrogenase deficiency
   (v) 20,22-desmolase deficiency
   (vi) Corticosterone methyl oxidase deficiency (Types I and II)
4. Miscellaneous
  a. Syndrome of inappropriate ADH secretion
  b. Bartter's syndrome
  c   Familial hyporeninaemic hypoaldosteronism

Ambiguous genitalia at birth:[15]
1. Genetic females (karyotype 46XX)
  a. Increased endogenous fetal androgen production
   (i) 21-hydroxylase deficiency
   (ii) 11β-hydroxylase deficiency
   (iii) 3β-hydroxysteroid dehydrogenase deficiency
   (iv) Androgen secreting tumour
  b. Exogenous androgens
   (i) Maternal injestion of progestins or androgens in pregnancy
      (iatrogenic)
   (ii) Maternal androgen secreting tumour
   (iii) Maternal 21-hydroxylase deficiency
  c. Nonhormonal female pseudohermaphroditism
   (i) Urogenital malformations
   (ii) Prominent clitoris of prematurity
   (iii) Associated with dysmorphic syndromes
2. Genetic males (karyotpe 46XY)
  a. Decreased fetal androgen biosynthesis
   (i) 20,22-desmolase deficiency
   (ii) 3β-hydroxysteroid dehydrogenase deficiency
   (iii) 17,20-desmolase deficiency
   (iv) 17α-hydroxylase deficiency
   (v) 17β-hydroxysteroid dehydrogenase deficiency
   (vi) Leydig cell unresponsiveness to HCG and LH
  b. Defective peripheral androgen metabolism
   (i) 5α-reductase deficiency
   (ii) Androgen receptor and post-receptor defects (complete and
      incomplete testicular feminisation)
  c. Exogenous maternal oestrogen
      Maternal injection (iatrogenic)

    d. Nonhormonal male pseudohermaphroditism
       Urogenital malformations
    e. Deficient synthesis or action of MIF
3. Chromosome abnormalities
    Genetic mosaics
       46XY/45X
       46XY/46XX

Treatment of hyponatraemia due to a lack of mineralocorticoid activity is relatively simple and life saving. In the case of ambiguous genitalia the need to reach a decision on the sex for rearing the child is often not treated with the urgency it deserves. It is, however, extremely important for the parents that the child has a definite sex assigned to it in order for the child to be accepted by them and their relatives.

Table 9.5 Main clinical features of the individual inherited disorders of steroid biosynthesis

Deficient enzyme	Ambiguous genitalia M	F	Salt loss	Hypertension	Pubertal development	Post natal virilisation
20,22-desmolase	+	−	+	−	Absent, needs induction	−
3β-hydroxysteroid dehydrogenase	+/−	+/−	+	−	May need induction	−
17α-hydroxylase	+	−	−	+	Absent, needs induction	−
21-hydroxylase	−	+	+/−	−	Early or normal	+ if undertreated
11β-hydroxylase	−	+/−	−	+/−	Early or normal	+ if undertreated
Corticosterone methyl oxidase (Type I)	−	−	+	−	Normal	−
Corticosterone methyl oxidase (Type II)	−	−	+	−	Normal	−
17,20-desmolase	+	−	−	−	Absent, needs induction	
17β-hydroxysteroid dehydrogenase	+	−	−	−	Normal age F to M gender change	
α-reductase	+	−	−	−	Normal age variable F to M gender change	

Table 9.5 summarizes the main signs and symptoms of each of the specific steroid biosynthetic disorders and each individual disorder is discussed in detail below. In most cases the disorders are extremely rare and the presentation variable; information in Table 9.5 should be treated with this knowledge.

20,22 (cholesterol) desmolase deficiency (adrenal hyperplasia I, McKusick 20171)

The conversion of cholesterol to pregnenolone is the initial step in the synthesis of all types of steroids. Patients present in severe adrenal crisis and rarely survive infancy. Males have ambiguous genitalia, usually severe with complete feminization, and it is likely that the enzyme deficiency is present in all steroid synthesizing tissues.

The condition is very rare but cases are probably missed because of neonatal death. Inheritance is probably autosomal recessive based on the small numbers of reported cases. Approximately half of all reported cases are from Japan.

At post mortem the adrenal cells are enlarged and fllled with lipid staining material consisting of choloesterol and cholesterol esters. The action of 20,22-desmolase involves at least three steps which possibly are sited in a single enzyme complex. Different variants of this disorder are theoretically possible from defects in the three steps. Where biochemical investigation has been performed, reduction in cortisol, aldosterone and the urinary metabolites of the sex hormones have been found. Some patients have been described with evidence of some testosterone biosynthesis and male internal genitalia.

3-hydroxysteroid dehydrogenase, $\Delta^{5,4}$ oxosteroid isomerase deficiency (Adrenal hyperplasia II, McKusick 20181. EC 1.1.1.145)

The conversion of Δ^5 to Δ^4 steroids is catalyzed by 3β-hydroxysteroid dehydrogenase, $\Delta^{5,4}$ oxosteroid dehydrogenase (3β-HSD). This enzyme which is almost certainly a complex is believed to have a number of isoenzymes[3] with different specificities for C21 or C19 steroids. The enzyme in different organs, adrenal, gonad and liver may be under separate genetic control and this together with the existence of partial deficiencies are possible explanations of the varying clinical and biochemical presentation of these cases.[16] Contrary to what might be predicted the steroids progesterone and 17OHP are often elevated in 3β-HSD deficiency, though to a much lower extent than the equivalent steroids pregnenolone and 17-hydroxypregnenolone. Pregnanetriol, the main urine metabolite of 17OHP, may be increased in the urine and it is obvious that simplistic investigation of these patients with measurement of plasma 17OHP and/or urine pregnanetriol can lead to the mistaken diagnosis of 21-hydroxylase deficiency. Hence it is mandatory in all cases of suspected steroid biosynthetic disorders to obtain estimations of several different steroids and to do repeated investigations where necessary.

Clinically the patients present with disturbances of electrolyte and water balance and ambiguous genitalia. The severity of hyponatraemia is variable, some cases appear to produce no cortisol or aldosterone and are resistant to treatment, usually dying early. Other cases appear to be able to synthesise small amounts of cortisol and aldosterone and respond more favourably to therapy. Patients with apparently normal mineralocorticoid production, and who do not have salt loss, have also been described. Milder cases can present in late childhood and in puberty. In the male a variable degree of masculinisation of the external genitalia is found, possibly due to variable amounts of residual testosterone production or to the action of DHA, a weak androgen which is produced in excess. This latter steroid is probably the cause of the mild masculinisation of females with 3β-HSD deficiency.

17α-hydroxylase deficiency (Adrenal hyperplasia V, McKusick 20211 EC 1.14.99.9)

17α-hydoxylase catalyses the conversion of pregnenolone and progesterone to their respective 17α-hydroxy derivatives. This step is the branch point in the pathway to synthesis of the glucocorticoids and sex steroids: the mineralocorticoids are not hydroxylated on the 17 carbon, the enzyme being absent in the zona glomerulosa. Males present with ambiguous genitalia and females later in life with delayed puberty. ACTH stimulation of the adrenal increases the synthesis of 11-deoxycorticosterone and deoxycorticosterone. The former is a weak mineralocorticoid and causes a hypokalaemic alkalosis and hypertension, while the latter has glucocorticoid activity and compensates in part for the decreased cortisol.

One unusual feature found in 17α-hydroxylase deficiency is the combination of low levels of aldosterone and renin together with high levels of the aldosterone precursor 18-hydroxycorticosterone. Renin and aldosterone secretion are suppressed by the sodium retention and hypokalaemia caused by 11-deoxycorticosterone. The elevated 18-hydroxycorticosterone at first seems to suggest a separate defect in the zona glomerulosa but there is evidence for the production of this steroid in the other adrenocortical zones under the influence of ACTH. Glucocorticoid therapy suppresses the release of ACTH and results in reduction in the secretion of 11-deoxycorticosterone, corticosterone and 18-hydroxycorticosterone while renin and aldosterone secretion are normalised.

The deficiency of 17α-hydroxylase is inherited as an autosomal recessive and is rare. It does not appear to be linked to HLA.

21-hydroxylase deficiency (Adrenal hyperplasia III, McKusick 20191 EC 1.14.99.10)

21-hydroxylase deficiency is one of the most common inborn errors of metabolism and is found at a much higher frequency than all the other disorders of steroid biosynthesis. There are several different clinical presentations covering the entire age range, although the majority of cases are diagnosed in infancy. In the neonatal period female patients classically present with virilisation with or without associated salt loss; male patients at this age present with salt loss. Patients with salt loss can also present later in infancy and breast feeding has been shown to delay the clinical presentation of neonates with salt loss despite biochemical evidence of severe hyponatraemia. Other patients who appear normal at birth present with virilisation or precocious puberty in childhood or acne, hirsutism, menstrual disturbances and infertility in the adult female. A number of asymptomatic individuals with the biochemical stigmata have been discovered on the basis of HLA typing (see later). All forms are inherited in an autosomal recessive mode.

The frequency of the neonatal form of 21-hydroxylase deficiency appears variable. In Caucasian communities the incidence in the more recent surveys lies between 1:5000 and 1:15 000 births; this gives a gene frequency of between 1:35 and 1:61. Very high incidences have been reported among the Yupik Eskimos in Alaska with a frequency of 1:500 and in other Alaskan Eskimos at a frequency of 1:1500. The proportion of patients with salt loss is approximately 66%,[17] although in the Yupik Eskimos all cases appear to have salt loss. Information on the frequency of the late onset type is less certain but estimates of gene frequencies between 1:18 and 1:67 have been derived from studies of hirsute women.

The current approach to diagnosis relies heavily on the measurement of basal plasma 17OHP and less frequently androstenedione. ACTH stimulation tests are additionally helpful. There are a number of problems associated with reliance on single measurements[18] with both false positive and false negative results. This is particularly important when the investigation is undertaken early in patients who present with ambiguous genitalia when the probability of a false negative diagnosis is more frequent.

Biochemical defect in 21-hydroxylase deficiency

The variability of the clinical presentation of 21-hydroxylase deficiency, especially the differences between the salt losers and non-salt losers, requires explanation. Several hypotheses have been advanced:

1. The one enzyme hypothesis attempts to explain the variability as being caused by differing degrees of enzyme deficiency. In non-salt losers sufficient residual 21-hydroxylase activity remains to allow the production of aldosterone and thus prevent sodium loss. Included in this hypothesis

is the possibility that certain steroids, 17OHP and 16α-hydroxyprogesterone, might act on the renal tubule as antagonists to any aldosterone synthesized to increase sodium loss. Thus some patients who have normal plasma aldosterone concentrations might continue to lose sodium if they are unable to increase aldosterone production any further

2. The two enzyme hypothesis postulates that one 21-hydroxylase enzyme is specific for 17-hydroxysteroids and a second independent enzyme for the 17-deoxysteroids. Both enzymes are absent in salt losers and this theory would therefore require two independent but linked genetic defects: it is known that the gene coding for 21-hydroxylase is reduplicated on chromosome 6. Alternatively, if the 21-hydroxylase enzyme was dimeric with one subunit common to the enzyme in all three adrenal zones and the other subunit existing in two types specific for either the zona glomerulosa or the zona fasciculata and reticularis, then a defect in the common subunit would give rise to virilisation and salt loss, whereas a defect in the subunit in the zona fasciculata and reticularis would cause simple virilisation.

3. A third hypothesis is that the zona glomerulosa is physiologically a separate gland from the other two adrenocortical zones and is separately regulated. In simple virilising 21-hydroxylase deficiency the zona glomerulosa is normal, aldosterone production being preserved. On the other hand, both 17-hydroxy and 17-deoxy pathways are affected in the zona fasciculata and reticularis. Evidence for this hypothesis has been obtained from the study of plasma steroid concentrations after ACTH stimulation and sodium depletion,[18] together with additional information from patients with 11 and 17α-hydroxylase deficiency.

4. The finding in many patients of increased production of 21-deoxycortisol and pregnanetriolone (3α, 17α, 20α-trihydroxy-5-pregnan-one), which do not appear to be produced by normals even when stimulated with ACTH, gave rise to the hypothesis that the defect may not be a deficiency of 21-hydroxylase but rather aberrant 11β-hydroxylase which could act on 21-deoxysteroids.[3] This aberrant enzyme alters the normal sequence of hydroxylations. The resulting 11-hydroxysteroids are poor substrates for a normal 21-hydroxylase enzyme and may also inhibit the enzyme giving rise to the accumulation of 17OHP. The production of 21-deoxycortisol and pregnanetriolone precedes the accumulation of 17OHP and pregnanetriol in infants with 21-hydroxylase deficiency. Large quantities of pregnanetriolone are also found on patients with 11β-hydroxylase defects and an alternative explanation is that the pregnanetriolone is produced in the liver or peripherally.

None of these hypotheses is capable of explaining all the biochemical observations made in the many cases studied. It is likely that more than one factor is operating and 21-hydroxylase deficiency may well turn out to be a group of related disorders.

The late onset 21-hydroxylase deficiency is an allelic variant with symptoms presenting from late childhood to adulthood. In some cases symptoms are extremely mild or even absent and in these cases patients are usually identified in family studies using HLA typing and ACTH stimulation tests (see later). The three alleles which have been identified are normal, congenital or severe and late-onset or mild.[19,20] The various possible combinations of the alleles and the clinical outcome is shown in Table 9.6.

Table 9.6   Allelic variants of 21-hydroxylase

Genotype (After Ref. 19)	Genotype (After Ref. 20)	Clinical group	Symptoms
NN	nn	Normal	None
SN	Cn	Heterozygote	None
MN	Ln	Heterozygote	None
SS	CC	Classical neonatal	Neonatal virilization ± salt loss
MM	LL	Late onset/cryptic	Post natal virilisation, premature puberty, infertility
SM	CL	Late onset/cryptic double heterozygote	Hirsutism asymptomatic

S = 21-hydroxylase deficiency (Severe)
M = 21-hydroxylase deficiency (Mild)
C = 21-hydroxylase deficiency (Congenital)
L = 21-hydroxylase deficiency (Late onset)
N/n = normal

11β-hydroxylase deficiency (Adrenal hyperplasia IV, McKusick 20201 EC 1.14.15.4)

11β-hydroxylase catalyzes the conversion of 11-deoxycortisol and 11-deoxycorticosterone to cortisol and corticosterone respectively. There is considerable evidence for the existence of several isoenzymes of 11β-hydroxylase with different specificities[3] and that in particular the two reactions above are catalyzed by different isoenzymes. An additional isoenzyme appears to be able to hydroxylate C19 steroids. There is also evidence that one of the isoenzymes can hydroxylate both the 11 and 18 positions: a separate enzyme capable of hydroxylation of C18 also exists.[21] The complex, and as yet not clearly defined, nature of 11β-hydroxylase activity is one possible explanation for the variable clinical and biochemical presentation of patients with 11β-hydroxylase deficiency.

Though the second most common inborn error of steroid biosynthesis, 11β-hydroxylase deficiency was believed to occur in only 5% of cases. Recent studies have suggested, however, that the disorder is more frequent[22] and may account for up to 15% of cases. A higher incidence has been observed in Jews from North Africa and Turkey. 11β-hydroxylase deficiency is inherited as an autosomal recessive.

The classical presentation in females is with severe ambiguous genitalia and hypertension and in males with pseudoprecocious puberty or hypertension. It is clear, however, that, as with 21-hydroxylase deficiency, there is a wide spectrum of clinical presentation. The ambiguous genitalia in the female varies between mild clitoral hypertrophy to extreme masculinization with a penile urethra and fused labioscrotal folds. Some females presenting later in life do not have abnormal genitalia. Hypertension is not universally present and can be absent in patients with the more severe forms of androgen excess. Hypokalaemia is present in a minority of patients. Other presenting symptoms described in patients with 11β-hydroxylase deficiency include tall stature in both sexes, hirsutism and oligo- or amenorrhoea. Hyperpigmentation is a common but variable finding.

The biochemical diagnosis of 11β-hydroxylase deficiency depends on the finding of increased deoxycortisol in plasma and/or its metabolite tetrahydro-deoxycortisol in urine. The urine metabolite may take 3–4 weeks to appear in large quantities.[21] Zachman and colleagues[22] divided patients into clinically classical (severe) and mild groups and showed that tetrahydro-deoxycortisol was much lower in the latter. The tetrahydro metabolite of deoxycorticosterone was increased in the urine from the classical patients but absent from the mild group. In response to ACTH there was no increase in the excretion of either of these two steroid metabolites in the classical cases suggesting that the adrenal glands in these patients were already maximally stimulated by endogenous ACTH. On the other hand, while all the mild patients responded to ACTH with an increased excretion of tetrahydro-deoxycortisol, a subgroup (5 out of 12) did not show any rise in the excretion of tetrahydro-deoxycorticosterone. These findings indicate that the milder cases appear to have an incomplete defect and that at least two types of defect occur. In one the 11-hydroxylation of both 17-hydroxy and 17-deoxy steroids is affected, while in the other only the 11-hydroxylation of 17-hydroxy steroids is involved (11-deoxycortisol to cortisol). Investigation of obligate heterozygotes of 11β-hydroxylase deficiency reveals no biochemical abnormality in response to ACTH and it is unlikely that the milder variants represent the heterozygote state.

The cause of the hypertension in these patients remains to be elucidated. It has been postulated that increased plasma concentrations of deoxycorticosterone gave rise to hypertension, but patients with high concentrations of this steroid have been reported as being normotensive, while severely hypertensive patients with very mild elevation of plasma deoxycorticosterone have been found. Hypertension may present for the first time in later childhood. Nearly all patients with 11β-hydroxylase deficiency have evidence of volume expansion with low plasma renin and aldosterone even though hypertension is absent. Treatment with glucocorticoids reduces ACTH stimulation of the adrenal cortex, blood pressure falls in hypertensive patients and plasma renin rises. The renin activity in treated patients is significantly increased above controls either on a salt restricted or normal diet. Moderate salt loss occurs on sodium restriction and this suggests that patients treated with glucocorticoids are at potential risk in other situations which disturb sodium balance.[23] It has been proposed that the mineralocorticoid causing hypertension could be 18-hydroxy, 11-deoxycorticosterone because of the relationship between 18 and 11-hydroxylation.

17,20-desmolase deficiency (McKusick 30915)

17,20-desmolase converts the C21 steroids 17OHP and 17α-hydroxypregnenolone to androstenedione and dehydroepiandrosterone respectively. In the absence of this enzyme the sex steroids are not synthesized. This is a very rare disorder and all patients have presented with male pseudohermaphroditism. Diagnosis is established on the basis of increased urinary excretion of metabolites of 17OHP and the failure of ACTH and/or HCG to induce increases in plasma androstenedione and dehydroepiandrosterone concentrations.

Unlike other inherited disorders of steroid biosynthesis 17,20-desmolase deficiency is most likely to be X-linked. Evidence for this is based on the study of one family with two male cousins (children of sisters) and a maternal uncle being affected. Autosomal dominant inheritance has not, however, been ruled out.

17β-hydroxysteroid dehydrogenase deficiency (EC 1.1.1.64)

The conversion of androstenedione and oestrone to testosterone and oestradiol respectively is catalyzed by the enzyme 17β-hydroxysteroid dehydrogenase. Deficiency of this enzyme is a very rare disorder which presents with male pseudohermaphroditism. The gonadal enzyme only appears to be affected since peripheral conversion of androstenedione to testosterone is still present. The diagnosis can be made on the basis of an elevated androstenedione:testosterone ratio. In infants an HCG stimulation test will show a much greater rise in androstenedione than testosterone.

Genital virilisation occurs at puberty in the majority of patients which could be due to the androgen activity of androstenedione or its peripheral conversion to testosterone. In some patients there is a change in gender role from female to male. Gynaecomastia is found in a minority of cases. Inheritance is probably autosomal recessive.

Aldosterone biosynthetic defects (McKusick 20340 and 20341. EC 1.14.15.5)

Classically the conversion of corticosterone to aldosterone was believed to be a two stage procedure involving 18-hydroxylation followed by dehydrogenation. On the other hand Ulick[9] has produced evidence that two hydroxylation steps are involved catalyzed by a catechol methyl oxidase enzyme.

This produces 18-dihydrocorticosterone which is converted to aldosterone by the loss of water. Nomenclature for the inherited disorders of aldosterone biosynthesis depends on which of these two pathways is used. Alternative names used in the literature are 18-hydroxylase and 18-dehydrogenase deficiency or corticosterone methyl oxidase deficiency Type I and II (CMOD Type I and CMOD Type II). The latter are now preferred.

The clinical presentation of the two varieties of CMOD are essentially the same. Patients present with failure to thrive, dehydration, hyponatraemia and hyperkalaemia. A few patients can present later in childhood with failure to grow and/or postural hypotension. Family studies have revealed asymptomatic patients, while in others the symptoms may be transitory. In CMOD Type I patients may present with intermittent pyrexia.

The diagnosis depends to a large extent on the elimination of other causes of hyponatraemia (see p. 340) and in particular other steroid biosynthetic disorders which cause salt wasting. Resistance to the action of aldosterone (pseudohypoaldosteronism) must also be excluded. Clinically helpful distinguishing features are absence of virilisation or other signs of androgen excess, normal blood pressure and the absence of pigmentation. Biochemically the diagnosis depends on the measurement of plasma aldosterone concentration and renin activity and urinary metabolites of aldosterone, its precursors deoxycorticosterone and corticosterone and their 18-hydroxy derivatives.[24] Plasma aldosterone concentrations may be low or normal in the presence of increased plasma renin activity. Interpretation of the urinary steroid patterns in these cases is complicated by variations in metabolism due to age and disturbances of sodium homeostasis. Thus excretion patterns may be different in sodium replete and deplete states. The main findings are decreased tetrahydroaldosterone and increases in various corticosterone metabolites. It has been suggested that tetrahydro, 18-hydroxy, 11-dehydro-corticosterone is useful in distinguishing the two types of CMOD but this remains to be proven. CMOD can be distinguished from pseudohypoaldosteronism by the increased excretion of tetrahydroaldosterone in the latter disorder.

Both types of CMOD are inherited as autosomal recessive disorders with both males and females affected. There is a considerable difference in incidence; CMOD Type I is very rare while CMOD Type II is more frequent with a particularly high incidence in Iranian Jews.

5α-reductase deficiency (McKusick 26460)

In order for testosterone to exert some of its biological actions, reduction of the 4–5 double bond in the A-ring of the steroid nucleus by the enzyme 5α-reductase is required to produce dihydrotestosterone (DHT). In females DHT is essentially derived from the peripheral conversion of testosterone and androstenedione, whereas in adult males 50% of circulating DHT is produced in the testis. In the fetus and neonate the relative contribution of testis and peripheral testosterone conversion is not known. DHT is required for the normal formation of male external genitalia and in 5α-reductase deficiency male neonates will present with pseudohermaphroditism. Clinically the patients have female external genitalia with clitoral hypertrophy and normal male internal genitalia with testes, epididymides etc. A vaginal pouch may be present. (A similar clinical picture is produced by deficiency of the intracellular receptor protein which is required for DHT action. These syndromes will not be discussed here, interested readers should consult Ref. 25).

At puberty patients show a variable degree of masculinisation; in some cases virilisation is so complete that the patients, reared as females, convert to a male gender role. Female breast development is absent.

In plasma, normal or high concentrations of testosterone are present, with a low plasma DHT and increased plasma testosterone: DHT ratio. The urine shows a reduction in the excretion of 5α-metabolites. In children an HCG stimulation test may be required to demonstrate these changes. Direct measurement of 5α-reductase is possible in skin biopsies from the genital area or fibroblasts grown from them. Studies have shown more than one type of defect; the majority of patients have much reduced enzyme activity, whereas other cases appear to have an unstable enzyme present in normal quantity or reduced to approximately 50%. This suggests that 5α-reductase deficiency is a genetically heterogeneous disorder.

The disease is inherited as an autosomal recessive with a particularly high frequency in the Republic of Santo Domingo where it has been extensively studied. Sufficient cases are known for investigation of heterozygotes of both sexes and homozygous affected females. No evidence of any endocrinological abnormality of development or reproduction has been found.

THERAPY

The therapy of disorders of steroid biosynthesis can be divided into two distinct stages; the management of the neonatal presentation with ambiguous genitalia and/or salt loss and the subsequent endocrinological, surgical and psychological management of these patients and others presenting with signs and symptoms later in life.

When patients present with salt loss, treatment with intravenous saline and mineralocorticoid replacement is urgently required to re-establish normal plasma volume and sodium homeostasis. A blood sample should be taken prior to treatment with glucocorticoids for the measurement of plasma steroid concentrations and, in addition, a random or, where possible, a timed collection of urine should be obtained. If this is not done, or additional investigations are required, then abnormal steroid metabolism can be revealed on stimulation of the adrenal cortex with exogenous ACTH even while the patient is being given glucocorticoid. The management of the pseudohermaphroditism depends on several factors including the specific diagnosis, genotypic sex and degree of genital ambiguity. There is an urgent need for a full evaluation since correctly treated females with 21-hydroxylase and 11β-hydroxylase deficiencies (accounting for the great majority of cases) can attain normal adulthood wiih full reproductive capacity. Male patients with severe degrees of feminisation are probably best reared as females after appropriate surgical correction but it should be remembered that patients with 5α-reductase deficiency and 17β-hydroxy-steroid dehydrogenase deficiency can undergo successful female to male conversion at puberty without medical interference.

The long term endocrinological management involves replacement of the missing steroids and the suppression of the production of other steroids with unwanted effects. Several different glucocorticoids have been used but the best one, and the optimum dosage regime, are still a matter of debate. The logical approach would appear to be to use exogenous cortisol to mimic the natural circadian rhythm. However, cortisol has a relatively short half life in vivo and may not suppress ACTH secretion unless given in large doses or several times during the day. Large doses of cortisol cause stunting of growth and Cushingoid features to develop. Longer acting synthetic glucocorticoids may therefore be more effective. Aldosterone is relatively insoluble and mineralocorticoid replacement is usually with 9 α-fluorohydro-cortisone (fludrocortisone) though occasionally deoxycorticosterone acetate (DOCA) in depot form may be required.

Assessment of the efficiency of gluco- and mineralocorticoid replacement is complicated by the close interrelationship of the two groups of steroids and their control. There is a need to ensure that replacement steroids are given neither in inadequate nor excessive amounts. Glucocorticoid activity has been assessed by the measurement of urinary ketosteroids and preg-nanetriol, plasma 17OHP, 17α-hydroxypregnenolone, androstenendione, testosterone and dehydroepiandrosterone and salivary 17OHP, androstene-dione and testosterone. There is some dispute as to the value of these biochemical parameters in assessing control and it has been suggested that clinical evaluation remains the optimum method for monitoring therapy.[26] Urine measurements are difficult to use in the assessment of overtreatment and give an integrated measure of adrenal activity over the period of collec-tion, usually 24 hours. Single plasma steroid estimations give information relevant only to one point in time. What is required is a method which allows repeated estimation of adrenal activity throughout the 24 hour period and preferably when the patient is in his normal environment. The meas-urement of steroids in saliva[27] or in dried blood spots collected onto absorbent paper[28] allow this to be done and glucocorticoid replacement to be optimised. The most useful individual steroids to measure in monitoring glucocorticoid replacement in 21-hydroxylase deficiency are 17OHP and androstenedione.

With the development of plasma renin activity measurements it became possible to assess the efficacy of mineralocorticoid therapy. Elevated plasma renin activity was found in salt losing and non-salt losing 21-hydroxylase deficient patients, reflecting reduction in body sodium: suppression of the plasma renin activity to normal levels has been shown to decrease ACTH secretion and improve management of glucocorticoid therapy as well as ensuring adequate sodium balance.[29] It should be noted that the method for the measurement of plasma renin activity (PRA) depends on adequate synthesis of the renin substrate, angiotensinogen. The synthesis of this α_2-macroglobulin by the liver is regulated in part by glucocorticoids and is lowered in adrenal insufficiency. Thus a decrease in PRA can reflect alteration in renin substrate as well as a reduction in renin concentration.[30]

HLA AND DISORDERS OF STEROID BIOSYNTHESIS

The Major Histocompatibility Complex is a group of genes located on the short arm of chromosome 6. Included in this group are the HLA (human leucocyte antigen) genes and structural genes for the complement components C2, C4A, C4B and properdin factor B(Bf). The HLA complex consists of at least seven loci which are in order from the centromere DP, DQ, DR, D, B, C and A. A large number of alleles occur at the HLA loci; currently 23, 47, 8, 19 and 16 have been definitely or provisionally allocated to A, B, C, D and DR respectively. HLA genes are expressed codominantly, with one haplotype being inherited from each parent. The genes for C2A, C2B and Bf are located between the HLA loci B and DR.

A linkage between HLA and 21-hydroxylase deficiency has been established. As a consequence of this discovery a large number of families with 21-hydroxylase deficiency have been studied and the gene has been mapped close to the HLA-B locus with recombination suggesting at least two genes, one between HLA-B and D/DR and the other on the centromere side of the HLA D/DR locus.[31] Genetic linkage disequilibrium (non-random association of alleles) has been described with increased frequencies of HLA-Bw47 being found in Caucasians with classical 21-hydroxylase deficiency while HLA-B14 and DR1 are associated with late onset 21-hydroxylase deficiency. The alleles for HLA-B8 and DR3 are decreased in frequency. Extended haplotypes of the Major Histocompatability Complex, including several rare alleles, and the closely located gene for the erythrocyte enzyme glyoxylase I appear to be highly conserved in patients with 21-hydroxylase deficiency over a wide geographical distribution, suggesting that this part of chromosome 6 is very stable.

Recent studies with DNA probes have allowed the mapping of human 21-hydroxylase genes.[32] Two genes 21OHA and 21OHB have been localized adjacent to the genes for C4B and C4A (Fig. 9.7). Both these genes are thus between HLA-B and D/DR. The existence of an additional gene or genes for 21-hydroxylase on the other side of HLA-D/DR, as suggested by family studies, remains to be resolved. Preliminary data has suggested that 21-

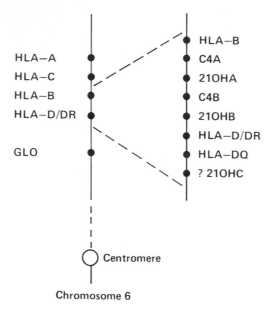

Fig. 9.7 Diagrammatic representation of the short arm of chromosome 6 showing the location of the genes for 21-hydroxylase.

hydroxylase is in some cases due to the deletion of 21OHA, the adjacent C4A and part of the HLA-B locus, converting HLA-B13 to B47.[33]

No linkage with HLA has been found in patients studied with 11β-hydroxylase and 17α-hydroxylase deficiency. On the other hand studies of patients with CMOD Type II suggest that a linkage with HLA remains a possibility.

PRENATAL DIAGNOSIS AND TREATMENT

The prenatal diagnosis of 21-hydroxylase deficiency has been accomplished in several different centres using the measurement of 17OHP in amniotic fluid, by HLA typing of fetal cells or both.[34] The comparison of the use of HLA typing and 17OHP concentration gave discordant results in 2 out of 17 pregnancies tested with the amniotic fluid 17OHP concentration correctly predicting a normal fetus. In the other 15 cases the predictions from the 2 methods agreed and the outcome being 12 normal and 3 affected pregnancies. Thus simple HLA typing alone should not be relied upon for prenatal diagnosis. The discrepancies arise from genetic recombination whose frequency is not known.

The role of prenatal diagnosis in 21-hydroxylase deficiency has been questioned. With current therapy the patient can expect an essentially normal life with possible exception of the most severely affected females. It is not known whether the late onset or cryptic forms of 21-hydroxylase deficiency demonstrate high amniotic fluid 17OHP concentrations and these patients may therefore be at risk from unnecessary termination of pregnancy. It has been argued that antenatal diagnosis allows early treatment of affected fetuses after birth but it is relatively easy to establish a diagnosis in the first 2–3 days of life if the neonate is known to be at risk and the additional problems of amniocentesis can be avoided. There is as yet no antenatal treatment to prevent virilisation.

Antenatal diagnosis of 11β-hydroxylase deficiency has been achieved by measurement of 11-deoxycortisol and tetrahydrocortisol in amniotic fluid.[35]

Prenatal diagnosis by amniotic fluid sampling takes place too late to prevent the genital abnormalities by any form of treatment. Treatment with glucocorticoid earlier in pregnancy has been attempted in 'at risk' pregnancies and some reduction in the severity of masculinisation compared to the respective siblings has been obtained in two females.[36]

SCREENING FOR 21-HYDROXYLASE DEFICIENCY

The development of a method for the determination of 17OHP in blood spots collected onto absorbent paper led to the proposal to add 21-hydroxylase deficiency to the neonatal screening programme for inborn errors of metabolism.[37] These programmes have now been established in a number of different countries. The need for screening for 21-hydroxylase deficiency is based on retrospective analysis of the presentation and age at diagnosis of individual clinics.[38] This type of approach inevitably includes patients who presented at times when the pathology of the disease was less well understood or when the diagnosis was less easy to establish. The most severely affected infants are likely to present early and the patients most at risk are almost inevitably the salt losers. Judgement on whether screening for 21-hydroxylase deficiency should be adopted should be reserved until a properly controlled study has been undertaken. One possible exception to this is where the disorder has a high frequency and where access to modern medical care is restricted.

HETEROZYGOTE DETECTION

As with prenatal diagnosis, heterozygote detection has been carried out using steroid assays and/or HLA typing in 21-hydroxylase deficiency[18]. Heterozygotes identified on the basis of HLA typing show an increased production of 17OHP in response to ACTH.

REFERENCES

1 Munro Neville A, O'Hare M J 1982 The human adrenal cortex. Springer Verlag, Berlin, ch 4, p 16–34
2 Symington T 1969 Functional pathology of the human adrenal gland. E and S Livingstone, Edinburgh, ch 2 and 3, p 5–28

3 Finkelstein M, Shaeffer J M 1979 Inborn errors of steroid biosynthesis. Physiological Reviews 59: 353–406
4 Wilson J D, Griffin J C, George F W, Leshin M 1981 The role of gonadal steroids in sexual differentiation. Recent Progress in Hormone Research 37: 1–33
5 Saenger P 1984 Abnormal sex differentiation. Journal of Pediatrics 104: 1–17
6 Anderson D C 1980 The adrenal androgen-stimulating hormone does not exist. Lancet ii: 454–456
7 Hornby P J 1985 The regulation of adrenocortical function by control of growth and structure. In: Anderson D C, Winter J (eds) The adrenal cortex. Butterworth, London, ch 1, p 1–31
8 Briggs M H, Brotherton J 1971 Steroid biochemistry and pharmacology. Academic Press, London. ch 1 Nomenclature of steroids, p 1–22
9 Ulick S 1976 Diagnosis and nomenclature of the disorders of the terminal portion of the aldosterone biosynthetic pathway. Journal of Clinical Endocrinology and Metabolism 43: 92–96
10 Price D A, Close G C, Fielding B 1983 Age of appearance of circadian rhythm in salivary cortisol values in infancy. Archives of Disease in Childhood 58: 454–456
11 Weinkove C, Anderson D C 1985 Interaction between adrenal cortex and medulla. In: Anderson D C, Winter J (eds) The adrenal cortex. Butterworth, London, ch 10, p 208–234.
12 Biglieri E G, Wajchenberg B L, Malerbi D A, Okada H, Leme C E, Kater C E 1981 The zonal origins of the mineralocorticoid hormones in the 21-hydroxylation deficiency of congenital adrenal hyperplasia. Journal of Clinical Endocrinology and Metabolism 53: 964–969
13 Paterson R E 1971 Metabolism of adrenal steroids. In: Christy N P (ed) The human adrenal cortex. Harper and Row, New York, ch 4, p 87–189
14 Wachtel S S 1983 H-Y Antigen and the biology of sex determination. Grune and Stratton, New York
15 Addison G M, Chard C R, Price D A 1984 Steroid hormone metabolism. In: Hicks J M, Boeckx R L (eds) Pediatric clinical chemistry. W B Saunders, New York, ch 9, 240–294
16 de Perretti E, Forest M G 1982 Pitfalls in the etiological diagnosis of congenital adrenal hyperplasia in the early neonatal period. Hormone Research 16: 10–22
17 Fife D, Rappaport E B 1983 Prevalence of salt losing among adrenal hyperplasia patients. Clinical Endocrinology 18: 259–264
18 New M I, Dupont B, Grumbach K, Levine S 1983 Congenital adrenal hyperplasia and related conditions. In: Stanbury J B, Wyngaarden J B Fredrickson D S, Goldstein J L, Brown M S (eds) The metabolic basis of inherited disease, 5th edn. McGraw Hill, New York, ch 47, p 973–1000
19 Kohn B, Levine L S, Pollack M S et al 1982 Late onset steroid 21-hydroxylase deficiency: a variant of classical congenital adrenal hyperplasia. Journal of Clinical Endocrinology and Metabolism 55: 817–827
20 Roitman A, Stivel M, Zamir R, Kaufman H, Pertzelan A, Laron Z 1982 Late-onset type of 21-hydroxylase deficiency in childhood. Israel Journal of Medical Sciences 18: 763–768
21 Honour J W, Anderson J M, Shackleton C H L 1983 Difficulties in the diagnosis of congenital adrenal hyperplasia in early infancy: the 11β-hydroxylase defect. Acta Endocrinologica 103: 101–109
22 Zachmann M, Tassinari D, Prader A 1983 Clinical and biochemical variability of congenital adrenal hyperplasia due to 11β-hydroxylase deficiency: a study of 25 patients. Journal of Clinical Endocrinology and Metabolism 56: 222–229
23 Zadik Z, Kahana L, Kaufman H, Benderli A, Hachberg Z 1984 Salt loss in hypertensive form of congenital adrenal hyperplasia (11β-hydroxylase deficiency). Journal of Clinical Endocrinology and Metabolism 58: 384–388
24 Honour J W, Dillon M J, Shackleton C H L 1982 Analysis of steroids in urine for differentiation of pseudohypoaldosteronism and aldosterone biosynthetic defect. Journal of Clinical Endocrinology and Metabolism 54: 325–331
25 Wilson J D, Griffin J E, Leshin M, McDonald P C 1983 The androgen resistance syndromes: 5α-reductase deficiency, testicular feminization and related disorders. In: Stanbury J B, Wyngaarden J B, Fredrickson D S, Goldstein J L, Brown M S (eds) The

metabolic basis of inherited disease, 5th edn. McGraw Hill, New York, ch 48, p 1001–1026

26 Hendricks S A, Lippe B M, Kaplan S A, Lavin N, Mayes D 1982 Urinary and serum concentrations in the management of congenital adrenal hyperplasia: lack of physiologic correlations. American Journal of Diseases of Children 136: 229–232

27 Hughes I A, Read G F 1982 Simultaneous plasma and salivary measurement as an index of control in congenital adrenal hyperplasia: a longitudinal study. Hormone Research 16: 142–150

28 Solyom J 1981 Blood spot 17α-hydroxyprogesterone radioimmunoassay in the follow-up of congenital adrenal hyperplasia. Clinical Endocrinology 14: 547–553

29 Rosler A, Levine L S, Schneider B, Novogroder M, New M I, 1977 The interrelationship of sodium balance, plasma renin activity and ACTH in congenital adrenal hyperplasia. Journal of Clinical Endocrinology and Metabolism 45: 500–512

30 Rosenthal S M, Reid I A, Kaplan S L, Grumbach M M 1983 Renin substrate depletion in salt losing virilizing adrenal hyperplasia: low plasma renin activity despite increased renin concentration. Journal of Pediatrics 102: 80–82

31 Dupont B, Pollack M S, Levine L S, O'Neill G J, Hawkins B R, New M I 1980 Congenital adrenal hyperplasia. In: Terasaki P I (ed) Histocompatability Testing 1980. UCLA Tissue Typing Laboratory, Los Angeles, p 693–706

32 Carroll M C, Cambell R, Porter R R 1985 The mapping of 21-hydroxylase genes adjacent to complement C4 genes in HLA the Major Histocompatibility Complex in man. Proceedings of the National Academy of Sciences (USA) 82: 521–525

33 Bodmer J, Bodmer W, 1984 Histocompatibility Immunology Today 5: 251–254

34 Forest M G, Betuel H, Couillin P, Boue A 1981 Prenatal diagnosis of congenital adrenal hyperplasia deficiency due to 21-hydroxylase deficiency by steroid analysis in the amniotic fluid of mid pregnancy: comparison with HLA typing in 17 pregnancies at risk for CAH. Prenatal Diagnosis 1: 197–207

35 Rosler A, Leiberman E, Rosenmann A, Ben-Uzilio R, Weidemfeld J 1979 Prenatal diagnosis of 11β-hydroxylase deficiency congenital adrenal hyperplasia. Journal of Clinical Endocrinology and Metabolism 49: 546–551

36 David M, Forest M G 1984 Prenatal treatment of congenital adrenal hyperplasia from 21-hydroxylase deficiency. Journal of Pediatrics 105: 799–803

37 Pang S, Hotchkiss J, Drash A L, Levine L S, New M I 1977 Microfilter paper method for 17-hydroxyprogesterone radioimmunoassay and its application for rapid screening for congenital adrenal hyperplasia. Journal of Clinical Endocrinology and Metabolism 45: 1003–1008

38 Lebovitz R M, Pauli R M, Laxova R, 1984 Delayed diagnosis in congenital adrenal hyperplasia: need for newborn screening. American Journal of Diseases of Children 138: 571–573

Lipid disorders

PLASMA LIPOPROTEINS

General introduction

The lipoproteins of plasma form a complex system for the transport of hydrophobic lipids, notably cholesterol esters and triglycerides, in a water-soluble form, between the tissues.

The varying proportions of lipid to protein in these macromolecular complexes produce a wide range of physical properties and the classification and identification of lipoproteins depend on these variations in properties. The two most commonly used systems of nomenclature are based on *a*. hydrated density and *b*. electrical charge. By either method lipoproteins

Table 10.1 Properties of lipoproteins

Ultracentrifugal behaviour	Chylomicrons	Very low density lipoproteins	Low density lipoproteins	High density lipoproteins
Electrophoretic mobility	origin	pre β	β	α
Composition: proteins %	<2	12	25	50
lipid %	98	88	75	50
major lipid	triglyceride	triglyceride	cholesterol	cholesterol or phospholipid
Major apoprotein	A, C, B48	C, B100, E	B100	A
Major function	Transport of exogenous triglyceride	Transport of endogenous triglyceride	Transport of cholesterol to peripheral tissues	Transport of cholesterol from peripheral tissues
Origin	Intestine	Intestine and liver	Metabolism of VLDL	Liver and intestine

Abbreviations: VLDL, LDL, IDL, HDL — Very low, low, intermediate, high density lipoproteins respectively; apo — apolipoprotein; FC — free cholesterol; CE — cholesterol ester; PL — phospholipid; LPL — lipoprotein lipase; LCAT — lecithin cholesterol acyl transferase; AcCoA — acetyl coenzyme A; HMG CoA — 3-hydroxy 3-methylglutaryl coenzyme A; ACAT — acyl CoA: cholesterol acyltransferase.

naturally fall into four major classes named according to their behaviour in the ultracentrifuge, or on electrophoresis (see Table 10.1).

The bulk of the lipoprotein is made up of a hydrophobic core of cholesterol esters and triglycerides, surrounded by a membrane-like structure containing free cholesterol and phospholipids in which the proteins 'float'. These proteins are known as apolipoproteins or, more simply, apoproteins. As the proportion of triglyceride, in particular, decreases, so the density of the particle increases. The amount of protein therefore in high density lipoprotein is approximately 50% whereas that in very low density lipoprotein is as low as 12% (see Table 10.1).

Whereas it was originally thought that the apoproteins served only a structural role, stabilising and solubilising the lipid core of the lipoprotein, it is now known that their functions extend to include enzyme modulation and receptor recognition.

At this time, 13 human plasma apoproteins have been identified and characterised. Of these, six have had their primary structure determined, apo AI, apo AII, apo CI, apo CII, apo CIII and apo E, and the importance of self-association and mixed association of apoproteins has been recognised.

Table 10.2 shows the major apoproteins, their occurrence within lipoprotein classes, molecular weights and, where known with certainty, the physiological functions.

Table 10.2 Properties and occurrence of the major apoproteins

Apoprotein	Major lipoprotein fraction	Molecular weight	Function
AI	HDL	28 300	Cofactor for LCAT
AII	HDL	17 000	Structural protein of HDL
B100	VLDL, LDL	ca 549 000	Interaction with LDL receptor
B48	Chylomicrons	ca 265 000	Structural protein and receptor binding of chylomicron remnants
CI	VLDL, HDL	6331	—
CII	VLDL, HDL	8837	Cofactor for lipoprotein lipase
$CIII_{0,1,2}$	VLDL, HDL	8764	—
$E_{2,3,4}$	VLDL, HDL	33 000	Receptor binding

Biosynthesis and metabolism of lipoproteins

Triglyceride-rich lipoproteins

Triglyceride-rich lipoproteins are secreted as chylomicrons and VLDL by the small intestine and the liver respectively (Fig. 10.1). Those produced by the liver are VLDL, containing apo B100 and those from the small

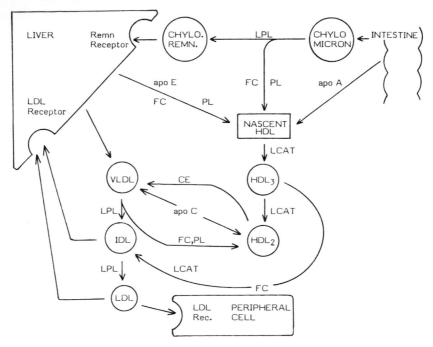

Fig. 10.1 Lipoprotein metabolism. For abbreviations see footnotes (p. 358)

intestine are chylomicrons which contain apo B48. After circulation to peripheral tissues they are hydrolysed by the triglyceride hydrolases (EC 3.1.1.3), lipoprotein lipase (EC 3.1.1.34) and hepatic lipase, to give smaller intermediate density lipoproteins (IDL), which can be further hydrolysed to produce LDL, and chylomicron remnants.

Both of these products, LDL and chylomicron remnants, are removed from the circulation by specific receptor systems. The liver has a receptor for chylomicron remnants which recognises the apo E carried on the surface of the remnant particles, along with apo B48. The high affinity LDL receptor, on the other hand, occurs widely in peripheral cells, such as fibroblasts, endothelial cells, smooth muscle cells, liver cells, and recognises both apo B100 and apo E. Circulating LDL is bound to the cell surface receptor (Fig. 10.2). Endocytosis then takes place and the particle is broken down by lysosomal enzymes, including an acid lipase, liberating free cholesterol and amino acids. This free cholesterol operates at three levels within the cell. First, it suppresses the activity of 3-hydroxy 3-methylglutaryl coenzyme A reductase (EC 1.1.1.88) which controls the rate-determining step in cholesterol biosynthesis. Secondly, it stimulates the re-esterification of free cholesterol by activation of the enzyme acyl-CoA:cholesterol acyltransferase (EC 2.3.1.26). The overall result of this re-esterification process is to shift the balance of fatty acids in the cholesteryl esters from a poly-

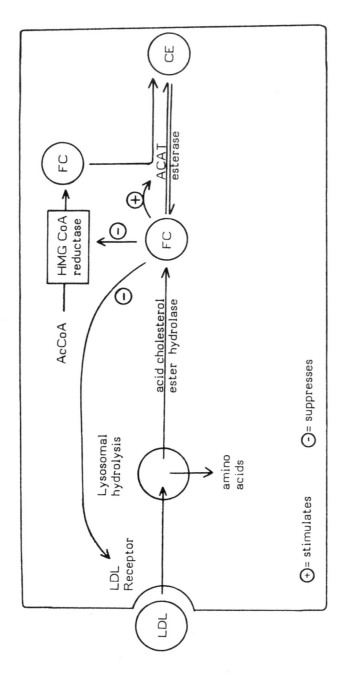

Fig. 10.2 LDL receptor pathway. For abbreviations see footnotes (p. 358)

unsaturated to a more saturated form. The third effect of the cellular free cholesterol is to suppress the formation of the LDL receptor itself. Thus, a delicate control of free cholesterol levels within the cell is maintained.

High density lipoproteins

The biosynthesis and metabolism of high density lipoprotein (HDL) is complicated by the polydispersity of the HDL particle itself (Fig. 10.1). It contains two major subfractions, HDL_2 and HDL_3, differing slightly in size and composition. The lipid and apoprotein components of HDL are derived from the catabolism of both VLDL and chylomicrons, as well as being synthesised directly by both liver and intestine. Hepatic HDL contains mainly apo E, whereas that from the intestine contains apo A. The newly-synthesised (nascent) HDL is disc-shaped, and contains no esterified cholesterol. On reaction with the plasma cholesterol-esterifying enzyme, lecithin cholesterol acyltransferase (EC 2.3.1.43) the discs are converted into the mature spherical particle, HDL_3, which then acquires apo C and phospholipid released during the lipolysis of triglyceride-rich lipoproteins. The product of this reaction is HDL_2 which releases some of its cholesterol esters and apo C back to triglyceride-rich lipoproteins.

HDL appears to be involved in reverse cholesterol transport from the peripheral tissues to the liver, a process which be may be important in explaining the inverse correlation which exists between HDL-cholesterol concentration and prevalence of premature cardiovascular disease.

Role of lipoproteins and their components as enzyme regulators

Two of the major enzymes of lipoprotein metabolism, lipoprotein lipase and lecithin cholesterol acyltransferase, have specific requirements for an apoprotein regulator.

Lipoprotein lipase is the enzyme responsible for the lipolytic breakdown of triglyceride-rich lipoproteins on the endothelial surface. A specific requirement for LPL activity is the presence of apo CII, which is found with the other C apoproteins in chylomicrons, VLDL and also HDL. It has been reported that apo CIII, at least in vitro, inhibits LPL activity but this has not been confirmed in vivo.

LCAT, which catalyses cholesterol esterification in plasma, is only active in the presence of apoprotein AI, one of the major apoproteins of HDL. It has been reported that apo CI also activates LCAT, though it appears to operate through a different mechanism from apo AI.

It can be seen therefore that the metabolism of lipoproteins is closely related to the spectrum of apolipoproteins which they contain. Previous classifications of lipoprotein disorders have been based almost entirely on the lipid content of lipoproteins. Although this has served a useful purpose by identifying many of the lipoprotein abnormalities observed, the underlying biochemical problem has frequently remained unsolved. More recent work has shown that considerable information can be derived by studying apoprotein abnormalities.

In this chapter therefore, the importance of the apolipoproteins in disorders of lipoprotein metabolism will be stressed wherever possible.

Laboratory investigation of lipoprotein disorders

Many of the techniques required for the analysis of lipoproteins and apoproteins are sophisticated and therefore unlikely to be available in all but the best-equipped clinical laboratories. Details of methodology are beyond the scope of this article but numerous texts are available which describe the relevant experimental methods.[1,2,3,4]

For a full lipoprotein analysis an ultracentrifuge is usually required,[1] though nowadays it is possible to separate most of the lipoproteins by differential precipitation,[2] using polyanions etc. This method is commonly employed for the isolation of HDL using heparin, sodium phosphotungstate or dextran sulphate.

Electrophoresis may be used for the qualitative analysis of lipoproteins,[3] and for apoprotein analysis it is mandatory. Polyacrylamide gel is the support medium of choice and if this is combined with isoelectric focusing a very powerful tool for the analysis of apoprotein isoforms is available.[4] This can be used in conjunction with a scanning device so that a semi-quantitative analysis of the apoprotein distribution can be obtained.

For a truly quantitative analysis of apoproteins it is usually necessary to resort to some form of immunoassay. Many methods have been described, including radial immunodiffusion, electroimmunoassay, radioimmunoassay and immunonephelometry (Table 10.3). All have their relative advantages and disadvantages but one common factor is that they all require specific

Table 10.3   Immunological procedures for apoprotein assay

Type of assay	Advantage or disadvantage	Apoproteins assayed	Typical references
Radial immunodiffusion RID	Simple, cheap, no automation, small numbers	AI, AII, B, CI	5
Electroimmunoassay EIA	Simple, cheap, no automation, large amount of antibody	AI, AII, B, CI, CII, CIII, E	6
Radioimmunoassay RIA	Very sensitive, specific, time-consuming, large numbers	AI, AII, B, CII, CIII, E	7
Immunonephelometric assay INA	Large numbers, may be automated, similar sensitivity to EIA, RID. large amount of antibody	AI, AII, B	8

antibodies to the desired apoprotein. Many antibodies, both poly- and monoclonal are now commercially available, some in the form of assay kits, but often it falls to the laboratory to develop its own antisera. Thus these analytical procedures may be available only in those laboratories with a strong research interest.

The analysis of the lipid content of serum and lipoproteins is usually less of a problem as most laboratories have efficient working methods available for the assay of cholesterol and triglycerides.

The estimation of enzymatic activity for any of the lipid-metabolising enzymes and the investigation of cell receptor function using tissue culture are specialised techniques and their availability will therefore be limited.

Molecular genetics and lipoprotein disorders

The analysis of apolipoprotein genes is still in its infancy. The genes for apo AI and apo CIII have been sequenced. They are both on chromosome 2 and coded for by opposite DNA strands. In the disease characterised by the absence of apo AI and apo CIII the defect responsible was found to be an abnormal insertion of DNA in the coding region of the gene for apo AI. Similarly an alteration in the apo CIII gene has been shown to be present in a high proportion of hypertriglyceridaemic patients.

The genes for apo E and apo CII are on chromosome 19. Extensive studies on the apo E gene have revealed mutations coding for altered amino-acid composition in several apo E polymorphs, some of which are responsible for the phenotype III with its greatly increased atherosclerotic risk. Analysis of apoprotein genes has already shown great potential for assessing the role of genetic factors in lipoprotein disorders, making early therapeutic intervention possible.

CLASSIFICATION OF LIPOPROTEIN DISORDERS

Most of the well-defined disorders involving lipoproteins can be divided into two groups.
1. Those in which there is a defect of either *a*. an apoprotein which is intimately involved in the synthesis or metabolism of lipoproteins, or *b*. a cell receptor which recognises a specific apoprotein.
2. Those in which there is a defect in an enzyme concerned with lipoprotein metabolism.

Table 10.4 lists these disorders according to the protein or enzymic defect and also indicates, where known, the type of dyslipoproteinaemia which is most likely to be manifested. In two relatively common inherited disorders, primary hypertriglyceridaemia and combined hyperlipidaemia, the defect is unknown. In Table 10.4, therefore, they are not placed in either of the two main categories.

The order of the diseases as shown in Table 10.4 takes no account of their relative incidence, and lipoprotein disorders which arise secondarily to other

Table 10.4 Classification of lipoprotein disorders

	Defect	Disorder
Structural	Apoprotein AI	Tangier (20540); Fish-eye; apo AI deficiency apo AI variants (Milano) (Marburg) (Munster) (Giessen) Apo AI + Apo CIII deficiency
	Apoprotein B48 +apoprotein B100	Abetalipoproteinaemia (20010); familial hypobetalipoproteinaemia (14595)
	Apoprotein B100 alone	Abetalipoproteinaemia (normotriglyceridaemic)
	Apoprotein CII	Chylomicronaemia—Type I* or Type V (14465)
	Apoprotein E	Type III (14450) and Type V
	LDL receptor	familial hypercholesterolaemia—Type IIa (14389, 14440)
	Remnant receptor	Type III
Enzymic	Lipoprotein lipase	Chylomicronaemia—Type I (23860)
	Hepatic lipase	Type III
	LCAT	LCAT deficiency (24590)
	Lysosomal cholesteryl-ester hydrolase	Wolman (27800); cholesterol ester storage disease (21500)
Defect unknown		Primary hypertriglyceridaemia—Type IV (15560) and V Combined hyperlipidaemia—Type IIb (14425)

* Type refers to the Fredrickson classification of hyperlipoproteinaemias (Table 10.5).
Numbers in parentheses refer to the McKusick classification of inherited diseases.[11]

major metabolic diseases are excluded, even though the profile of lipids generated may be similar, if not identical, to that in primary dyslipoproteinaemias.

Because there is often an intricate interrelationship between several lipoproteins and their apoproteins, there is frequently an overlap of biochemical signs so that the more widely-used Fredrickson classification[9,10] (Table 10.5) is unable to identify clearly the underlying metabolic lesion.

Table 10.6 indicates the primary inherited defect which can be considered when a major plasma lipid (cholesterol and triglyceride) level is abnormal. It has to be emphasised that often more than one molecular defect can give expression to a particular lipoprotein phenotype. Because of the rarity of many of these disorders, all other possible causes of a lipid abnormality should first be excluded.

DEFECTS INVOLVING APOPROTEINS—APOPROTEIN A

Tangier disease (Analphalipoproteinaemia)

This rare disorder was first described by Fredrickson in 1961 following its discovery in two inhabitants of Tangier island, Virginia.

Table 10.5   Classification of hyperlipoproteinaemias* Fredrickson (1967); WHO (1970)

Lipoprotein abnormality	Phenotype expressed**
Raised chylomicrons (chylomicronaemia)	Type I
Raised LDL (hypercholesterolaemia)	Type IIa
Raised LDL and VLDL (combined hyperlipidaemia)	Type IIb
Raised IDL (broad beta disease: beta VLDL)	Type III
Raised VLDL (hypertriglyceridaemia)	Type IV
Raised chylomicrons and VLDL (chylomicronaemia and hypertriglyceridaemia)	Type V

  * Several lipoprotein disorders have come to be named according to this classification. Although the system leaves much to be desired, it has become a working framework for identifying some of the primary disorders of lipoprotein metabolism. This system will therefore be used for those disorders which fall naturally into one of these categories, whilst accepting that ultimately a more specific definition, identifying the underlying apoprotein or metabolic defect, could be used.
 ** The phenotype expressed may arise for a variety of reasons. It is thus a classification of the lipoprotein status of the patient's plasma, rather than the underlying genetic abnormality of the patient.

Table 10.6   Relationship between laboratory findings and molecular defect

Laboratory findings	Disease phenotype	Major lipoprotein abnormality	Molecular defect if known
Raised cholesterol	Type IIa	LDL and apo B raised	LDL receptor absent or defective
Raised triglyceride	Type I	Chylomicrons raised	LPL or apo CII absent or decreased
	Type IV	VLDL raised	?
	Type V	Chylomicrons and VLDL raised	?
			apo CII deficiency
	Fish eye disease	LDL triglyceride raised	?
Raised cholesterol and triglyceride	Type IIb	VLDL and LDL raised	?
	Type III	VLDL raised apo E2 raised Chylomicron remnants raised IDL raised	apo E2 homozygosity Remnant receptor defect Hepatic lipase deficient
	Cholesterol ester storage disease	VLDL and LDL raised HDL decreased	CE hydrolase deficiency
	LCAT deficiency	VLDL raised Absence of CE	Absence of LCAT
Decreased cholesterol	Abetalipoproteinaemia	Absence of VLDL LDL and chylomicrons	Absence of apo B
	Hypobetalipo- proteinaemia	Decrease in VLDL LDL and chylomicrons	Decrease in apo B
	Tangier disease	Absence of HDL	Absence of apo A

Clinical symptoms

The disease is characterised by the presence of enlarged orange tonsils. Even after tonsillectomy, residual tonsillar tissue may be detected in the pharynx. There is often corneal opacity but without impairment of vision. Hepatosplenomegaly is fairly common, as is peripheral neuropathy. Anaemia (often haemolytic) occurs in many cases and thrombocytopenia may be present. The mucosa of the colon and rectum is frequently discoloured.

Histology shows excessive deposition of cholesterol esters in the reticuloendothelial system, particularly in the macrophages and Schwann cells. This is most evident in the tonsils, bone marrow, intestine, nerves, liver and spleen.

Biochemical signs

Characteristically there is marked plasma hypocholesterolaemia (less than 2.6 mmol/l) due to decreased levels of cholesterol esters. Plasma triglycerides may be elevated by the presence of chylomicrons and raised LDL-triglycerides. The most striking feature is, however, the almost complete absence of HDL. The levels of plasma apo AI and apo AII are, as expected, very much reduced to less than 10% of normal values. This is almost certainly due to rapid catabolism of apo AI, apo AII and HDL and a possible slight reduction in synthesis rates of apo AI and apo AII.

Despite the absent HDL fraction, premature atherosclerosis is not considered to be a complication of Tangier disease.

Inheritance and incidence

The disease is transmitted in an autosomally recessive manner. All the symptoms so far described are therefore typical of the homozygous subject. It is extremely rare, and approximately 90% of cases so far described are of Caucasian origin. It is possible that the disease may be more common than it would seem from the small number of cases so far described, since often the symptoms may be mild and may therefore pass unnoticed. The only prominent clinical sign is the enlarged orange tonsil.

Molecular defect and metabolic disorder

It is not known for certain what is the primary cause of the HDL deficiency in Tangier disease. Assmann and his co-workers believe that there may be a structural defect in apo AI. There is a small amount of precursor protein resembling pro-apo AI in the HDL infranatant (d > 1.21 g/ml) after ultracentrifugation. This protein is indistinguishable from the pro-apo AI of normal subjects. It is possible then that there may be a defect in the proteolysis of pro-apo AI, leading to the absence of apo AI in Tangier plasma. Infusion of labelled normal apo AI and apo AII into Tangier patients has yielded conflicting results. Although the catabolic rate is much greater than normal, it is not clear whether the infused apoproteins can combine to form normal HDL in Tangier subjects.

Zannis and his group have suggested there may be an inability to convert secreted apo AI into the mature plasma form.

Investigation

In the few cases where tonsil changes are not present, differential diagnosis is sometimes necessary to distinguish Tangier disease from, for example, chronic liver disease, biliary cirrhosis, lipid or mucopolysaccharide storage diseases, hypo- and hyperlipoproteinaemias and LCAT deficiency. This can be effectively achieved by histology of liver biopsies or rectal mucosa and by measurement of HDL.

Treatment

No specific treatment is possible. Infusion of normal HDL offers no solution as the half-life of HDL is drastically reduced, and normal apolipoproteins may not be re-incorporated into Tangier HDL.

Partial alleviation of symptoms is possible by introducing a low-cholesterol diet, thereby reducing the storage of dietary cholesterol as cholesteryl esters. A low fat diet is unnecessary as fat transport appears to be normal. If haemolytic anaemia is present, a low carbohydrate diet will reduce the possibility of increased red cell fragility. As diabetes mellitus may develop in old age, weight control is advisable from an early stage.

Hypoalphalipoproteinaemia

This is a rare and heterogeneous condition which includes patients heterozygous for Tangier disease. The clinical symptoms of Tangier disease are not apparent. Biochemically levels of HDL are approximately half those of normal subjects and the ratio of apo AI to apo AII is normal. Diagnosis must be confirmed by exclusion of other causes, e.g. obesity, diabetes mellitus, hypertriglyceridaemia, and by detection of the condition in other family members.

Variants of apoprotein AI

Structural variants of apoprotein AI have been detected by the technique of isoelectric focusing. The clinical implication of such structural differences is not apparent as in some cases, e.g. apo AI Marburg and apo AI Munster, there is no functional difference from normal, but in others e.g. apo AI Milano, there is a marked reduction of HDL level, but giving none of the clinical symptoms of Tangier disease.

It is likely that isoelectric focusing will reveal many such structural variants though their clinical manifestations may be difficult to assess.

Apoproteins AI and CIII deficiency

This is a condition recently described which is symptomatically distinct from Tangier disease, presenting with severe premature arterial disease, skin and tendon xanthomas, and corneal cloudiness. HDL levels are very low, but LDL is higher than in Tangier disease and apo AI and apo CIII levels are very low.

The molecular defects involve a DNA insertion in the apo AI gene, and alteration in the apo CIII gene, which are very close to each other and coded for by opposite DNA strands.

Fish-eye disease

This very rare condition, where the eyes resemble those of 'boiled fish' was first described in 1979. The clinical symptoms are dense corneal opacity with marked visual impairment, in contrast to Tangier disease, and atherosclerosis in old age.

Biochemically there is a 90% reduction in plasma HDL-cholesterol, but with normal amounts of total cholesterol. Hypertriglyceridaemia, particularly in the LDL fraction of plasma, is apparent. LCAT and cholesteryl ester levels appear to be normal, in contrast to LCAT deficiency. Apoproteins AI and AII are reduced to approximately 15 and 10% of normal values respectively.

DEFECTS INVOLVING APOPROTEINS—APOPROTEIN B

Abetalipoproteinaemia

This disorder was first described by Bassen and Kornzweig in 1950.

Clinical symptoms

Fat malabsorption is present from birth. Jejunal biopsy reveals normal villi in contrast to coeliac disease. Effects which occur secondarily to malabsorption e.g. anaemia, occur in some children but they can be easily treated.

Biochemical signs

There is a marked plasma hypocholesterolaemia (0.6–3 mmol/l) characterised by a lack of all apo B-containing lipoproteins (chylomicrons, VLDL, LDL) both in plasma and in intestinal mucosa, the synthesis site of chylomicrons. Plasma triglyceride levels are also characteristically low, usually less than 0.4 mmol/l. The remaining plasma lipids and apoproteins are carried exclusively by the HDL fraction which is present in about half the normal concentration. Apo AI and apo AII are reduced to 40% of normal levels and apo CIII-1 is absent. The phospholipid fraction of HDL is grossly abnormal. The lecithin: sphingomyelin ratio is much reduced and the fatty acid composition of these phospholipids is abnormal.

Inheritance and incidence

This very rare disease is inherited in an autosomally recessive manner. The obligate heterozygotes are unaffected clinically and their lipid profile is not grossly abnormal. Abetalipoproteinaemia has been reported from several countries though 23% are of Jewish extraction. Although 71% of affected subjects are males, a sex linkage has not been proven. Family studies show that consanguinity is present in about half the reported cases.

Molecular defect and metabolic disorder

The classical feature of this disease is the complete lack of apoprotein B (both apo B48 and apo B100) in both plasma and intestinal mucosa. It is possible that the gene coding for apoprotein B is defective.

Cholesterol-feeding experiments in abetalipoproteinaemia have shown that cholesterol absorption is negligible although sterol excretion is high and bile acid synthesis normal. Whole body synthesis of cholesterol is however higher than normal, in all probability as a compensatory mechanism for the malabsorption. Diagnosis of abetalipoproteinaemia is dependent on the demonstration of the absence of apoprotein B in plasma by immunoassay.

Treatment

In order to counteract the gastrointestinal symptoms a low fat diet is recommended. There is controversy over the use of medium-chain triglycerides as an alternative calorie source. Supplements of the fat-soluble vitamins A and K are necessary and pharmacologic doses of vitamin E are now thought to be important for correction of some retinal and neuromuscular abnormalities.

Hypobetalipoproteinaemia

The homozygous form of this disease is clinically and biochemically indistinguishable from abetalipoproteinaemia. However, this variant is incompletely recessive. Heterozygotes have reduced levels of plasma LDL, occasionally overlapping the normal range, and may have mild clinical signs and symptoms.

Treatment of the heterozygous form is unnecessary, but the homozygote requires similar dietary manipulations to those used for abetalipoproteinaemia.

Normotriglyceridaemic abetalipoproteinaemia

This condition is very rare and represents a variant of classical abetalipoproteinaemia.

The clinical symptoms of the disease are always milder than in typical abetalipoproteinaemia. Biochemically only apo B100 is absent, which means that chylomicron synthesis can take place, though VLDL and LDL are absent. This confirms that apo B48 and apo B100 are under separate genetic control and that chylomicron apo B48 is not a precursor of LDL apoprotein B100. The mode of inheritance is unknown.

DEFECTS INVOLVING APOPROTEINS—APOPROTEIN CII

Apoprotein CII deficiency

This recently discovered disorder bears some similarities to lipoprotein lipase deficiency and presents with the Type V phenotype.

Clinical symptoms

There is gross plasma lipaemia from an early age, which is often accompanied by lipaemia retinalis, haemolytic anaemia and bouts of acute abdominal pain due to pancreatitis. Red cell survival is reduced and diabetes mellitus often develops, which may or may not be insulin-dependent. Despite diabetic control, the lipaemia persists. In the few cases so far described, there is apparently no detectable xanthomata or hepatomegaly, in contrast to lipoprotein lipase deficiency. Information on potential clinical complications is necessarily sparse.

Biochemical signs

Massive hypertriglyceridaemia results from the presence of chylomicrons and elevated levels of VLDL. Polyacrylamide gel electrophoresis, or isoelectric focusing, of VLDL proteins reveals a complete absence of apo CII, which is confirmed by immunological tests. The triglyceride-rich lipoproteins from patients will not activate normal lipoprotein lipase, but addition of apo CII by infusion of normal plasma will cause a temporary clearance of lipaemia.

Inheritance and incidence

The disease in inherited in an autosomally recessive fashion. Heterozygotes, with 30–50% of normal levels of apo CII, show effective clearing of lipaemia. The number of subjects so far described is very small.

Molecular defect and metabolic disorder

The absence of apoprotein CII from the plasma of subjects with this disorder can almost certainly be traced to a defect in the gene coding for the synthesis of apo CII. A preliminary analysis of the gene has been carried out recently.[12] Studies on fragments of the apo CII molecule have revealed that a short section of the polypeptide chain (amino acids 55–78) is necessary for complete activation of lipoprotein lipase. The use of such fragments obtained synthetically may have therapeutic value. Clearance of lipaemia can be effected by the addition of as little as 10% of the normal level of apo CII, even in homozygotes.

Treatment

The only suggested treatment to date is a low-fat diet, to alleviate the pancreatitis. Generally, subjects live well into middle-age in spite of the gross hypertriglyceridaemia.

DEFECTS INVOLVING APOPROTEINS—APOPROTEIN E

Apoprotein E exists in three different isoforms, apo E2, E3 and E4 which are controlled by three alleles at a single genetic locus, thus giving expression to six phenotypes, three homozygous and three heterozygous.[13] Apo E3 and apo E4 are considered to be 'normal' apo E isoforms, and apo E2 'abnormal'.

Apoprotein E-2 homozygosity

1% of the population is homozygous for apo E2 and 1–2% of those present with overt Type III hyperlipoproteinaemia.

Clinical symptoms

The Type III phenotype normally presents with coronary heart disease, peripheral arterial disease, intermittent claudication, xanthomatosis (characteristically yellowish lipid deposits in the palmar creases) and tuberoeruptive xanthomas on the elbows. Other forms of xanthomata and corneal arcus are much less common. Approximately half the subjects have hyperuricaemia and abnormal glucose tolerance.

Biochemical signs

The dysbetalipoproteinaemia which usually accompanies apo E2 homozygosity is characterised by the presence of abnormal cholesterol-rich VLDL showing a broad, β-migrating band on electrophoresis. Ratios of

VLDL cholesterol to total triglyceride greater than 0.69 (SI units) or VLDL cholesterol to VLDL triglyceride over 0.97 are both very good indicators of the condition. The best criterion, however, is apo E2 homozygosity in association with the clinical findings.

Inheritance and incidence

The mode of inheritance of Type III hyperlipoproteinaemia is still not clear though the evidence suggests autosomally dominant transmission. Apo E2 homozygosity exists in about 1% of the population though most of those do not progress to the classical Type III phenotype which probably requires the presence of additional genetic factors producing hyperlipidaemia, or secondary diseases which have the same effect.

Molecular defect and metabolic disorder

The accumulation of β-VLDL in the plasma, characteristic of dysbeta-lipoproteinaemia and Type III hyperlipoproteinaemia is due to defective removal of chylomicron remnants and IDL. The reason for this lies in the primary structure of the apo E. It is thought that the three alleles arise from point mutations in the structural gene for apo E. Amino-acid interchanges take place at two positions in the peptide chain. Thus in apo E2, two cysteine residues occur at these positions, in apo E3, one cysteine and one arginine, and in apo E4, two arginine residues. Apo E2 binds much less avidly to the hepatic remnant receptor than either apo E3 or E4. Remnants are not removed from the circulation for catabolism and therefore accumulate. The defective binding is caused by the cysteine. If lysine is substituted binding is increased.

Diagnosis and treatment

Apo E2 homozygosity can only be demonstrated by isoelectric focusing of the VLDL proteins. The Type III phenotype can be confirmed by the clinical findings (particularly the palmar crease xanthomas) coupled with demonstration of the presence of β-VLDL. Type III hyperlipoproteinaemia responds well to dietary modification. Fat restriction with a high polyunsaturated content, low cholesterol and low alcohol will all be beneficial. Lipid-lowering drugs (excluding cholestyramine) are usually effective. Cholesterol and triglyceride levels will possibly normalise, but β-VLDL will always persist.

Other aberrations of apoprotein E

In Type V hyperlipoproteinaemia, there is often an increased abundance of individuals with apo E4 (53% of subjects compared with 15% in the normal population). It is possible that other genetic disturbances may be required for the full manifestation of the hypertriglyceridaemia character-istic of Type V.

Complete absence of apoprotein E has been shown in one kindred. The clinical picture is that of Type III hyperlipoproteinaemia i.e. β-VLDL is present due to impaired hepatic removal of remnant particles.

DEFECTS OF RECEPTOR FUNCTION—LDL RECEPTOR

Familial hypercholesterolaemia

In Fredrickson's classification, this is expressed as the Type IIa phenotype. There is a characteristic elevation of cholesterol concentration in the LDL (β) fraction of serum.

Clinical symptoms

Hypercholesterolaemia is evident within the first decade of life. The more frequently found heterozygotes present with arcus corneae and xanthomas during the second decade and clinical coronary heart disease is shown by the fourth decade. Homozygotes have similar symptoms much earlier and death usually ensues before the age of 30 years. Yellow/orange cutaneous xanthomas may be present even at birth, and certainly by the fourth year. Tendon xanthomas and arcus accompanied by generalised atheroma are present during childhood. Coronary, cerebral and peripheral vessels are all affected, and infiltration of the aortic valve is common.

Biochemical signs

There is a specific elevation of LDL-cholesterol which causes the total serum cholesterol concentration to be greater than 9 mmol/l in hetero-zygotes and 15 mmol/l in homozygotes. LDL-cholesterol is twice the normal level in heterozygotes and approximately six times normal in homo-zygotes. There is no apparent abnormality in composition or structure of the LDL. Thus LDL obtained from a homozygote is metabolised normally when injected into a normal individual, and it will suppress the activity of the major cholesterol synthesising enzyme HMG CoA reductase just as normal LDL would.

Inheritance and incidence

Familial hypercholesterolaemia is transmitted in an autosomally dominant manner by a single mutant allele. The rare homozygote is affected much more severely than the heterozygote. The gene is highly penetrant: over 90% of all carriers have LDL cholesterol concentrations greater than the

95 percentile value of the normal population. The gene frequency has been calculated at 1:500 in Caucasians in U.S.A., and as high as 1:200 in London where approximately one person per million is homozygous. The premature death of undiagnosed individuals might explain the small number of homozygotes found in relation to the gene frequency. Thus it is among the most common of the simply inherited human genetic disorders.

Molecular defect and metabolic disorder

The molecular defect in familial hypercholesterolaemia has been described in detail by Goldstein and Brown.[14] There is an absence or deficiency of the high affinity receptor for LDL on the liver or peripheral cell surface. In the extreme case of homozygotes, the so called receptor-negative subjects, there is a total absence of receptor function. Thus the binding and internalisation of LDL is prevented. There is no suppression of HMG CoA reductase or activation of intracellular cholesterol esterification. Catabolism of LDL therefore does not occur, leading to massive build-up in plasma and to deposition in the arterial wall, producing premature atherosclerosis.

The receptor-deficient heterozygotes have approximately half the normal number of receptors and consequently half their normal function. Thus the accumulation of LDL is not so severe as in the homozygotes.

In a third, much rarer, sub-group, binding takes place but there is no internalisation, thus all the characteristics of the homozygous receptor-negative syndrome exist.

Diagnosis

The homozygous form of familial hypercholesterolaemia is characterised by plasma cholesterol levels in excess of 15 mmol/l. Cutaneous xanthomas and juvenile atherosclerosis are present from an early age. In the heterozygote, it is important to establish the cause of the hypercholesterolaemia, which is usually greater than 9 mmol/l, as hyperbetalipoproteinaemia (raised LDL-cholesterol levels). Tendon xanthomas are usually present and family studies should show vertical transmission of hypercholesterolaemia and xanthomatosis. Many young heterozygotes have no tendon xanthomas but do have hypercholesterolaemia; in fact it is important to note that only about 1 patient in 20 with hypercholesterolaemia has the heterozygous familial type. In many symptomatic patients the disease is multifactorial in origin and polygenic in inheritance.

Neonatal diagnosis is possible by measuring the LDL-cholesterol level in the cord blood of babies born to parents who are known to carry the hypercholesterolaemia gene.[15] General screening is not informative, as most babies with raised LDL-cholesterol level do not have familial hypercholesterolaemia.

Prenatal diagnosis of homozygotes is possible since normal amniotic fluid cells have LDL-receptor function.[16]

Treatment

It has recently been shown that administration of the bile-acid binding resin cholestyramine actually stimulates the synthesis of the high-affinity LDL receptor. This allows more LDL to be internalised and metabolised. Thus plasma levels are kept under more strict control. Similarly promising work on the inhibition of cholesterol synthesis using compactin or mevinolin has shown that LDL-cholesterol levels can be significantly reduced in heterozygotes.[17]

In receptor-negative homozygous familial hypercholesterolaemia, receptor synthesis cannot be stimulated. Dietary treatment of all types of hyper-cholesterolaemia consists of reduction of cholesterol intake (300 mg/24 h in adults or 150 mg/24 h in children), and an increase in the polyunsaturated/saturated fat ratio. This should produce a slight fall in plasma cholesterol level which, in heterozygotes, may be enhanced by the use of the anion exchange resins cholestyramine or colestipol, to bind bile salts in the intestinal lumen and thus increase the excretion of cholesterol. The addition of nicotinic acid may be helpful.[18]

More drastic treatment of the homozygous form has been used. For example, a portocaval shunt has been carried out with some success and in heterozygotes a partial ilial by-pass has been shown to have comparable success to cholestyramine therapy. Plasmapheresis on a twice weekly basis has been shown to be effective in some cases.[19]

DEFECTS OF RECEPTOR FUNCTION—REMNANT RECEPTOR

It seems probable that the hepatic remnant receptor specifically removes IDL and chylomicron remnants by recognition of apo B48 and apo E. A deficiency in this receptor will therefore lead to a marked increase in triglyceride-rich remnant particles and a clinical picture characteristic of Type III hyperlipoproteinaemia.

The same effect is produced by a deficiency in hepatic lipase, an enzyme which has many similar properties to lipoprotein lipase, though not requiring a protein cofactor.

DEFECTS INVOLVING ENZYME FUNCTION

Lipoprotein lipase deficiency

This rare disease, first described in 1939, exhibits the Fredrickson Type I phenotype and is characterised by pronounced fasting chylomicronaemia.

Clinical symptoms

The disease usually presents in childhood and is often accompanied by pain in the epigastrium or mid-abdominal region. There is massive chylomicronaemia due to deficient fat absorption. About half the patients have papulo-eruptive xanthomas in skin creases or pressure areas. Foam cells are present in bone marrow, spleen and liver, and hepatosplenomegaly is frequent, particularly in periods of high fat intake. The liver and spleen may be tender and pancreatitis is often present.

Lipaemia retinalis accompanies the severe chylomicronaemia. Glucose tolerance is normal, in contrast to many other hypertriglyceridaemias. There is no apparent tendency for premature atherosclerosis.

Biochemical signs

Dietary chylomicrons persist even in the fasting state due to the lack, or severe deficiency, of lipoprotein lipase in extrahepatic tissues. Levels of apo CII, the co-factor required for the full activity of the lipase, are normal. In apo CII deficiency, which can also be expressed as the Type I phenotype, there is a normal level of lipoprotein lipase but with inefficient activation.

Inheritance and incidence

The disease has an autosomal recessive inheritance and heterozygotes are indistinguishable from normal. It is very rare and has been found in Caucasians, Chinese and Negroes.

Molecular defect and metabolic disorder

The reason for the low or absent lipoprotein lipase activity on the capillary endothelium is not clear.

Diagnosis and treatment

On a regular diet, there is marked fasting chylomicronaemia. Standing plasma overnight in a refrigerator characteristically produces a creamy layer over a clear plasma. Serum triglycerides can reach levels of 20 mmol/l or more due solely to the presence of chylomicrons. Cholesterol levels are usually normal except in very severe cases of hypertriglyceridaemia. LDL and HDL levels are usually slightly reduced and remain so, even on treatment.

A diet very low in fat (40–60 g/24 h) is usually recommended; if calorie supplementation is needed, medium chain triglycerides may be effective since they are absorbed directly into the portal circulation, without chylomicron synthesis.

Severe hypertriglyceridaemia with an apparent Type I pattern will often arise secondarily to other disease e.g. pancreatitis, uncontrolled diabetes mellitus, paraproteinaemia etc. but will always disappear on treatment of the primary cause.

Lecithin cholesterol acyltransferase deficiency

The deficiency of this enzyme, which is responsible for cholesterol esterification in plasma, was first recognised in 1966 in western Norway. It is rare, having been described in only seven families.

Clinical symptoms

The earliest sign is proteinuria at 3–4 years followed by corneal opacity at puberty. Haemolytic anaemia is normally present in the third decade. Hyperlipidaemia is characteristic and eventually renal failure ensues. There is usually evidence of early atherosclerosis. Foam cells are present in the bone marrow though platelets are normal.

Biochemical signs

Elevations in total plasma cholesterol and triglycerides are usual. The ratio of cholesteryl ester to free cholesterol is invariably low. Since one of the substrates of this enzyme is lecithin, plasma levels of the phospholipid are elevated. Levels of lysolecithin are correspondingly reduced.

In spite of hypertriglyceridaemia, there is no pre-β band on electrophoresis, the VLDL migrating as β-VLDL. All the lipoproteins are very heterogenous: thus both the LDL and HDL particles contain a high proportion of disc-like particles and the HDL concentration is only one third of the normal level. 75% of the total plasma apo AI (which is usually found in HDL) appears in the fraction of density greater than 1.21 g/ml. This may be a reflection of the unstable nature of the HDL fraction, which is disrupted by ultracentrifugation.

Molecular defect and metabolic disorder

All the biochemical features of this disease are caused by the lack or severe deficiency of LCAT, which normally esterifies free cholesterol in plasma. At the same time lecithin is not converted to lysolecithin. The lack of this enzyme therefore prevents the lipoprotein-maturing process which accompanies cholesterol esterification. The normal spherical lipoprotein particles are not produced.

Inheritance and incidence

LCAT deficiency is probably inherited recessively and it appears to be caused by a single gene defect. In western Norway the gene frequency is 2%, but few cases have been described elsewhere.

Treatment

Dietary fat restriction will reduce elevated levels of LDL and may prevent kidney damage. Renal transplantation has been done, but without effect on LCAT activity.

Cholesterol ester hydrolase deficiency

The deficiency of acid cholesterol ester hydrolase (EC 3.1.1.13) (see Fig. 10.2) results in two diseases which differ clinically only in degree. Wolman's disease, first described in 1956, is considerably more severe, being invariably fatal within months of birth. Cholesterol ester storage disease (CESD) is a more benign form of Wolman's disease and can be detected in adulthood.

Clinical symptoms

Both diseases show massive accumulation of lysosomal cholesterol esters and triglycerides. Wolman's disease presents very early with gastrointestinal symptoms, steatorrhea and hepatosplenomegaly. There is marked adrenal calcification and tissue lipid storage which is characteristic. Anaemia develops within six weeks of birth and increases in severity. Foam cells are present in the bone marrow.

The clinical symptoms in CESD are less pronounced than in Wolman's disease. Hepatomegaly occurs with occasional splenomegaly, oesophageal varices and hepatic fibrosis. Premature atherosclerosis is likely.

Biochemical signs

In Wolman's disease, the plasma cholesterol and triglyceride levels are often normal. Liver lipids however show an elevated level of cholesterol esters.

Inheritance and incidence

Both diseases are probably autosomally recessive in inheritance and rare. There is an unexplained preponderance of females with CESD. Wolman heterozygotes can be detected by assay of the enzyme acid cholesteryl ester hydrolase in cultured fibroblasts.

Molecular defect and metabolic disorder

The major defect is a marked decrease in activity of acid cholesteryl ester hydrolase in several cells, notably Kupffer cells, liver and spleen macrophages, leucocytes, lymphocytes and fibroblasts. Thus all these cells accumulate large quantities of cholesteryl esters and triglycerides. The enzyme plays a crucial role in the intracellular catabolism of LDL. It is thought that Wolman's disease and CESD are two allelic disorders involving mutations at the gene locus for the hydrolase.

Diagnosis and treatment

Wolman's disease has characteristic hepatosplenomegaly accompanied by GI symptoms and failure to thrive. X-ray detection of adrenal calcification is strongly suggestive. Definitive diagnosis can be achieved by enzyme assay in cultured fibroblasts. The similar, though less severe, symptoms of CESD can be confirmed by enzyme assay in cultured cells. No therapy is known to be effective in either disease.

DISORDERS WITH UNKNOWN PRIMARY DEFECTS

Primary hypertriglyceridaemia

According to the degree of severity this disease may be expressed phenotypically as Type IV or Type V in the Fredrickson classification.

Clinical symptoms

In the milder Type IV phenotype, specific clinical features are few. Associations have been seen with obesity, impaired glucose tolerance, insulin resistance, hyperinsulinism and hyperuricaemia. Premature coronary heart disease may occur. Xanthomas are not normally seen. Confirmation of familial inheritance is necessary.

In Type V hyperlipoproteinaemia, when plasma triglyceride levels are grossly elevated, all of the aforementioned symptoms may be present, together with those features characteristic of chylomicronaemia, e.g. eruptive xanthomas, hepatosplenomegaly, abdominal pain (with or without pancreatitis), foam cells in the bone marrow and other organs. Type V rarely occurs in children, in contrast to Type I, and lipoprotein lipase activity is normal.

Both forms of primary hypertriglyceridaemia often occur secondarily to other stimuli e.g. diabetes mellitus, alcohol abuse, oral contraceptive usage.

Biochemical signs

Plasma levels of triglycerides are elevated moderately in Type IV and grossly in Type V hyperlipoproteinaemia. There is no clear cut-off point between the two, as chylomicronaemia may be induced in Type IV subjects by a high carbohydrate diet, or alcohol. Only VLDL is elevated in Type IV, but in Type V chylomicrons are present and LDL levels are characteristically low. In both disorders, HDL is reduced.

Inheritance and incidence

Primary hypertriglyceridaemia is autosomally dominantly transmitted though it is not expressed early in life. The Type IV heterozygote frequency according to the Seattle study is 1:100,[20] but the fully expressed Type V disease is very much rarer. Relatives of Type V subjects often have the Type IV phenotype.

Molecular defect and metabolic disorder

The defect in hypertriglyceridaemia is not clear. There may be overproduction, or inefficient catabolism, of triglyceride-rich lipoproteins. There is some evidence in support of both mechanisms. Recent work suggests that there is a reduced level of apo CIII-0 relative to apo CIII-1 and CIII-2 in Type V. The relevance of an increase in sialylated forms of apo CIII is obscure.

Diagnosis and treatment

Hypertriglyceridaemia is characteristic. In Type IV plasma triglyceride levels may reach 10 mmol/l with a mean of 5 mmol/l, caused by an increase in the VLDL fraction (or pre-β band on electrophoresis). This is only confirmed if family members are affected. The disease is often not expressed until the third decade.

The Type V phenotype has much higher levels of plasma triglyceride, usually greater than 11 mmol/l. Chylomicrons are present in addition to elevated levels of VLDL. Cholesterol levels may be slightly raised and it is sometimes necessary to use ultracentrifugation and electrophoresis to distinguish this disease from Type III hyperlipoproteinaemia. If the Type V pattern arises before the age of 20 years it is important to exclude lipoprotein lipase or apo CII deficiencies.

Carbohydrate restriction will reduce levels of VLDL and if chylomicrons are present fat restriction will be necessary. Effective drug therapy for Type IV uses clofibrate analogues, bezafibrate for example, and for Type V nicotinic acid, or its derivatives.

Combined hyperlipidaemia

This complex disease is expressed in the Fredrickson classification as Type IIb but patterns of lipid elevation vary greatly in affected members of the same family.

Clinical symptoms

The disease is often accompanied by an increased frequency of obesity, hyperinsulinaemia and abnormal glucose tolerance. Coronary heart disease is very common. Expression of the disease normally occurs in the third decade but 10–20% of affected children show elevated plasma lipid levels.

Biochemical signs

The disease is characterised by increased levels of both VLDL (pre-β) and LDL (β) fractions. Affected members of the same family may have elevations in either or both of these lipoproteins.

There is therefore a modest rise in both cholesterol and triglyceride levels.

Inheritance and incidence

The disease is thought to be transmitted in an autosomally dominant manner. The phenotype IIb is fairly common, occurring in about 3% of an apparently healthy London population.[21] In Seattle, 11% of the survivors of myocardial infarction aged under 60 years expressed the IIb phenotype. It is possible for the phenotypic expression to vary not only within a family but sometimes within an individual, when sampled on different occasions.

Molecular defect and metabolic disorder

Recent evidence suggests that the underlying defect may be the increased synthesis of apo B which results in overproduction of VLDL particles. This may be coupled with decreased catabolism of LDL. There appears to be no defect in LDL receptor function in Type IIb.

Diagnosis and treatment

In the true phenotype IIb both plasma cholesterol and triglycerides are modestly elevated, but the diagnosis is complete only if relatives are checked and found to include various types of hyperlipidaemia as described above.

Treatment for combined hyperlipidaemia is based on the normal regimes for reduction of plasma levels of cholesterol and triglycerides. Dietary modification, low cholesterol and high polyunsaturated fat, coupled if necessary with the use of clofibrate analogues, is often effective.

REFERENCES

1 Havel R J, Eder H A, Bragdon J H 1955 The distribution and chemical composition of ultracentrifugally separated lipoproteins in human serum. Journal of Clinical Investigation 34: 1345–1353
2 Burstein M, Legmann P 1982 Lipoprotein precipitation. Clarkson T B, Kritchevsky D, Pollak O J (eds) Monographs on atherosclerosis, Vol 11. Karger, Basel.

3 Neuback W, Wieland H, Habernicht A, Muller P, Baggio G, Seidel D 1977 Improved assessment of plasma lipoprotein patterns. III Direct measurement of lipoproteins after gel electrophoresis. Clinical Chemistry 23: 1269–1300

4 Ghiselli G, Gregg R E, Zech L A, Schaefer E J, Brewer H B Jr 1982 Phenotype study of apolipoprotein E isoforms in hyperlipoproteinaemia patients. Lancet ii: 405–407

5 Cheung A C, Albers J J 1977 The measurement of apolipoprotein AI and AII levels in men and women by immunoassay. Journal of Clinical Investigation 60: 43–50

6 Curry M D, Gustafson A, Alaupovic P, McConathy W J 1978 Electroimmunoassay, radioimmunoassay and radial immunodiffusion assay evaluated for quantification of human apolipoprotein B. Clinical Chemistry 24: 280–286

7 Durrington P N, Whitcher J T, Warren C, Bolton C H, Hartog M 1976 A comparison of methods for the immunoassay of serum apolipoprotein B in man. Clinica Chimica Acta 71: 95–108

8 Rosseneu M, Vercaemst R, Vinaimont M, Van Tornout P, Henderson L O, Herbert P N 1981 Quantitative determination of human plasma apolipoprotein AI by immunonephelometry. Clinical Chemistry 27: 856–859

9 Fredrickson D S, Levy R I, Lees R S 1969 Fat transport in lipoproteins—an integrated approach to mechanisms and disorders. New England Journal of Medicine 276: 34–44, 94–103, 148–156, 215–226, 273–281

10 Beaumont J L, Carlson L A, Cooper G R, Fefjar Z, Fredrickson D S, Strasser T 1970 Classification of hyperlipidaemias and hyperlipoproteinaemias. Bulletin of the World Health Organisation 43: 891–915

11 McKusick V A 1983 Mendelian inheritance in man, 6th edn. Johns Hopkins University Press, Baltimore

12 Fojo S S, Law S W, Sprecher D L, Gregg R E, Baggio G, Brewer H B Jr 1984 Analysis of the apo CII gene in apo CII deficient patients. Biochemical and Biophysical Research Communications 124: 308–314.

13 Zannis V I, Breslow J L, Utermann G et al 1982 Proposed nomenclature of apo E isoproteins, apo E genotypes, and phenotypes. Journal of Lipid Research 23: 911–914

14 Brown M S, Goldstein J L 1977 Familial hypercholesterolaemia: model for genetic receptor disease. Harvey Lectures 73: 163–201

15 Kwiterovitch P O, Levy R I, Fredrickson D S 1973 Neonatal diagnosis of familial Type II hyperlipoproteinaemia. Lancet i: 118–122

16 Goldstein J L, Harrod M J E, Brown M S 1974 Homozygous familial hypercholesterolaemia: specificity of the biochemical defect in cultured cells and feasibility of prenatal detection. American Journal of Human Genetics 26: 199–206

17 Goldstein J L, Brown M S 1982 Lipoprotein receptors: genetic defence against atherosclerosis. Clinical Research 30: 417–426

18 Kane J P, Malloy M J, Tun P et al 1981 Normalisation of low-density lipoprotein levels in heterozygous familial hypercholesterolaemia with a combined drug regime. New England Journal of Medicine 304: 251–258

19 Thompson G, Kilpatrick D, Oakley C, Steiner R, Myant N 1978 Reversal of cholesterol accumulation in familial hypercholesterolaemia by long-term plasma exchange. Circulation 58:Suppl II–71

20 Goldstein J L, Schrott H G, Hazzard W R, Bierman E L, Motulsky A G 1973 Hyperlipidemia in coronary heart disease. Genetic analysis of lipid levels in 176 families and delineation of a new genetic disorder, combined hyperlipidemia. Journal of Clinical Investigation 52: 1544–1568

21 Lewis B, Chait A, Wootton I D P et al 1974 Frequency of risk factors for ischaemic heart disease in a healthy British population. Lancet i: 141–146

11

P. J. Aggett

Metal disorders

INTRODUCTION

The metabolism of inorganic elements is influenced by their solubility and oxidation state at physiological conditions. Since anions are water soluble and are able also to cross lipid membranes easily, they are absorbed readily by the intestine and do not need any vascular transport proteins to mediate their systemic dispersal. This mobility means that the metabolic pathways for anionic elements are hard to regulate and their whole body homeostasis depends on their excretion and conservation by the kidneys. In contrast cations need carrier mechanisms to cross the cell membranes which they encounter during their absorption by the intestine and their uptake by tissues; additionally, since most metal cations (with the exceptions of sodium, potassium, and to a lesser extent of calcium and magnesium) are poorly soluble under physiological conditions they require specific transport proteins to carry them via the circulation to their respective uptake mechanisms in body tissues. Subsequently intracellular ligands impose a metabolic compartmentation which controls the transfer of metals to their functional sites and their sequestration in depots which may act either as stores, or as a means of preventing the tissue damage which unregulated accumulations of reactive metals (e.g. copper, iron, and zinc) can cause.

Such a sequence of mediated mechanisms for the absorption, transport, cellular uptake, storage, and excretion of cations has an overall selectivity which minimises competition between elements for their ultimate functional sites and provides a variety of stages at which homeostatic control can be achieved. For example, the absorption of customary dietary intakes of iron, and high intakes of zinc, are regulated by sequestration mechanisms in the intestinal mucosa; at normal dietary intakes of zinc homeostasis is achieved by resecretion of the metal into the intestinal lumen, and whole body homeostasis of copper is mediated by hepatobilary secretion of the element in a chemical form which is presumed to impede its reabsorption. The essential alkaline earth and alkali metals are soluble in body fluids and they are subject to renal homeostasis.

In man, inherited defects affecting the metabolism of iron, copper, zinc and magnesium have been described, as has a defect arising from impaired utilisation of molybdenum. Collectively these defects represent abnormalities of all the metabolic mechanisms outlined above.

IRON

Haem iron and inorganic iron are taken up by separate mechanisms from the intestinal lumen. Within the enterocyte haem oxygenase releases the haem iron which thereafter forms a common pool with its inorganic counterpart. The transfer of iron from the mucosa is controlled by the enterocytic protein apoferritin which binds and sequesters the metal as ferritin. This is lost into the intestinal lumen when the mucosal cell is desquamated. The mucosal content of apoferritin is regulated, possibly by the iron content of reticuloendothelial cells (monocytes and macrophages) in the lamnia propria. There may also be a homeostatic mechanism whereby endogenous iron is resecreted into the intestinal lumen.

After its transfer across the intestinal epithelium iron is incorporated, as the Fe (III) state, into the glycoprotein transferrin for transport in the circulation to tissues such as the liver and erythroid cells of the bone marrow. At these sites transferrin binds with receptors on the cell membranes, and either releases its iron immediately or, more probably, the entire complex is endocytosed and the iron is released intracellularly for incorporation into haem and apoproteins. The residual apotransferrin is recycled.

Normally adults contain 4–5 g of iron of which 0.5–1.0 g is stored intracellularly in the form of water soluble ferritin. Denaturation of ferritin by lysosomal enzymes produces the insoluble iron depot haemosiderin; many intermediate degradation products can exist and are particularly evident in tissues with chronic iron overload.

Hereditary (idiopathic) haemochromatosis (McKusick 23520)

In hereditary haemochromatosis an excessive amount, 20–40 g, of iron accumulates in the body causing extensive tissue damage.[1,2] The precise abnormality is not known, but the intestinal homeostasis of iron is ineffective and absorption of the metal is inappropriately high for the degree of iron overload: small intestinal mucosal biopsies from patients with hereditary haemochromatosis accumulate, in vitro, larger amounts of iron than do similar biopsies from patients with secondary iron overload. Furthermore, and again in contrast to individuals with secondary iron overload, the intestinal mucosa and the reticuloendothelial system of patients have a low content of iron and ferritin. These observations are consistent with the possible defect in idiopathic haemochromatosis being an impaired uptake of iron into the reticuloendothelial system with consequent impaired regulation of the intestinal transfer and uptake of iron. Pathogeneses of hereditary haemochromatosis based on abnormalities of transferrin and ferritin have been proposed but these seem unlikely, especially as genetic mapping has located the locus for the allele causing hereditary haemochromatosis on the short arm of chromosome 6 whereas those for transferrin and for the light protein subunits of ferritin are on chromosomes 3 and 19 respectively.

The defect is inherited as an autosomal recessive characteristic and there is a close linkage of the affected allele with the HLA.A locus on chromosome 6.[3] The gene frequency is approximately 1:20 of the population; any race can be affected although it is more common in whites of Celtic origin. In homozygotes there is a variable penetrance of the abnormality and nine times as many men as women present with the disease. This difference has been attributed to the protective loss of iron during menstruation and pregnancy.

Clinical features

Patients usually present between 40 and 60 years of age but presentations in children and in premenopausal women have been reported.

The increased body burden of iron becomes distributed in all organs and tissues except for the gut mucosa and reticuloendothelial system. At first the metal is accumulated in ferritin and then in haemosiderin within lysosomes. Subsequent degeneration of these vesicles releases acid hydrolases and iron, which cause cellular damage and degeneration. The onset of symptoms is insiduous and individuals may present with any combination of the features below:

Asymptomatic

Pigmentation (skin, lips, tongue, buccal mucosa, conjunctiva, scars, external genitalia)	(90%)
Loss of body hair, ichthyosis, dermal atrophy, Koilonychia	(50%)
Hepatomegaly	(95%)
Splenomegaly	(50%)
Jaundice	(10%)
Hepatocellular carcinoma, cholangiocarcinoma	(30%)
Anorexia, lethargy, malaise, confusion, weakness	(45%)
Vertigo, loss of auditory acuity, peripheral neuropathy, retinopathy	(15%)
Weight loss, vomiting	(45%)
Abdominal pain	(30%)
Chondrocalcinosis (knees), bone demineralisation	(25–75%)
Chronic arthropathy 2nd-3rd mcp joints and proximal interphalangeal joints	(30%)
Cardiomegaly	(20–30%)
Cardiomyopathy, ECG changes, dysrythmias, conduction abnormalities, cardiac failure, constrictive pericarditis	

| Diabetes mellitus | (60%) |
| Pituitary damage, testicular atrophy, gynaecomastia | (50%) |

Loss of libido, impotence, ammenorrhoea,
   hypoparathyroidism, adrenocortical insufficiency,
   hypothyroidism, low serum somatostatin,
   hypoprolactinaemia.

(The figures in parentheses indicate approximate percentage of patients in whom the features appear.)

Skin pigmentation is initially dusky brown and is due to increased melanin production which is more marked on scars, exposed skin, and the external genitalia. Later, as haemosiderin accumulates in the corium and vascular endothelium, and around the sweat glands, the skin becomes slate-grey.

The liver mass is increased and hepatocellular necrosis leads to variable clinical and biochemical indications of hepatic damage. Hepatic fibrosis may progress to frank cirrhosis, and the subsequent development of portal hypertension leads to an increase in the usually moderate degree of splenomegaly.

Chondrocalcinosis may arise from the inhibitory effect of iron on pyrophosphatase activity, as a result pyrophosphate is deposited in articular cartilage. The arthropathy of the hand differs from that of rheumatoid arthritis by the absence of ulnar deviation of the fingers.

Many patients have a low voltage ECG with ventricular ectopics, and sustained supraventricular tachycardias; the T waves may become flattened or inverted. Myocardial involvement can be a poor prognostic sign but some features including failure and angina pectoris frequently improve with adequate treatment. Echo-cardiography can provide evidence of the increased ventricular mass, end systolic and end diastolic diameters of secondary cardiomegaly. There is an increased susceptibility to cardiac arrythmias in alcoholic patients and during the initiation of treatment by phlebotomy.

Abdominal pain is a common phenomenon but no definitive cause may be found; identified precipitants include ascites, peptic ulceration, pancreatitis, cholecystitis, nephrolithiasis, and peritonitis.

Although iron deposits extensively damage the pancreatic acinar cells, exocrine pancreatic insufficiency is unusual. In contrast two thirds of cases have reduced secretion of insulin, and an impaired glucose tolerance which may be exacerbated by hepatic dysfunction. It is possible that a linkage of the HLA haplotypes with a susceptibility to insulin dependent diabetes mellitus may contribute partially to the incidence of this disorder in hereditary haemochromatosis. Other endocrine anomalies may arise from damage to the pituitary gland since the low circulating levels of gonadotrophins do not respond to exogenous releasing factors.

Older patients may have a risk as high as 1 in 3 of developing hepatocellular carcinoma; this risk is increased in patients with cirrhosis and is not reduced by subsequent venesection therapy.[2] Cholangiocarcinoma is much rarer, additionally patients with hereditary haemochromatosis may have an increased chance of developing neoplasia at other sites such as the rectum, bronchus, pancreas and gallbladder.[2] The development of malignancy is often heralded by weight loss, fever and a sudden fall in the plasma concentrations of iron and ferritin.

Diagnosis

Since the clinical manifestations of herediatary haemothromatosis are so protean, diagnosis depends on a high degree of suspiscion and on the thorough screening of asymptomatic relatives for the disorder. The most valuable laboratory investigations are those used to assess the body burden of iron. The serum iron concentration is elevated above the accepted reference range (10–25 μmol/l), in many cases to over 40 μmol/l. The serum transferrin is more than 60% saturated with a concomitant fall in iron binding capacity. Normally serum ferritin concentrations are less than 200 μg/l and 300 μg/l in women and men respectively; in untreated hereditary haemochromatosis the levels commonly exceed 1000 μg/l. Occasionally some ambiguity arises from elevations of serum ferritin and iron in patients with secondary iron overload or hepatic necrosis. Conversely complicating factors such as stress, infection and malignancy in patients with haemochromatosis may lower plasma iron concentrations into the physiological range. When investigating patients and screening their relatives these problems can often be avoided by repeating these investigations three times at weekly intervals. Another uncertainty may arise from the possible failure of hepatic or cardiac isoferritins to react with an immunoassay developed against splenic or placental ferritin. Consequently, early iron overload may occur without any increase in the immunodetectable serum ferritin. If any of these assessments of iron overload are abnormal a percutaneous needle biopsy of the liver should be taken for histological examination and determination of the iron content. The latter is usually less than 150 μg (2.7 μmol)/100 mg dry weight or 25 μg (0.45 μmol)/100 mg wet weight of liver, but is grossly elevated to more than 1000 μg/100 mg dry weight in hereditary haemochromatosis. Since the overload of iron increases with age an improved interpretation of the hepatic iron content can be achieved, especially in young adults, by an hepatic iron/age index.[4] On light microscopy the hepatic parenchyma shows periportal accumulation of iron with tissue damage, the Kupffer cells are spared.

Increasing experience with analyses of plasma, and hepatic biopsies, has reduced the need to use indirect means of assessing iron overload such as measuring the urinary iron excretion following administration of the chelator

Desferroxamine (e.g. a diagnostic threshold of 8 mg/24 h urine after 500 mg i.m. of the compound).[1] Determination of hepatic density by computerised axial tomography may be a useful way to assess the iron content of the liver if hepatic biopsy is precluded. The role of nuclear magnetic resonance in assessing the iron load of the liver has not been fully evaluated.

Other causes of iron overload (see below) can usually be distinguished by the clinical history and hepatic histology (e.g. whether or not the Kupffer cells are involved); and few produce the degree of overload seen in an untreated patient with idiopathic haemochromatosis.

The causes of iron overload are:

1. Idiopathic or hereditary haemochromatosis

2. Secondary iron overload
   a. Alcoholic liver disease and cirrhosis
   b. Fermented beverages with high iron content (Bantu siderosis)
   c. Ingestion of medicinal iron
   d. Post portacaval anastomosis
   e. Chronic anaemia
      (i) transfusion overload
      (ii) ineffective erythropoiesis
      (iii) sideroblastic anaemias
      (iv) thalassaemia major, sickle cell anaemia
      (v) other haemolytic anaemias, hypoplastic anaemias
   f. Porphyria cutanea tarda
   g. Transferrin deficiency

Screening

Once a case has been diagnosed, heterozygotes and other homozygotes should be sought amongst as many relatives as possible including uncles, aunts and cousins. Initially the serum iron, transferrin and iron binding capacity, and serum ferritin should be assayed. Since one or other of these values are elevated in a quarter of heterozygotes as well as in homozygotes, determining the HLA haplotypes of the proband and the family pedigree is of considerable value in planning further investigations such as liver biopsy.[3] If a relative has no haplotype in common with the patient's then their risk of being homozygous for idiopathic haemochromatosis is very small, there is a greater chance that relatives who share a single A or B type with the index case are heterozygous, whereas it is highly likely that those with both A and B types in common with the index case are homozygous for the haemochromatosis gene.[3] There is no known effective screening procedure for the general population.

Treatment

The cornerstone of treatment is to reduce the body burden of iron and to minimise acute iron toxicity. The most effective therapy is phlebotomy; about 200–250 mg of iron would be lost with 250 ml of blood. This volume of blood can be withdrawn twice weekly and should therefore reduce the iron overload by 20–25 g a year. Since most patients have an estimated overload of about 40 g of iron this treatment would be needed regularly for two years. However the frequency of venesection may have to be curtailed if the patient develops cardiac failure, which may be induced by hypovolaemia and anaemia, or arrythmias. During initial therapy mobilisation of iron may exacerbate cardiac dysrythmias, this hazard can be minimised by simultaneous administration of chelators such as desferroxamine (4–8 mg slowly i.v. per 24 hours)[1] or calcium diethylene triamine pentaacetate (DTPA). Although these agents are useful in the management of secondary iron overload they are unsuitable for routine treatment in hereditary haemachromatosis because they cannot match the loss of iron induced by phlebotomy and they have the inconvenience of needing to be given parenterally.

The haemoglobin concentration falls after regular venesection is started; it may then increase again. With adequate treatment the plasma iron and ferritin fall gradually and achieve normal levels when the overload has been removed. Serial determinations of haemoglobin to ascertain tolerance of the blood loss, and of serum iron and ferritin to assess residual iron overload, are suitable monitors of treatment. A haemoglobin of 10–11 g/dl, a serum iron of 10 μmol/l and a serum ferritin less than 200 μg/l, are indications that the iron burden is adequately reduced and for stopping frequent phlebotomy; the frequency of subsequent phlebotomies is adjusted to maintain these iron and ferritin values. Most patients need six or less venesections annually.

Phlebotomy considerably improves the prognosis and life expectancy in idiopathic haemochromatosis,[1,2] before its introduction most patients died from diabetes mellitus. However, although phlebotomy improves glucose tolerance in almost half of patients, hepatic fibrosis and portal hypertension, hypogonadism, and arthropathy persist despite treatment, persistent cardiomyopathy and hepatic dysfunction indicate a poor prognosis. The risk of malignancy was mentioned earlier.

Idiopathic neonatal iron storage disease (McKusick 23110)

In this rare condition increased lysosomal storage of iron and resultant tissue and organ damage occur in a similar pattern to haemochromatosis.[5] The liver is the most severely affected organ, and biochemical evidence of gross iron overload is present. Affected children die by 4 months of age.

Congenital atransferrinaemia (McKusick 20930)

This very rare entity appears to be inherited as an autosomal recessive defect.[6] Patients present in early childhood with a hypochromic microcytic and iron resistant anaemia, a low serum iron with a low iron binding concentration caused by a very low or absent serum transferrin.

These children also have a systemic iron overload which spares the bone marrow. It is not clear if this overload arises from dietary iron or from that administered in blood transfusions. Intravenous infusions of human transferrin can be beneficial but there are no reports on their extended use.

Other causes of hypotransferrinaemia such as infection, nephrotic syndrome, protein losing enteropathies, hepatic disease and malignancy can be excluded easily. A similar syndrome arises in autoimmune atransferrinaemia[7] but in this condition gross secondary haemochromatosis is associated with an increased total iron binding capacity secondary to the incorporation of iron in a circulating immune-complex of transferrin.

Impaired uptake of iron by reticuloendothelial cells (McKusick 20610)

In a brother and sister an iron resistant hypochromic microcytic anaemia was associated with a high plasma iron concentration and a saturated transferrin or iron binding capacity.[8] Whereas the hepatocytes were laden with iron the liver and bone marrow reticuloendothelial cells had none. These manifestations may be caused by impaired translocation of iron into the reticuloendothelial cells secondary to a defect in either the binding of transferrin to the cell membrane receptors or the subsequent translocation of the iron into the cells. An acquired analogous defect with an autoimmune aetiology has been reported in an adult woman.[9]

COPPER

The daily dietary intake of copper in adults is between 1 and 5 mg. Following its intestinal absorption the metal is transported in the portal circulation bound to albumin, and, to a lesser extent, by free amino acids. These complexes are cleared rapidly by the liver which has a pivotal role in the metabolism of copper. There are at least three discrete hepatic pools of copper; one pool is that destined for homeostatic secretion in the bile, another comprises the newly synthesised glycoprotein caeruloplasmin and the third is a presumed hepatic store of copper. Additionally the liver may contain, as well as its cupro-enzymes, a pool of copper associated with a low molecular weight protein called metallothionein. Metallothionein is involved principally with the metabolism of zinc but copper can displace zinc from the protein. Caeruloplasmin is secreted into the systemic circulation where 90–95% of copper is in this form. Caeruloplasmin may have several physiological roles; its oxidase activity facilitates the incorporation of iron into transferrin, and may also serve as a plasma biogenic amine oxidase and as an anti-oxidant. In addition, since membrane receptors for the endocytosis of caeruloplasmin exist, and because the protein is able to donate copper to apoenzymes, it seems probable that caeruloplasmin has a specific transport role for the element. Some examples of cupro-enzyme activities are shown in Table 11.1.

Table 11.1 Copper dependent enzyme activities

Enzyme	Activity
Amine oxidases	Amine and polyamine oxidation
Cytochrome-c-oxidase	Mitochondrial oxidative phosphorylation
Dopamine-β-hydroxylase	Synthesis of catecholamines
Tyrosinase	Tyrosine → dopa → dopaquinone and melanin
Superoxide dismutase	Cytosolic antioxidant $ZO_2^- + H_2O \rightarrow H_2O_2 + O_2$
Lysyl oxidase (and related enzymes)	Condensation of amino acids → cross-linkages of elastin and collagen
Caeruloplasmin	Multiple oxidase activities, copper transport

Wilson's disease (hepato-lenticular degeneration, McKusick 27790)

This condition is a copper toxicosis arising from an excessive accumulation of the metal in the body. Initially this occurs in the liver, but then all other tissues become involved.[10] The, as yet uncharacterised, basic defect occurs in the liver and is associated simultaneously with impaired biliary secretion of copper and with defective incorporation of the metal into apocaeruloplasmin. The similarity of hepatic copper deposition in Wilson's disease with that in the neonate has stimulated the proposal that the fundamental error may be that of an altered controller gene which fails to switch the metabolism of copper in the fetus to that of extrauterine life. The true incidence of Wilson's disease is unknown but has been reported to vary between 1:200 000 and 1:30 000. This variability may occur because the diagnosis is so often missed.

Clinical features and pathogenesis

The onset of symptoms is variable, a chronic insidious presentation is well known but many of these patients have a history of transient icteric episodes which have been attributed to varieties of 'hepatitis'; and a sudden onset with haemolysis and hepatic and renal failure secondary to an acute release of free copper from the liver is often overlooked.[11] The factors which influence the release of non-caeruloplasmin bound copper from the liver are unknown but intercurrent infections or similar stresses may contribute. It is clearly important to consider Wilson's disease in anybody with recurrent jaundice or haemolysis.

The many features of Wilson's disease are shown below:

Asymptomatic
Hepatic
   transient hepatitis with intercurrent infections,
   subacute, acute or chronic hepatitis,
   cryptogenic cirrhosis,
   hepatosplenomegaly, portal hypertension, oesophageal varices,
   fulminant hepatic failure (encephalopathy)
Neurological
   clumsiness, deteriorating handwriting and school
   performance, ataxia, fine tremor,
   dysarthria, dysphagia, dystonia,
   spasticity, athetosis, muscle spasms,
   coarse flapping tremor at wrists and shoulders,
   peripheral neuropathy, epilepsy (partial or generalised),
   pseudo-bulbar palsy (death),
   'schizophrenia', fatuous drooling facies,
   non specific EEG abnormalities
Ophthalmic
   Kayser-Fleischer rings, sunflower cataract,
   strabismus, xerophthalmia,
   impaired visual accuity, pallor of disc, night blindness
Haematological
   acute haemolysis, haemolytic anaemia, thrombocytopenia,
   leucopenia, pancytopenia, coagulation defects, bruising,
   intravascular coagulation
Renal
   renal tubular acidosis, concentration defect,
   amino aciduria, phosphaturia, hypercalcuria, uricosuria,
   acute renal failure,
   renal stones
Skeletal
   osteoporosis, patchy osteosclerosis, osteophytes, cysts in
   long bones, spontaneous fractures, osteomalacia,
   chondrocalcinosis, osteoarthritis, chondromalacia patellae,
   osteochondritis dissecans, chondrocalcinosis
   arthritis, morning stiffness
Endocrine
   amenorrhoea, increased incidence of miscarriages,
   gynaecomastia
Abdominal pain, colic
Bacterial peritonitis
Blue lanulae of finger nails

40% of cases have hepatic features—such patients are usually, but not exclusively, children and young adults; 35% have neurological sequelae—

these are rare but not unknown before adolescence; 12% have endocrine or haematological complications; 10% have neuropsychiatric disease and may have been admitted to psychiatric care before the underlying disorder had been recognised. The insidious and protean manifestations of Wilson's disease are best emphasised by the aphorism attributed to Walshe that, 'there is no such thing as a typical patient with Wilson's disease'.

All patients have hepatic involvement irrespective of their initial presentation. The youngest reported age of presentation is 4 years, but hepatocellular damage has been detected in an asymptomatic one year old sibling of a known case.

In spite of the possible gross neurological disabilities the patients' intellect is relatively spared until late in the course of the disease and many have a distressing insight into their deterioration. The Kayser-Fleischer rings and sunflower cataracts are caused by the deposition of copper in Descemets membrane and beneath the lens capsule respectively; both may be detectable only by slit-lamp microscopic examination. The Kayser-Fleischer rings are brown-green discolorations which appear first at the upper limbus and then at the inferior limbus before they meet bi-laterally to encircle the cornea (Fig. 11.1). Rarely only one cornea may be affected. Patients with neurological involvement usually have Kayser-Fleischer rings but the converse is not true; furthermore these rings are absent in many patients

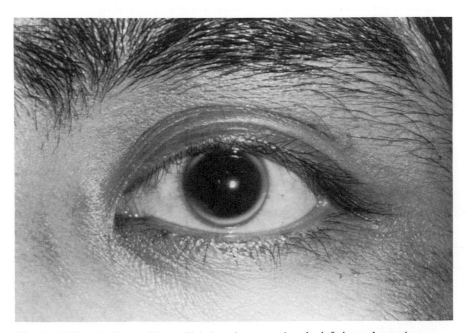

Fig. 11.1 Wilson's disease: Kayser-Fleischer ring; note that the inferior and superior depositions have met laterally but have not yet fused medially. Reproduced with permission of Department of Medical Illustration, University of Aberdeen.

with hepatic involvement, especially those who present with acute hepatic disease.

Laboratory findings

In most patients the plasma copper concentration is reduced below 10 μmol/l (reference range 10–25 μmol/l), and is accompanied by hypo-caeruloplasminaemia of less than 200 mg/l (reference range 300–400 mg/l). However, in 15% of cases the plasma caeruloplasmin may be in the lower end of the customary reference range. Sometimes subnormal caeuroplasmin concentrations in patients may be elevated into the lower reaches of the healthy range by factors such as pregnancy, ingestion of oestrogens and during the acute phase reaction to intercurrent infections or stress. Since in Wilson's disease much of the plasma pool of copper is not bound to caeruloplasmin the urinary excretion of copper is grossly elevated to over 100 μg in 24 hours compared with that seen in health of less than 50 μg/24 h.

Percutaneous needle biopsy of the liver is the essential investigation because it enables histological examination of the hepatic parenchyma and, more importantly, direct determination of the tissue content of copper. The histological changes are often nonspecific features of hepatocellular degener-ation with steatosis, glycogen deposition, ballooned nuclei and pleomorphic mitochondria, sometimes copper rich lipofuscin granules may be evident.[12] Piecemeal necrosis, diffuse fibrosis and micronudular cirrhosis can develop. The intracellular and lobular distribution of copper in Wilson's disease can differ from the more periportal distribution of copper overload seen in cholestatic syndromes and Indian childhood cirrhosis, but this difference is not sufficiently specific to aid diagnosis. Furthermore, in Wilson's disease, and especially in young patients, the copper is distributed diffusely in the hepatocytic cytoplasm and is rarely congregated with cytoplasmic and lysosomal granules; consequently, it may be undetectable histochemically, even though its concentration is excessive. This emphasises the need of an accurate determination of the copper content of the liver for diagnosis; usually in Wilson's disease the copper content exceeds 250 μg (3.9 μmol)/g dry weight compared with normal levels of less than 50 μg (0.8 μmol)/g dry weight.

A study of the hepatic uptake and resecretion of a radioisotope of copper (^{64}Cu or ^{67}Cu) will provide evidence of impaired caeruloplasmin synthesis by showing the failure of radio-copper to reappear in the plasma four to six hours after its administration[13] and is especially valuable when hepatic biopsy is contraindicated, or if a suspected patient does not have hypocaeruloplasminaemia.

In most instances the above investigations and the clinical picture enable the correct diagnosis to be made. Other causes of hypocaeruloplasminaemia such as malnutrition, malabsorption, protein losing enteropathies and proteinuria can be excluded easily. Secondary copper accumulation occurs in cholestasis, primary biliary cirrhosis, and chronic active hepatitis and other conditions which prevent the hepatobiliary excretion of copper. In many of these conditions, microscopically detectable Kayser-Fleischer rings may develop but, apart from Wilson's disease, macroscopic rings have only been reported in a monoclonal gammopathy. Neurological sequelae and basal ganglia lesions have developed in chronic cholestatic syndromes,[14] but in these instances plasma copper and caeruloplasmin concentrations are not depressed and the hypercupraemia and liver copper concentrations seldom approach those of Wilson's disease. If any doubt about the diagnosis remains, radiocopper studies would be helpful.[13] In Indian childhood cirrhosis hepatic copper levels are similar to those of Wilson's disease but these children have normal plasma levels of copper and caeruloplasmin.

One difficult differential diagnosis arises when Wilson's disease presents as fulminant hepatic failure with a rapid onset of icterus, encephalopathy, coagulopathy, renal failure and, as a result of hepatic necrosis, a serum copper which is within the normal range. In these circumstances, the serum caeruloplasmin is uninterpretable whatever its level. Although these patients will probably have a raised urinary copper, other features which should alert one to the possibility of Wilson's disease are the inappropriately small elevations, if any, in the serum aminotransferase and alkaline phosphatase activities.[11] Wilson's disease should also be considered in any patient with an occult encephalopathy.

Ancillary investigations will indicate the extent of deranged renal and hepatic function, should help establish the degree of involvement of the myocardium, skeleton, joints and other tissues and will exclude other possible diagnoses. Cerebral ventricular dilatation, cortical atrophy and degeneration of the basal ganglia can be assessed by computerised axial tomography which can also be used to monitor the resolution with therapy of the basal ganglia lesions.

Once a case has been identified all family members, including cousins, should be screened. The serum caeruloplasmin concentrations of the patient's unaffected parents (i.e. presumed heterozygotes) should indicate the serum caeruloplasmin concentrations to expect in the heterozygous members of the family. About 10% of heterozygotes have hypocaeruloplasminaemia and if anyone is found with a low caeruloplasmin concentration radio-copper studies or, more preferably, a hepatic biopsy for the determination of the hepatic copper content, or both, are needed to detect asymptomatic homozygotes.

Heterozygotes have been considered free of any risk of copper toxicosis but recently a number of heterozygous children have been reported to have hypocupraemia, hypocaeruloplasminaemia, non specific EEG abnormalities and an increased body burden of copper as evidenced by a cupruresis induced by D-penicillamine.[15]

Treatment

The life long treatment is aimed at reducing the amount of copper in the body and, if necessary, at preventing the toxic effects of free copper in the tissues and circulation. The most successful agent in this respect is the chelator D-penicillamine (dimethylcysteine)[16] in daily doses of 0.75–3 g given in three divided doses half an hour before meals. Side effects are less frequent with D-penicillamine than with the earlier mixed D and L-penicillamine preparations. If side effects do develop, the agent should be withdrawn and reintroduced in a reduced dosage; tolerance to gradually increasing doses can be improved by giving prednisolone simultaneously. Chelation therapy may induce pyridoxine deficiency and supplements of this vitamin should be given. D-penicillamine like many other chelators is non-specific and as effective de-coppering is achieved it will chelate other metals, and may, for example, induce zinc deficiency as the cupuresis diminishes. Normally, however, D-penicillamine therapy is reasonably safe and has been used throughout pregnancy.[17] If the more serious side effects of D-penicillamine preclude its continued use, alternative agents are the polyamine chelator trien (triethylene tetra amine)[16] and unithiol.

The efficacy and dosage of treatment can be assessed by monitoring the urinary excretion of copper,[15] which, as a rule of thumb, can be maintained at up to 5 mg of copper per day. Clinical resolution may be slow, neurological abnormalities may take up to two years to improve, but the eventual degree of resolution is frequently rewarding. Kayser-Fleischer rings disappear in the reverse sequence to their development. Hepatic cirrhosis and portal hypertension do not resolve, but hepatocellular carcinoma is rare; the resolution of other hepatic lesions can be monitored biochemically and by annual or appropriately frequent liver biopsies to check the histological appearance and the diminution of the copper content of the organ. With effective treatment the plasma caeruloplasmin and copper concentrations may actually increase, but not to within the physiological range.

The management of a presentation with acute copper toxicity is not easy. Approaches to reducing the free copper in the circulation need to be integrated with the management of any hepatic and renal failure and have included peritoneal dialysis with albumin or D-penicillamine added to the dialysate, intravenous infusions of albumin and plasma exchange. Haemodialysis is less useful. If such interventions and standard supportive treatment are unsuccessful in managing acute or fulminant hepatic failure then hepatic transplantation may have to be considered.[18]

Large oral doses of zinc (100 mg of elemental zinc per 24 hours) are also a potentially valuable adjunct to chelation therapy in Wilson's disease.[19] This has been attributed to the induction of metallothionein in the gut mucosa by zinc, which then sequesters copper and thereby blocks its absorption; but it is not known if oral zinc alone alters the defective metabolism of copper in Wilson's disease similarly.

Familial hypocaeruloplasminaemia (McKusick 14599)

An asymptomatic kindred with an autosomal recessive hypocaeruloplasminaemia (i.e. less than 21 mg/l or 23 mg/l in men and women respectively) has been reported[20] in which affected individuals also had low serum copper concentrations but a normal urinary excretion of copper and, most importantly, normal hepatic histology and content of copper.

Menkes' disease (Synonyms: Kinky hair disease, Trichopoliodystrophy McKusick 30940)

Menkes' disease is an X-linked recessive syndrome of overt copper deficiency in which systemic compartmentation of copper is grossly disturbed. The content of copper in the brain and liver is greatly reduced whereas that of the kidneys, spleen, pancreas, intestinal mucosa, lung, skin, muscle and, in utero, the placenta are elevated. Most of this excess copper is associated with metallothionein, but since the locus for this protein is on chromosome 16 this phenomenon is probably secondary to the basic inborn error of metabolism.

The role of copper in Menkes' disease[21] was first suspected because of the syndrome's similarity to symptomatic copper deficiency in sheep, and was then confirmed by the demonstration in affected boys of hypocupraemia, hypocaeruloplasminaemia and low hepatic copper concentrations. Although the intestinal absorption of copper is impaired by the retention of the metal in the intestinal mucosa, parenteral administration of copper has no significant therapeutic effect, even though it may increase circulating levels of caeruloplasmin. This does improve the uptake of copper by other tissues but there is a defect which impairs the subsequent incorporation of copper into cuproenzymes thereby creating a paradoxical condition of functional copper deficiency in organs which have an abundance of the element.

Clinical features and their pathogeneses[21,22]

The clinical features are summarised below:

Placid expressionless 'cherubic' face, frontal and occipital bossing, micrognathia, 'cupid's bow lip', gingival hyperplasia, high arched palate
Scalp, hair and eyebrows: sparse, depigmented, brittle stubbly hair—twisted on long axis (pili torti), irregular calibre (monilethrix), nodelike fracture points (trichorrhexis nodosa)
Pale skin, non-specific seborrhoeic dermatosis, skin laxity
Failure to thrive, dysphagia, hiatus hernia, oesophageal reflux, vomiting haematemesis, loose frequent stools, delayed eruption of teeth
Hypothermia, lethargy, apnoea
Arterial and venous tortuosity and dilatations, fragmentation of internal elastic lamina, subdural haematomata and intracranial haemorrhages
Developmental arrest and regression: hypotonia, spasticity with hyper-

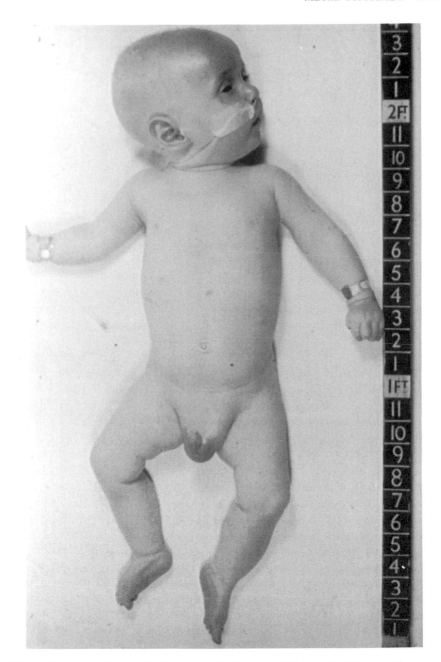

Fig. 11.2 Menkes' disease; this boy has typically abnormal hair, a placid facies and micrognathia. Note also the inguinal hernia, his hypotonic posture and the use of a nasogastric tube to manage the infant's poor feeding. Reproduced with permission of Dr J Wilson, Hospital for Sick Children, London

reflexia, focal and generalised epilepsy, retinal degeneration, optic atrophy, blindness, microcysts in pigment epithelium, cataracts
Inguinal herniae, undescended testes
Hydroureter and hydronephrosis, urinary reflux, bladder trabeculation and diverticulae
Skeletal anomalies: wormian bones in skull, periosteal thickening and scorbutic changes, (metaphyseal cupping flared anterior ends of the ribs), delayed skeletal maturation, osteophytes, spurring, osteoporosis, spontaneous fractures, pectus excavatum, clubbed feet

The condition affects all races and has a calculated prevalence at birth of 1:35 000. Most cases present by two months of age. Presenting features include the slowing of development and the loss of milestones—such as smiling and social responsiveness—which had already been achieved, convulsions, apnoea, infections and failure to thrive. Although the boys may seem normal at birth, many have non-specific neonatal histories of low Apgar scores, hypotonia, hypothermia, preterm delivery and prolonged jaundice. Initially the hair may be normal but the characteristic changes are usually evident by the time of presentation (Fig. 11.2). During the first two weeks of life the plasma concentrations of copper and caeruloplasmin may be normal or elevated, they then fall to levels encountered in normal neonates but, in contradistinction to healthy children, these levels do not show the subsequent normal increase towards the physiological range.

Many of the clinical features can be related to reduced cuproenzyme activities. Low activities and histochemical staining for dopamine-β-hydroxylase and cytochrome-C-oxidase occur in several tissues, including the brain which also has a decreased content of unsaturated fatty acids. Many tissues including muscle, brain and liver exhibit increased lipofuscin and degenerative intracellular changes. Focal cerebral and cerebellar degeneration, with diffuse loss of neurones and non specific axonal changes, may be secondary both to these biochemical abnormalities and to an impaired vascular supply caused by arterial damage. As well as contributing to the vascular changes, defective formation of connective tissue is responsible for the skeletal, dermal, urogenital tract anomalies and, with prolonged survival, pulmonary emphysema.

The affected hair (Fig. 11.3) has a low copper and pigment content, and an increased content of free sulphydryl groups despite a normal amino acid composition.

If untreated, most cases die by the third year of life. They develop intracranial haemorrhages, increasingly uncontrollable fits, gross failure to thrive and overwhelming infections such as bronchopneumonia, meningitis and septicaemia.

A mild form of the condition has been reported. In this boy the hair abnormalities were less marked and his development had progressed to the extent that he was able to walk and thus display cerebellar ataxia and choreoathetosis.[23]

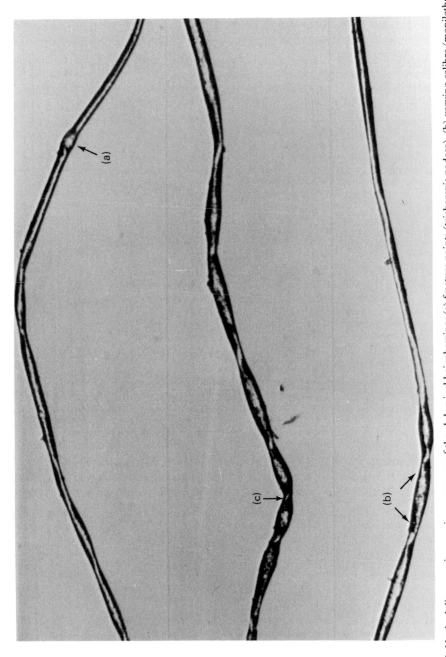

Fig. 11.3 Menkes' disease: microscopic appearance of the abdominal hair showing; (a) fracture points (trichorexis nodosa), (b) varying calibre (monilethrix) and (c) longitudinal twisting (pili torti). Reproduced with permission of Dr B Lake, Hospital for Sick Children, London.

Laboratory investigations

Once Menkes' disease has been suspected on the basis of the clinical picture it can be established by the hypocupraemia (less than 10 μmol/l) and hypocaeruloplasminaemia (less than 20 mg/dl). Further confirmatory investigations include determination of the abnormally low copper content of a needle biopsy of the liver, the usual range in early infancy being 50–150 μg/g (0.2–2.4 μmol/g) dry weight, and the assessment of the increased uptake and retention of copper in vitro by lymphocyte cultures.[24]

Radiography and other clinical chemical investigations would demonstrate the presence of skeletal, vascular, urogenital, and biochemical abnormalities. Anaemia and neutropenia do not occur in Menkes' disease although they occur in other forms of copper deficiency.

Prognosis

There is no effective treatment of Menkes' disease; parenteral copper salts (e.g. Cu-EDTA, Cu-nitrilotriacetate, and Cu(II)-L-Histidine$_2$ complexes) correct the hypocupraemia and hypocaeruloplasminaemia and induce a cupruresis. They also prolong life and modify some features, but, since they do not successfully alter the neurological anomalies such treatment has now been generally abandoned.

Detection of heterozygotes and antenatal screening

Since Menkes' disease is an X-linked defect some heterozygotes can be detected because they exhibit lyonisation and have some features of the disorder. Patchy suntanning may occur in whites and one black mother had areas of depigmented skin. Abnormal scalp hair occurs in many heterozygotes, as does altered lymphocytic metabolism of copper. A typical Menkes' syndrome has been described in the sister of one case.[25]

Antenatal diagnosis in at risk pregnancies is aided by determining the sex of the fetus and, if it is male, by then measuring the uptake and retention of copper in vitro by cultured amniotic cells.[23] This is a technique which is best referred to a specialist laboratory. The discovery of a high copper content in chorionic villus biopsies may in time prove a more convenient and useful discriminant for antenatal diagnosis.

Other neurological abnormalities associated with copper metabolism

Other neurological syndromes have been described in which the aetiological role of deranged copper metabolism is less clear than in Wilson's disease or Menkes' disease. These include syndromes resembling the neurological manifestations of Wilson's disease[26,27] but with a copper metabolism which was inconsistent with that diagnosis, and an X-linked neurological syndrome of progressive retardation, hypotonia and athetosis with inconstant changes of copper metabolism.[28]

ZINC

Acrodermatitis enteropathica (McKusick 20110)

This rare autosomal recessive condition comprises a systemic zinc deficiency syndrome[29,30] secondary to a defect in the intestinal absorption of the metal.

Clinical features

The clinical features are summarised below:

Neuropsychiatric: depression, paranoia, apathy, impaired abstract thought, anorexia, cerebellar ataxia, tremor, reversible cerebral atrophy, hoarseness
Dermatological: periorificial, oral and extensor dermatitis, icthyosis (vesicular-bullous, pustular, hyperkeratotic and acneiform) stomatitis, glossitis paronychia, nail dystrophy, Beau lines, alopecia, hair: fine and brittle, trichonodosis, shaft varying calibre, tapered tips
Ophthalmological: blepharitis, conjunctivitis, keratopathy, photophobia, corneal opacities, impaired dark adaptation
Gastrointestinal: loose frequent watery stools, infection, disaccharide intolerance
Growth retardation, failure to thrive, weight loss
Recurrent infections: impaired blast response, moniliasis, fungaemia, impaired chemotaxis

The protean and relatively non-specific features of acrodermatitis enteropathica arise from the fundamental role of zinc in cellular metabolism. All the major metabolic pathways contain a zinc dependent enzyme; additionally zinc is involved with nucleic acid and protein synthesis, the regulation of cell division, cytoskeletal function, antioxidant activity, the stabilisation of macromolecules such as nerve growth factor and of polymers such as presecretory insulin granules, and the association of hormones with receptors both in the nucleus and on the cell membrane. Consequently it is not always possible to ascribe clinical features to the loss of a specific biochemical function. Furthermore, the features of zinc deficiency can be modified by the supply of other nutrients or factors whose metabolism has been deranged. For example, reducing the protein intake ameliorates the neuropsychiatric consequences of zinc deprivation and, in animal models, increased supplies of vitamin E compounds and of unsaturated fatty acids correct anomalies resulting from membrane instability and disturbed metabolism of linolenic acid.

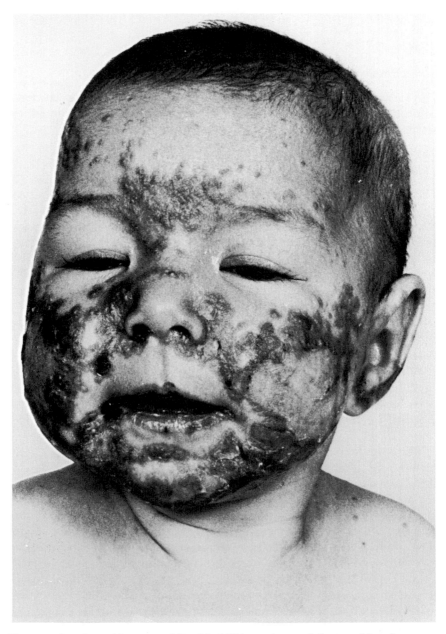

Fig. 11.4 Acrodermatitis enteropathica: this child has a characteristic stomatitis and an extensive symmetrical dermatitis involving the naso-labial folds, the nostrils and the auricles. Reproduced with permission of Dr P Milla.

Acrodermatitis enteropathica usually presents in infancy.[30,31,32] Babies fed on infant formula develop the syndrome sooner than those fed human breast milk in whom problems do not appear until solids and alternative formulae are introduced. This difference arises from the better availability for intestinal absorption of zinc in human milk than from the other products.

The earliest recognised feature is the symmetrical, circumorificial, retroauricular and acral dermatitis which may extend to involve the cheeks, trunk and limbs (Fig. 11.4 and 11.5). Older patients may complain of swelling and pain or tingling in the fingers and feet before the rash appears at these sites. Failure to thrive, anorexia and irritability are the other major presenting features, as was the frequent passage of watery stools until an improved awareness of the condition facilitated earlier diagnosis.

The clinical features deteriorate during infections and physiological stress, at times of anabolic demand such as the growth spurts of early childhood, and early puberty. Males are less vulnerable to zinc deficiency after puberty but women may experience relapses during menstruation and pregnancy. Miscarriages, congenital skeletal defects and anencephaly have been reported in the pregnancies of affected women but adequate zinc supplementation antenatally and, ideally, before conception obviates this risk.

Some cases present in adolescence or adulthood with chronic skin disorders, neuropsychiatric features or a history of abnormal pregnancies.[32]

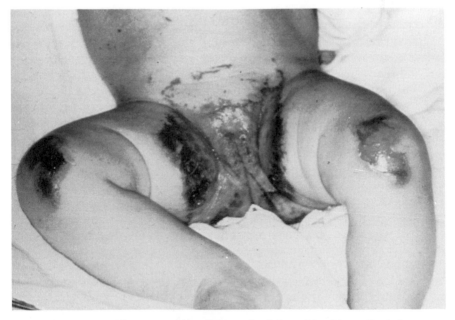

Fig. 11.5 Acrodermatitis enteropathica: severe perineal dermatitis with satellite lesions on the abdomen. The rash has also been precipitated by frictional trauma on both knees. Reproduced with permission of Dr P Milla.

Laboratory investigations

The major laboratory finding is a reduced plasma zinc concentration, but this is not invariable. Some patients may have clinical features of zinc deficiency in the presence of a plasma zinc concentration within the reference range (9–20 μmol/l). This reflects the maintenance of the small plasma zinc pool by zinc released from tissues which are being catabolised as a consequence of zinc deprivation.

Other biochemical changes, such as low serum alkaline phosphatase activity, raised blood ammonia, hypobetalipoproteinaemia, an altered fatty acid profile in the serum and skin, with reduced 18:1 and 20:4 levels and increased concentrations of 18:2 and trienes, illustrate the diverse metabolic roles of zinc.

Diagnosis

This depends on recognising the clinical features and observing their resolution and later deterioration after the introduction and subsequent withdrawal of oral zinc supplementation. Monitoring the plasma zinc concentrations and the activity of a zinc dependent enzyme (e.g. alkaline phosphatase) are valuable adjuncts to this approach. Plasma zinc concentrations alone are unreliable markers of zinc deficiency because they are reduced by a variety of other pathophysiological stresses and infections. The possibility of finding normal levels in symptomatic acrodermatitis enteropathica has been mentioned and it is noteworthy, also, that with the introduction of treatment plasma zinc concentrations may fall initially as new body tissue is synthesised and depletes the plasma zinc pool. This paradox, however, resolves when the deficiency is corrected. Hair zinc concentrations are of no value in the diagnosis and management of acrodermatitis enteropathica.

The differential diagnosis of the skin rash includes psoriasis, familial benign chronic pemphigus, congenital ichthyosiforn dermatitis, moniliasis, epidermolysis bullosa, and, in adults, necrolytic migratory erythema. Other important causes of zinc deficiency are protracted malabsorption states in which loss of endogenous zinc may also occur, the use of synthetic diets, and the development of zinc deficiency in ex-preterm neonates. In contrast to acrodermatitis enteropathica the latter infants can become symptomatic whilst being breast fed. Term infants and those on formulae are less often affected. The most convenient means of differentiating these patients from those with acrodermatitis enteropathica is to withdraw the zinc supplementation after three to six months and monitor the clinical response.

There is no known way of detecting carriers of acrodermatitis enteropathica.

Treatment

Between 35 and 100 mg of elemental zinc per 24 hours in divided doses is usually adequate. Zinc sulphate heptahydrate (50 mg, or 0.77 mmol, of elemental zinc in 220 mg) is used commonly but other salts such as the acetate (1 g contains 300 mg, or 4.6 mmol, of zinc) aspartate and gluconate can be used. Effervescent preparations are available and may be more palatable. The dose should be tailored to match the patient's progress; relatively larger doses are needed during accelerated growth and immediately following initiation of treatment. Whereas male patients may not need continued large doses of zinc after adolescence some supplements are still needed, and women should certainly be advised to maintain their supplements especially if they plan to become pregnant.

Before the pathophysiological role of zinc in acrodermatitis enteropathica was realised chelating agents such as 8-hydroxyquine derivatives were used therapeutically but these are no longer necessary.

With adequate zinc supplements the prognosis of the disorder is excellent.

Familial hyperzincaemia[33] (McKusick 19447)

One pedigree has been reported in which some members inherited, in an autosomal dominant fashion, plasma zinc concentrations up to five times normal (9–20 μmol/1). The additional zinc is associated with plasma albumin and affected individuals are asymptomatic.

MAGNESIUM

Primary hypomagnesaemia (McKusick 24130)

This rare defect arises from an inability of the intestinal mucosa to absorb magnesium from normal intraluminal concentrations of the metal, however at much higher intraluminal concentrations net intestinal absorption of magnesium is achieved.[34] Although the condition is inherited in an autosomal recessive fashion most of the reported cases have been male.

Clinical features[34,35]

Most affected infants were born at term and were apparently healthy during the initial 2–4 weeks of life, after which they became irritable, and developed sleeping and feeding difficulties. Non specific neurological features then appeared; these progressed through jitteriness and eye rolling, to hyperreactivity and disturbance, tetany with facial twitching and carpo-pedal spasm. Not surprisingly, Chvostek's and Trousseau's signs may be positive; generalised convulsions and opisthotonus may then develop. Some infants are hypotonic and areflexic. Other presentations include a protein losing enteropathy, hyponatraemia and peripheral oedema secondary to the hypomagnesaemia; one child presented with raised intracranial pressure, bulging fontanelles and an increased occipito-frontal circumference.

If untreated these children deteriorate rapidly, with impaired feeding and increasingly intractable fits resulting in death during infancy.

Laboratory findings

Affected babies are hypocalcaemic and hypomagnesaemic. The latter concentration is reduced markedly and is often less than 0.2 mmol/l (reference range 0.7–1.0 mmol/l). Hypokalaemia and hyponatraemia develop sometimes. Serum inorganic phosphorus concentrations are increased and circulating levels of parathormone are reduced. The hypocalcaemia responds variably to calcium supplements, it may be secondary to impaired secretion of endogenous parathormone or defective end organ responsiveness or both. Supplements of calcium and parathormone have no effect on the profound hypomagnesaemia. Functional abnormalities are reflected in a grossly but non specifically abnormal electro-encephalogram. Electro-cardiographic anomalies which include arrythmias, prolonged QT intervals, flat and inverted T waves, and U waves are probably due to the secondary hypocalcaemia and hypokalcaemia. Adequate supplements of magnesium rapidly correct all these metabolic anomalies.

Diagnosis

Hypomagnesaemia and a favourable clinical and biochemical response to magnesium therapy confirms the diagnosis. Other possible causes of magnesium deficiency such as primary hypoparathyroidism and aldosteronism, excessive urinary loss (including diuretic therapy), malabsorption states and enteropathies, exchange transfusions and magnesium loss secondary to acidosis can be excluded easily. Subsequently the diagnosis of primary hypomagnesaemia rests on the child's continuing dependence on magnesium supplements, or on the demonstration of impaired intestinal absorption of the metal.

Treatment

Intramuscular magnesium (0.4–0.75 mmol/kg per 24h) produces a rapid and gratifying clinical remission. Subsequently oral therapy is adequate, and the dose can be tailored to the clinical response. Supplements providing 1.5–2.0 mmol of elemental magnesium/kg body weight per 24h may be needed; this is about five times the customary dietary intake. To provide this extra magnesium, magnesium sulphate (4.1 mmol of magnesium in 1 g of $MgSO_4 7H_2O$) is suitable, alternative salts include magnesium chloride (4.9 mmol of elemental magnesium in 1 g) and magnesium acetate (4.66 mmol of magnesium in 1 g). Lactate, citrate and hydroxide salts are available also. Although oral supplements correct the clinical, EEG, ECG and most biochemical abnormalities, it is usually difficult to achieve normal serum

magnesium concentrations without inducing an undesirable secretory diarrhoea; this is probably an effect of the magnesium itself and it is not
ameliorated by using alternative salts of the element. It may be necessary
sometime after successful treatment to withdraw magnesium supplements
to establish the diagnosis, but once this has been achieved affected children
will probably need supplements indefinitely.

MOLYBDENUM

Congenital deficiency of molybdenum-pterin cofactor (McKusick 25215)

A molybdenum-pterin cofactor is required for the activities of sulphite
oxidase, aldehyde oxidase, and xanthine dehydrogenase. A probably autosomal recessively inherited defect in the synthesis of this cofactor leads to
impaired metabolism of sulphur amino acids and nucleotides.[36,37] (see
p. 118 and p. 223). These patients present as neonates; they have
dysmorphic features, feeding difficulties, bilateral dislocation of the lens,
hypertonicity or, less commonly, hypotonicity, mental retardation, cerebral
and cerebellar atrophy with encephalopathy, and generalised and partial
epilepsy. The biochemical anomalies include hypouricaemia, xanthinuria,
sulphituria, thiosulphaturia and a reduced urinary excretion of inorganic
sulphate. The activities of sulphite oxidase and xanthine dehydrogenase in
the liver are undetectable. The absence of sulphite oxidase activity in fibroblasts from these patients indicates a possible means of prenatal diagnosis.

No effective management of the disease has been developed and the prognosis is poor.

REFERENCES

1 Milder M S, Cook J D, Stray S, Finch C A 1980 Idiopathic hemochromatosis: an
   interim report. Medicine 59: 34–49
2 Bomford A, Williams R 1976 Longterm results of venesection therapy in idiopathic
   haemochromatosis. Quarterly Journal of Medicine 45: 611–623
3 Simon M, Bourel M, Genetet B, Fauchet R 1977 Idiopathic hemochromatosis:
   demonstration of recessive transmission and early detection by family HLA typing. New
   England Journal of Medicine 297: 1017–1021
4 Bassett M L, Halliday J W, Powell L 1986 Value of hepatic iron measurements in early
   haemochromatosis and determination of the critical iron level associated with fibrosis.
   Hepatology 6: 24–29
5 Goldfischer S, Grotsky H W, Chang C H et al 1981 Idiopathic neonatal iron storage
   involving the liver, pancreas, heart, and endocrine and exocrine glands. Hepatology
   1: 58–64
6 Goya N, Miyazaki S, Kodate S, Ushio B 1972 A family of congenital atransferrinemia.
   Blood 40: 239–245
7 Westerhausen M, Meuret G 1977 Transferrin-immune complex disease. Acta
   Haematologica 57: 96–101
8 Sahadi N T, Nathan D G, Diamond L K 1964 Iron deficiency anaemia associated with
   an error of iron metabolism in two siblings. Journal of Clinical Investigation
   43: 510–521
9 Hyman E S 1983 Acquired iron-deficiency anaemia due to impaired iron transport.
   Lancet 1: 91–94

10 Walshe J M 1962 Wilson's disease: the presenting symptoms. Archives of Disease in Childhood 37: 253–256

11 McCullough A J, Fleming C R, Thistle J L et al 1983 Diagnosis of Wilson's disease presenting as fulminant hepatic failure. Gastroenterology 84: 161–167

12 Goldfischer S, Popper H, Sternlieb I 1980 The significance of variations in the distribution of copper in liver disease. American Journal of Pathology 99: 715–730

13 Sternlieb I, Scheinberg I H 1979 The role of radiocopper in the diagnosis of Wilson's disease. Gastroenterology 77: 138–142

14 Smith A L, Danks D M 1978 Secondary copper accumulation with neurological damage in children with chronic liver disease. British Medical Journal 2: 1400–1401

15 Marecek Z, Nevsimalova S 1984 Biochemical and clinical changes in Wilson's disease heterozygotes. Journal of Inherited Metabolic Disease 7: 41–45

16 Walshe J M 1973 Copper chelation in patients with Wilson's disease. Quarterly Journal of Medicine 42: 441–452

17 Walshe J M 1977 Pregnancy in Wilson's disease. Quarterly Journal of Medicine 46: 73–83

18 Sternlieb I 1984 Wilson's disease: indications for liver transplants. Hepatology 4: 155–175

19 Hoogenraad T U, Van den Hamer C J A, Van Hattum J 1984 Effective treatment of Wilson's disease with oral zinc sulphate: two case reports. British Medical Journal 289: 273–276

20 Edwards C Q, Williams D M, Cartwright G E 1979 Hereditary hypoceruloplasminemia. Clinical Genetics 15: 311–316

21 Danks D M. Campbell P E, Stevens B J, Mayne V, Cartwright E 1972 Menkes' kinky hair syndrome: an inherited defect in copper absorption with widespread effects. Pediatrics 50: 188–201

22 Menkes J H, Alter M, Steigleder G K, Weakley D R, Sung J H 1962 A sex linked recessive disorder with retardation of growth, peculiar hair, and focal cerebral and cerebellar degeneration. Pediatrics 29: 764–779

23 Procopis P, Camakaris J, Danks D M 1981 A mild form of Menkes' steely hair syndrome. The Journal of Pediatrics 98: 97–98

24 Horn N 1981 Menkes' X linked disease: prenatal diagnosis of hemizygous males and heterozygous females. Prenatal Diagnosis 1: 107–120

25 Iwakawa Y, Niwa T, Tomita M 1979 Menkes' kinky hair syndrome: a report on an autopsy case and his female sibling with similar clinical manifestations. Brain Development 11: 260–266

26 Godwin-Austen R B, Robinson A, Evans K, Lascelles P T 1978 An unusual neurological disorder of copper metabolism clinically resembling Wilson's disease but biochemically a distinct entity. Journal of Neurological Sciences 39: 85–98

27 Willvonseder R, Goldstein N P, McCall J T, Yoss R E, Tauxe W N 1973 A hereditary disorder with dementia, spastic dysarthria, vertical eye movement paresis, gait disturbance, splenomegaly and abnormal copper metabolism. Neurology 23: 1039–1049

28 Haas R H, Robinson A, Evans K, Dubowitz V 1981 An X linked disease of the nervous system with disordered copper metabolism and features differing from Menkes' disease. Neurology 31: 852–859

29 Moynahan E J 1974 Acrodermatitis enteropathica: a lethal inherited human zinc-deficiency disorder. Lancet 2: 399–400

30 Neldner K H, Hambidge K M 1974 Zinc therapy of acrodermatitis enteropathica. New England Journal of Medicine 292: 879–882

31 Ginsburg R, Robertson A, Michel B 1976 Acrodermatitis enteropathica: abnormalities of fat metabolism and integumental ultrastructures in infants. Archives of Dermatology 112: 653–660

32 Olholm-Larsen P 1978 Untreated acrodermatitis enteropathica in adults. Dermatologica 156: 155–166

33 Failla M L, Van de Veerdonk M, Morgan W T, Smith J C 1982 Characterisation of zinc binding proteins of plasma in familial hyperzincaemia. Journal of Laboratory and Clinical Medicine 100: 943–952

34 Milla P J, Aggett P J, Wolff O H, Harries J T 1979 Studies in primary hypomagnesaemia: evidence for defective carrier mediated small intestinal transport of magnesium. Gut 20: 1028–1033

35 Paunier L, Radde I C, Kooh S U, Cohen P E, Fraser D 1968 Primary
   hypomagnesaemia with secondary hypocalcaemia in an infant. Pediatrics 41: 385–402
36 Johnson J L, Waud W R, Rajagopalan K V, Duran M, Bremer F A, Wadman S K
   1980 Errors of molybdenum metabolism. Combined deficiencies of sulphite oxidase and
   xanthine dehydrogenase in a patient lacking the molybdenum cofactor. Proceedings of
   the National Academy of Sciences (USA) 77: 3715–3719
37 Wadman S K, Duran M, Bremer F A et al 1983 Absence of hepatic molybdenum
   cofactor: an inborn error of metabolism leading to a combined deficiency of sulphite
   oxidase and xanthine dehydrogenase. Journal of Inherited Metabolic Disease 6 (suppl
   1): 78–83

Red cell disorders

INTRODUCTION

It is convenient to consider the mature, human red cell as comprising three components—membrane,[1] carbohydrate and associated metabolism, and haemoglobin. This triad omits innumerable enzymes known to be present in the cell but the majority of these are not involved in the cell's mature function and are considered redundant at the red-cell precursor stage following loss of the nucleus. The metabolism of mature red cells is restricted to anaerobic glycolysis (the Embden-Meyerhof pathway, EMP) and the pentose phosphate pathway (PPP) with its associated reactions. Within each of the three components inherited abnormalities are known; some are common, others are rare; some do not affect red-cell survival but many are associated with haemolytic disease. Mostly, the defects are located only in red cells but sometimes other tissues are affected.

DISORDERS OF THE RED-CELL MEMBRANE

Structure of the normal membrane

Red cells are unlike other cells in that the membrane has roughly equal proportions by weight of protein and lipid; the constituents of these two major fractions are shown in Tables 12.1 and 12.2.

Lipids (Table 12.1).

The phospholipids comprise approximately 60% by weight of total lipid of which some 60% is neutral, the remainder acidic. Approximately 23% of total lipid is cholesterol, almost all of it un-esterified. Free fatty acids, gangliosides, phosphatidate and lysolecithin are present in the membrane only in small amounts. The major phospholipids are the phosphatidyl esters of choline, ethanolamine and serine, together with sphingomyelin: these four together form the planar, hydrophobic bilayer within the interior of the membrane. The lipid bilayer is asymmetrical, with most of the sphin-

Table 12.1 Lipid constituents of the red-cell membrane. (All figures are % of total dry weight of total)

Neutral lipids	
Free cholesterol	20
Esterified cholesterol	2
Free fatty acids	2
Phospholipids	
Neutral	
Phosphatidylcholine	20
Sphingomyelin	15
Acidic	
Phosphatidyl ethanolamine	16
Phosphatidyl serine	4
Phosphatidate	2
Lysolecithin	4
Glycosphingolipids	
Neutral	
Globosides	13
Gangliosides	2
	100

Table 12.2 Protein constituents of the red-cell membrane*

Band number[†]	Name	Proportion (% by weight)	Integral (I) Peripheral (P)	Molecular weight (x10^5)
1 2 }	Spectrin	25	P	{ 2.4 2.2
2.1 2.2 2.3 2.6 }	Ankyrin	5	P	2.1 1.95 1.75 1.45
3	Anion exchange protein	25	I	0.93
4.1	—	4–5	P	0.80
4.2	—	4–5	P	0.72
4.3	—	0.5–1.0	P	0.45
5	Actin	4–5	P	0.45
6	GAPD	4–5	P	0.35
7	—	4–5	P	0.29
8	—	1.2	P	0.23
GPA	Glycophorin A	1.5 }		≈ 0.31
GPB	Glycophorin B	0.5 }	I	≈ 0.23
GPC	Glycophorin C	0.3 }		0.29

* Based on Lux[1]
† Nomenclature based on electrophoretic and other studies[2,3]

gomyelin and phosphatidylcholine located on the outer half of the bilayer and the bulk (approximately 80%) of the phosphatidylethanolamine and all the phosphatidylserine lying on the inner half. Cholesterol is distributed throughout the bilayer and, unlike the phospholipids, exchanges with plasma cholesterol. The planar configuration of cholesterol allows it physically to enter the hydrophobic lipid domain and its non-polar character permits it to stay there. It affects membrane fluidity so that its presence increases the surface area of the cell and its removal diminishes the cell area. Such changes of surface area have consequences for cell shape; for example, removal of enough cholesterol from the membrane will reduce the surface area of the cell sufficiently to convert a normal discocyte into a microspherocyte.

Proteins (Table 12.2).

Electrophoresis on polyacrylamide gel in sodium dodecyl sulphate will identify 10 to 12 major membrane proteins which are of two general types, integral and peripheral.[2,3] Integral proteins enter or span the membrane and their hydrophobic regions interact with the inner hydrophobic lipid domain. The two major integral proteins, the glycophorins and the anion exchange channel protein (protein 3), have end carbohydrate regions which lie on the external membrane surface, a non-polar region in the central lipid bilayer, and a polar region in the internal hydrophilic domain. By contrast, peripheral proteins lie on the surface of the membrane bound to integral proteins and to the polar phospholipid heads. Most of the peripheral proteins are attached to the cytoplasmic surface either as enzymes e.g. glyceraldehyde-3-phosphate dehydrogenase (protein 6), or as the protein constituents of the cytoskeleton.

The cytoskeleton is an unordered, flexible, two-dimensional network anchored on the inner surface of the membrane and directly associated with the shape, strength and flexibility of the cell. Its relevance to cell shape is established because isolated cytoskeletons retain the form of the parent cells; its role in preserving cell flexibility is suggested by the increased cell rigidity which occurs with abnormalities of the cytoskeletal constituents. Biophysical data show that a flexible protein network linked to a lipid bilayer will yield a biconcave disc shape. Short-term alterations of this shape, as in the microcirculation, are reversible, but severe constraints or congenital abnormalities of cytoskeletal proteins will yield permanently abnormal cell morphology.

The principal components of the cytoskeleton are spectrin, actin, protein 4.1 and ankyrin. *Spectrin* accounts for some two-thirds of the cytoskeletal weight and lies as an unsymmetrical network covering the entire cytoplasmic surface, while the other components pin down this network to the membrane (Fig. 12.1). It should be noted that parts of the other proteins— 3, 4.2 and 7—are also involved in the anchoring process. Spectrin functions

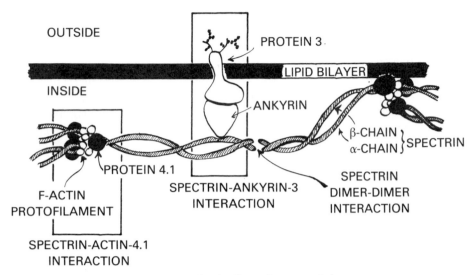

Fig. 12.1 Diagrammatic appearance of red-cell membrane cytoskeleton.

in two structurally different states α (or 1) and β (or 2); both are long (100 nm) polypeptides twisted together into dimer form which react head-to-head with other dimers to give tetramers. Branching occurs where each dimer strand reacts with a single strand from different dimers; in this way an unsymmetrical network is established. *Actin*, probably as F-actin, exists in short filamentous bundles bound weakly at their sides to the tails of spectrin dimers. *Protein 4.1* is a globular polypeptide sited near actin where it consolidates the weak actin-spectrin bond; it is also bound to membrane protein and/or lipid. *Ankyrin* is a protein complex bonded between the integral anion exchange channel (protein 3) of the membrane and the heads of spectrin dimers, where it provides the main anchor point for the network.

The cytoskeleton is the flexible network which is a determinant of red-cell shape and a major factor in shape changes. Acquired or hereditary abnormalities of the cytoskeleton will be manifested by shortened red-cell survival, abnormal cell morphology or both.

Hereditary spherocytosis (HS, McKusick 18290)

HS is transmitted as an autosomal dominant, although in some 25% of cases neither parent is apparently affected. It is associated with a haemolytic process of mild to moderate degree but occasionally is severe enough to be transfusion-dependent. When haemolysis is not compensated, anaemia is present. Moderate splenomegaly occurs and splenectomy, when practicable, resolves the anaemia. HS is the commonest haemolytic anaemia in subjects of northern European extraction (about 1:5000). However, the disorder is not peculiar to any ethnic group. HS is usually diagnosed in childhood, although there are notable exceptions.

Blood examination reveals the usual criteria of haemolysis; a low haemoglobin if anaemia is present, reticulocytosis and raised serum bilirubin, blood film showing polychromasia, anisocytosis and, notably, microspherocytes. The fresh blood osmotic fragility curve may indicate fragile cells; curves from blood incubated for 24 hours are more likely to demonstrate a shift towards fragile cells than with fresh blood. Incubation of sterile blood for 48 hours gives abnormal lysis, but when glucose is present lysis is reduced, even into the normal range (the autohaemolysis test). Dilute suspensions of red cells in acid-buffered glycerol solutions undergo more rapid and extensive lysis than do normal cells (the AGLT test). There is no specific diagnostic test for HS; the set of tests mentioned above, in the absence of an autoimmune process, the existence of affected family members and the beneficial effects of a splenectomy, together afford the definitive diagnosis.

There are two related and characteristic features of the red cells in HS. First, the membrane is inherently unstable and in vivo fragments are lost throughout the shortened life of the cell. As a consequence the surface area of the cells is diminished, without loss of contents, giving rise to microspherocytes in the old cohort of cells. Secondly, the process is gradual, reticulocytes and young red cells having normal morphology. The reticuloendothelial system, especially the spleen, plays a role in hastening this spontaneous sphering process. The sinusoids of the spleen are a poor environment for red cells although normal cells can survive many transits. In HS the transit time is prolonged as the sphering process proceeds and, since the environment is anyway adverse, sphering is hastened. Red cells become increasingly stiff and inflexible as the sphering process continues and the end-stage microspherocyte is particularly so; for this reason its time in the spleen is indefinitely prolonged and such cells are trapped. Splenectomy removes the trap and, although the spontaneous sphering process continues, it does so at a rate dependent only on the extent of the cellular defect in the cells. The result is a lengthening of red-cell life span and a disappearance of the signs of haemolysis.

The primary defect in HS is in the structural protein component of the membrane, the cytoskeleton (see above). The constituents of this skeleton are quantitatively normal in all but a few unusual cases and it is generally accepted that a qualitative abnormality exists in spectrin, the major structural component of the cytoskeleton. The precise nature of the defect is not known and most of the evidence is presently circumstantial. In a small number of patients with otherwise typical HS, the primary defect appears to be due to inadequate binding of a portion of the spectrin to protein 4.1: in others protein 4.2 appears to be deficient.

Hereditary elliptocytosis (HE, McKusick 13050 and 13060)

HE is genetically and clinically a heterogeneous disorder. It is inherited as an autosomal dominant but, unlike HS, the more common forms show greater penetrance. One of the genes is linked closely to the Rh locus on the short arm of chromosome 1. The disease is not uncommon and all ethnic groups are affected; in the United States the incidence is some 1:3000. In its commonest form HE is mild; patients with compensated haemolysis are not anaemic while in others anaemia may be mild or severe. Mostly the anaemia is mild to moderate. Splenomegaly is present only with marked haemolysis.

Normal blood films contain up to 10% elliptocyes; in patients with HE there can be more than 30% and up to 100% present. When haemolysis is severe, microspherocytes, poikilocytes and cell fragments are conspicuous. As in HS, the formation of elliptocytes is a gradual process, nucleated precursors are round while reticulocytes are intermediate in shape, being notably less ellipsoid than mature cells. In neonates with HE, elliptocytes are not prominent in the first few months of life. The presence of elliptocytes in normal blood and in somewhat larger numbers in hypochromic, microcytic and megaloblastic anaemias does not usually complicate a diagnosis of HE because of the markedly increased numbers of elliptocytes in this disease. The degree of elliptocytosis correlates poorly with the severity of the disease; in addition, there is variation not only between patients with the disorder but within individual patients.

The primary defect in HE, as in HS, resides in the cytoskeleton although less is known about the nature of the abnormality than with HS. Isolation of ghosts or cytoskeletons from intact red cells yields material which retains the ellipsoid shape of the parent cells. If poikilocytes are present in the peripheral blood, their characteristic shape is also retained in isolated ghosts and cytoskeletons. Intact elliptocytes and also cytoskeletons prepared from elliptocytes are mechanically and thermally fragile and purified spectrin is more sensitive to heat denaturation than spectrin from normal cells. Spectrin isolated from normal red cells at 0°C is substantially tetra- or oligomeric. Several recent studies of mild and severe cases of HE have shown an increased dimer content of isolated spectrin and this may implicate the dimer-tetramer association as being of primary significance in HE.

Hereditary stomatocytosis (McKusick 18500 and 18501)

Red cells which are cup- or bowl-shaped in wet preparations and have a longitudinal slit in place of the usual circular pallid area in dried blood films are called stomatocytes. They can be formed reversibly by mild treatment of normal red cells with different agents. They occur, also, in association with several unrelated disorders, namely, malignant disease, thalassaemia minor, alcoholic liver disease, infectious mononucleosis and GSH peroxidase deficiency. They are now recognised in connection with hereditary haemolytic anaemia in which there may be 10–40% stomatocytes present and a reticulocytosis of up to 40%.

The monovalent cation function of stomatocytes which are associated with a haemolytic anaemia has been studied in some detail. The characteristic properties are an increased water content (hydrocytosis), increased surface area and volume and marked abnormalities in Na^+ and K^+ content and flux. Thus, the intracellular Na^+ level is high and can be ten times normal while the K^+ is low. The total monovalent cation $(Na^+ + K^+)$ concentration is greater than normal and this is reflected in the large cell volume. Net leakage of both cations is abnormally high and for Na^+ is even faster than would be expected from the high intracellular concentration. Active transport is very rapid and the usual coupled ratio of $3Na^+:2K^+$ is considerably increased because of the relatively higher active flux of Na^+ over K^+. As a consequence of the enormously increased active flux, the rate of glucose consumption is high. The active transport mechanism lies in the red-cell membrane and the anomalous cation flux suggests a membrane abnormality; there is some evidence of an abnormal protein.

Hereditary pyropoikilocytosis (HP, McKusick 26614)

Poikilocytes (tear-drop cells) are present in a number of disparate haematological conditions such as iron-deficiency, thalassaemia, myelofibrosis and megaloblastic anaemia. They also arise from damage inflicted upon cells in vivo as in microangiopathic haemolytic anaemia. However, HP has been described as a discrete entity in three children with congenital haemolytic anaemia. The blood film showed marked spherocytosis, cells with budding projections and others triangular in shape. The cells were abnormally heat-sensitive and underwent fragmentation at a lower temperature (45°) than do normal cells (49°). In several respects there are similarities between HP and HE. The morphology of the cells in HP is not dissimilar to that in severe HE and in some forms of neonatal HE. In addition, the red cells of neonates with mild HE and poikilocytosis are thermally fragile and finally, some family members of patients with HP have mild HE.

DISORDERS OF THE EMBDEN-MEYERHOF PATHWAY (EMP)

Normal pathway

The EMP in normal red cells (Fig. 12.2) consumes glucose at a rate of 1–2 mmol/l of red cells per hour, producing intermediates of which five are particularly important in red cells (Table 12.3).

The pathway in red cells is singular in generating a high level of 2,3-diphosphoglycerate (*2,3-DPG*), whose function is to modulate the oxygen affinity of haemoglobin. Changes in the concentration of 2,3-DPG are observed to shift the oxygen dissociation curve (Fig. 12.3). A rise in ester

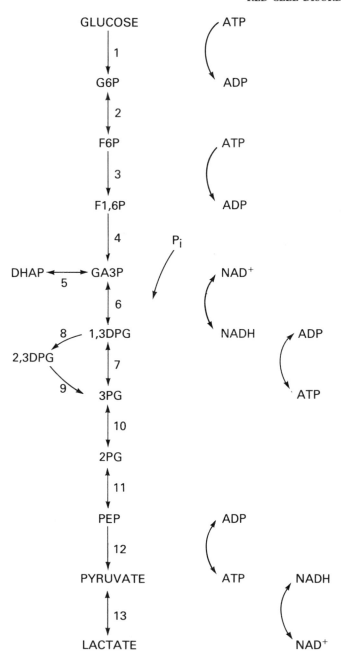

Fig. 12.2 The Embden-Meyerhof pathway (EMP). G6P, glucose-6-phosphate; F6P and F-1,6P, fructose-6-phosphate and 1,6-diphosphate; GA3P, glyceraldehyde 3-phosphate; DHAP, dihydroxyacetone phosphate; 1,3 DPG and 2,3-DPG, 1,3 and 2,3-diphosphoglycerate; 3PG, 3-phosphoglycerate; 2PG, 2-phosphoglycerate; PEP, phosphoenolpyruvate. 1, Hexokinase; 2, glucose isomerase; 3, phosphofructokinase; 4, aldolase; 5, triose phosphate isomerase; 7, phosphoglycerate kinase; 8, 2,3-DPG mutase; 9, 2,3-DPG phosphatase; 10, phosphoglyceromutase; 11, enolase; 12, pyruvate kinase; 13, lactic dehydrogenase.

Table 12.3 Levels of key red-cell intermediates

Intermediates	Concentration mmol/l
ATP	0.8–1.4
2,3-DPG	3–5
GSH	2.2
NAD$^+$(H)	0.03–0.07
NADP$^+$(H)	0.045

Units are referred to volume of packed red cells

concentration above normal (about 4 mmol) results in a rightward shift because of a decrease in oxygen affinity while a fall in ester concentration shifts the curve leftwards, increasing the oxygen affinity of haemoglobin. A second determinant of oxygen affinity is pH, a fall in pH producing a rightward shift of the curve (Bohr effect) and vice versa. The EMP is also pH-sensitive and the rate decreases with a fall in pH; this decreases the level of 2,3-DPG and so the level of this ester affects the dissociation curve in the opposite sense to the change in intracellular pH. Physiologically, the curve is positioned as shown in Fig. 12.3. Irregularities in the curve arise, therefore, with acid-base disturbances and conditions in which the 2,3-DPG level is abnormal, i.e. anaemia, hypoxia and congenital deficiencies of glycolysis. Abnormalities arise also in certain haemoglobinopathies when the affinity of the ester for haemoglobin is abnormal.

Red cells also contain a high concentration of *ATP* (Table 12.3) and this nucleotide, apart from its role in the EMP, is required in several reactions. Primarily, it serves to maintain active monovalent cation transport across the membrane via the sodium pump. The pump is generally similar, although slower, to that in other tissues and passes Na$^+$ and K$^+$ through the membrane, in the ratio of 3:2 respectively. However, calculation shows that only about a fifth of available ATP is used in this connection and the quantitative deployment of the remainder is not established. Some is required to extrude Ca^{2+} from cells against a steep concentration gradient by an active transport mechanism not dissimilar to the sodium pump. ATP is also involved in the biosynthesis of GSH (see later) and in the formation of PRPP (phosphoribosyl pyrophosphate) which can react with adenine to generate AMP (p. 427). Synthesis of ATP de novo does not occur in mature red cells except from adenine and, apart from its generation from ADP in the EMP, the only means of producing it is through the adenylate kinase reaction (p. 428). The bulk of available ATP appears to be required to maintain cell flexibility by a mechanism which is not understood; most of the evidence is derived either by depleting cells of ATP and demonstrating increased rigidity or by regenerating depleted ATP and observing a return of flexibility towards normal. Calcium is involved in this process; an excess of intracellular Ca^{2+} decreases flexibility which reverts to normal

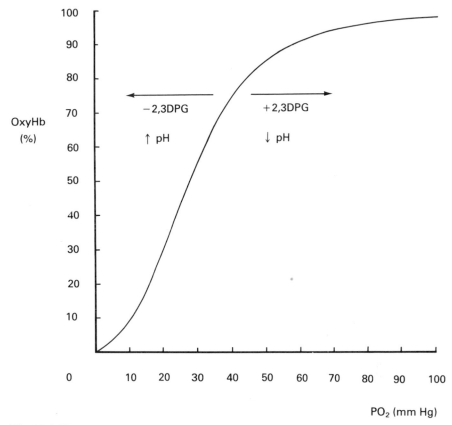

Fig. 12.3 Normal oxygen dissociation curve.

as the cation leaves the cell, but this can occur independently of the ATP level.

The third key intermediate in the EMP is $NAD^+/NADH$ which also operates as coenzyme in the principal route for methaemoglobin reduction (p. 440). The remaining two intermediates *GSH* and *$NADP^+/NADPH$*, are maintained by pentose phosphate pathway activity (p. 430).

The sole requirement of the EMP is a small, continuous source of glucose and this is available even in acute hypoglycaemia. Transport of glucose across the cell membrane is by facilitated diffusion, a rapid process involving a glucose carrier, and the intracellular glucose concentration follows the continuously changing plasma level when glucose is expressed in terms of cell or plasma water.

Abnormalities in the pathway

There are reports of low activity for every enzyme except phosphoglycerate mutase in the red-cell EMP and all deficiencies, with the exception of lactate dehydrogenase (LDH), are associated with a congenital haemolytic anaemia. All are rare and of even the commonest, pyruvate kinase (PK) deficiency, only some 300 cases are on record. All the deficiencies so far reported are due to a mutant enzyme present in normal concentration in young cells. The mutant may be unstable, the level declining with red-cell ageing, or it may have abnormal kinetics, or both; but the characteristic feature is a subnormal activity in the tested blood sample which indicates a glycolytic block and which results in a shortened red-cell life span. As a consequence haemolytic anaemia with a young red-cell population occurs, as demonstrated by the accompanying reticulocytosis. Peripheral reticulocytes carry vestigial Krebs cycle activity which fades with disappearance of the mitochondria during the few days of reticulocyte development into mature cells. While Krebs cycle activity persists it yields ATP which is supplementary to that from the EMP. On maturation this source dries up and the cell relies solely upon EMP activity; this can sustain the cell only as long as the declining activity of the variant enzyme permits. This mechanism has been studied in particular with PK deficiency, in which the peripheral blood can contain a large reticulocyte cohort, even up to 90%.

The expected laboratory and clinical findings are those of erythroid hyperplasia, reticulocytosis, jaundice and splenomegaly, with worsening of the anaemia by infections. Tissues other than blood may be affected and this can give rise to muscular or neurological complications. White cells are not affected functionally. Abnormalities of red-cell morphology tend to be non-specific with mild to moderate anisocytosis and poikilocytosis, polychromasia, fragmentation, crenated forms and occasional target cells and spherocytes. Treatment consists of blood transfusions as required, folate supplements and timely treatment of infections. Splenectomy has been carried out with some benefit and is considered where transfusion requirements are excessive. Unlike defects of the PPP (p. 427), oxidant drugs do not present a hazard to patients with EMP deficiencies.

A problem which arises in measuring enzyme activity in red cells from patients with a haemolytic process, or in red cells from neonates, is the presence of a cell population skewed towards young cells which contain higher enzyme activity. If the variant enzyme activity is sufficiently low, as with homozygotes, then there is usually no diagnostic problem. If, however, there is a partial deficiency, as with heterozygotes, and the measured activity is a resultant of the lowered variant enzyme activity and the raised activity due to young cells, values may be obtained which are in the normal range. There are two methods of resolving this problem. Either the suspected enzyme is assayed against a second age-dependent enzyme, to eliminate the effect of a young cell population, or data are acquired on enzyme activities in young, normal, red-cell populations.

Mutants of the EMP

Hexokinase (Hx, McKusick 23570)

The normal enzyme has the lowest capacity of the glycolytic enzymes with a decay rate which follows closely the decline in glycolytic activity as red cells age; as the rate-limiting enzyme it is regarded as the glycolytic pacemaker. Its activity in young red cells is approximately ten times that in old cells and consequently in determining Hx deficiency with reticulocyte-rich blood it is particularly important to allow for this effect. Hx deficiency was first described in 1964 in three patients with Fanconi's syndrome; curiously it was not associated with haemolytic anaemia and may have arisen through chromosome breaks. Since then hereditary Hx deficiency associated with a haemolytic anaemia and occurring as a primary defect has been reported in twelve patients. The level of Hx activity was within or below the normal range but the deficiency is revealed against normal reticulocyte-rich-blood. In several cases Hx deficiency resulted in diminished glucose consumption and low 2,3-DPG levels. The defect is inherited typically in an autosomal recessive manner.

Hx deficiency represents a further diagnostic problem which has arisen also with some cases of PK deficiency. Where a variant has a raised Km for glucose, assays with the excess substrate usually present may yield a normal result; whereas at a lower, physiological, substrate concentration a deficiency may be revealed. For this reason red-cell enzymes are assayed routinely at both low and high substrate levels.[4]

Glucose phosphate isomerase (GPI, McKusick 17240)

A considerable number of variants of GPI are reported but many are not associated with haemolytic anaemia, which is the sole clinical disorder known in association with variant GPI. Where anaemia is present it may be mild or severe. Osmotic fragility is near normal with increased autohaemolysis, only marginally reduced when glucose is present. White cells and platelets are usually normal and blood films show only those changes typical of nonspherocytic haemolytic anaemia. The deficiency occurs in an autosomal recessive manner and affects various ethnic groups.

Many of the variants can be characterised electrophoretically, by abnormal Km values or pH optimum curves. Those with low activity are thermolabile. The red-cell G6P level is raised in GPI deficiency, but the product F6P is near-normal. PPP activity is normal but recycling is notably restricted. ATP is usually low or normal.

Phosphofructokinase (PFK, McKusick 17185 and 23280)

This enzyme is an important regulator of red-cell glycolysis and is sensitive to a number of effectors. A red cell and muscle deficiency of PFK (Type

VII glycogen storage disease) is reported in three Japanese siblings having clinical histories compatible with muscle phosphorylase deficiency (McArdle's disease) and some evidence of haemolytic anaemia. Normal red cells contain two forms of PFK and one of them, with about 50% of the total activity, is immunologically indistinguishable from the muscle enzyme (see p. 15). The patients' red cells contained about 50% of normal PFK activity and the muscle component was missing. However, a patient is described with 60% activity of normal PFK, haemolytic anaemia, normal muscle enzyme activity and no muscular disorder. Despite the haemolytic anaemia, the osmotic fragility, autohaemolysis, red-cell Na^+, K^+ and Na^+ flux, together with lactate production were normal. The patient's mother and maternal grandmother showed a similar low red-cell activity but had no haemolytic anaemia. Following these reports a number of further cases of PFK deficiency have been described in association with haemolysis. Inheritance is autosomal recessive.

G6P and F6P levels are increased in PFK deficiency and it is suggested that these intermediates are diverted into the PPP, thereby increasing phosphoribosylpyrophosphate and purine and pyrimidine production. The suggestion arose because of hyperuricaemia and gout in a patient. 2,3-DPG is decreased in PFK deficiency while muscle glycogen storage is increased.

Aldolase (McKusick 20335)

Only a single case of aldolase deficiency is reported, in a mentally handicapped child with a mild haemolytic anaemia; both parents, who were first cousins, showed normal red-cell aldolase activity. The disease is presumed to involve deficiency of aldolase A, the red-cell enzyme, as opposed to Type B which is deficient in hereditary fructose intolerance (p. 49).

Triosephophosphate isomerase (TPI McKusick 27580)

TPI deficiency was first reported in an infant with chronic haemolytic anaemia and a progressive neuromuscular disorder. Red cell TPI activity in a surviving child was 10% of normal and this also was associated with haemolytic anaemia. Both parents showed intermediate heterozygote values but were without other haematological abnormalities. The same authors later reported another child, similar to their first case with both parents giving intermediate values; the two families were thought to be related. A number of other cases have been described. TPI deficiency follows an autosomal recessive pattern.

Such red-cell intermediates and pathways as have been determined show glucose consumption to be high even after correction for the young red-cell population present. The PPP is adequate, ATP normal or somewhat low and dihydroxyacetone phosphate (DHAP) inordinately high. F1,6P and glyceraldehyde-3-phosphate (GA3P) were also increased. It has been suggested that the high level of DHAP is toxic to red cells but the mechanism is unknown.

Glyceraldehyde-3-phosphate dehydrogenase (GA3PD, McKusick 13840)

Few cases of GA3PD deficiency are known. In one, where the activity was 20–30% of normal, the deficiency was accompanied by a compensated haemolytic anaemia. Where red-cell activity was diminished by 50% anaemia was not present. A large family is described in whom the deficiency occurred in association with hereditary spherocytosis.

Phosphoglycerokinase (PGK, McKusick 26170)

A moderate deficiency of PGK was first described in 1968 accompanied by a chronic haemolytic anaemia. Since then a number of other cases have been described and a sex-linked basis of transmission established. Female heterozygotes with a partial deficiency have two red-cell populations, one normal and the other PGK deficient, as in G6PD deficiency. ATP is somewhat low in this condition while 2,3-DPG is increased; lactate and pyruvate production are normal.

2,3-diphosphoglycerate mutase (2,3-DPGM, McKusick 22280)

The first unequivocal description of 2,3-DPGM deficiency is that of a German male infant with a severe and eventually fatal congenital haemolytic anaemia. Both parents, a sister and paternal grandmother were asymptomatic with red-cell activities 55–66% of normal and 2,3-DPG levels decreased by some 50%. Several other cases are described and a low 2,3-DPG level appears to be a common feature.

2,3-diphosphoglycerate phosphatase (2,3-DPGase)

Two unrelated cases are described in conjunction with a haemolytic anaemia. The 2,3-DPG concentration was normal but ATP and ADP were raised by 50% of normal.

Phosphoglycerate mutase (PGM)

PGM has not been reported as a deficiency state in the red cell.

Enolase

A single case has been reported of a 40-year-old woman with a haemolytic anaemia and 50% of normal red-cell enolase activity. The enzyme appeared to be kinetically normal but present in low concentration.[5]

Pyruvate kinase (PK, McKusick 26620)[6]

PK deficiency is the commonest of the EMP enzyme defects and was first described in 1961 in three males. Some 300 cases are now known affecting all ethnic groups. Heterozygotes have intermediate values of red-cell PK activity, usually with a normal blood film and without signs of haemolysis. Homozygotes show a marked reduction of PK activity (5–40% of normal) with an associated non-spherocytic haemolytic anaemia which may be mild or severe in different subjects and with reticulocyte counts that can be notably high following splenectomy. Both parents of severely affected patients usually have intermediate values of red-cell PK activity as do all offspring of a grossly-affected parent. This, together with the incidence of consanguinity in PK deficiency, indicates an autosomal recessive mode of inheritance. Affected patients have a different mutant gene from each parent, unless the parents are consanguinous, and their red cells contain two mutant proteins. It is now clear that the compound heterozygotes have many different mutant genes coding for different mutant PK proteins which differ notably in their physical properties; hence the marked differences in catalytic activity, kinetics, thermolability, electrophoretic mobility, pH optima and behaviour towards allosteric effectors. Those mutants which display clinical expression appear to share an instability which results in low residual activity, decreased affinity for PEP, decreased activation by F1,6P and increased inhibition by ATP.

Several secondary red-cell abnormalities occur in PK deficiency when associated with haemolytic anaemia. The most frequently recorded is an elevated 2,3-DPG level which arises through the glycolytic block distal to production of this ester. Other esters preceding the block are also raised but increased 2,3-DPG is important physiologically because the oxygen dissociation curve is shifted to the right, which serves to alleviate the anaemia. ATP is low, or low-normal, and the level measured is the sum of that produced by a stricken EMP and that which is available from the fading Krebs cycle contained in the reticulocytes. The total nicotinamide adenine dinucleotide level is low, although the $NAD^+/NADH$ ratio is normal, and glucose consumption is near the normal range, but it is low after correction for the young red-cell population present. The activity of the PPP is somewhat depressed relative to the EMP. The blood film shows bizarre crenation of many red cells which are also poorly flexible, as are PK-deficient reticulocytes.

Some PK mutants are described with normal activity when assayed with the excess substrate used in standard assays but subnormal activity in the presence of low substrate. In default of determining the Km value it is necessary in routine diagnosis to use both excess and low substrate concentrations.

Lactate dehydrogenase (LDH, McKusick 15010)

One case is reported in an elderly diabetic Japanese male without any other haematological abnormalities. Normal red cells contain four tetrameric isozymes of LDH made up of heart (H) and muscle (M) enzyme subunits. The four isozymes, H_4: H_3M: H_2M_2: HM_3 are present in the proportions 39:40:20:1, respectively. The patient's red cells contained only an M_4 enzyme together with raised levels of F1,6P, DHAP and GA3P, a low whole blood lactate and a normal pyruvate. Although DHAP was increased 10-fold the cells were not apparently affected; this is contrary to the suggestion (p. 425) that in TPI deficiency the raised level of DHAP is injurious to the cell. A brother of the five offspring of the propositus had red-cell LDH activities that were around 50% of the mean normal activity with a 50% lack of H_4.

DISORDERS OF THE PENTOSE PHOSPHATE PATHWAY (PPP)

In the mature, normal human red cell this pathway accounts for some 2% of consumed glucose although, under the influence of an electron acceptor such as methylene blue, it can be stimulated around 40-fold. The composition of the pathway and its connection with anaerobic glycolysis are shown in Fig. 12.4. The PPP serves two functions in red cells, it provides ribose-5-phosphate (R5P) which participates in the limited purine metabolism present in red cells, and reducing capacity is made available to counter oxidative assault.

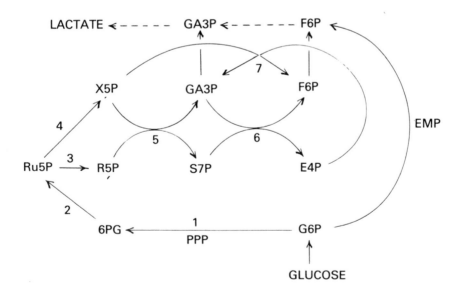

Fig. 12.4 The pentose phosphate pathway (PPP) and its connection with the EMP. G6P, glucose-6-phosphate; 6PG, 6-phosphogluconate; Ru5P, ribulose 5-phosphate; R5P, ribose 5-phosphate; S7P, sedoheptulose 7-phosphate; E4P, erythrose 4-phosphate; XRP, xylulose 5-phosphate; GA3P, glyceraldehyde 3-phosphate; F6P, fructose 6-phosphate. 1, Glucose-6-phosphate dehydrogenase; 2, 6-phosphogluconate dehydrogenase; 3, isomerase; 4, epimerase, 5,6, transketolase; 7, transaldolase.

Purine metabolism

R5P is a reactant in the formation of 5-phosphoribosyl-α-l-pyrophosphate (PPRP):

$$R5P + ATP \quad \underset{\text{synthetase}}{\xrightarrow{\hspace{1.5cm} PPRP \hspace{1.5cm}}} PPRP + AMP$$

PPRP is involved in two types of reaction. Firstly, in a combination with L-glutamine in the initial step of purine ring synthesis; this appears not to happen in mature red cells. Secondly, PPRP combines with adenine to form adenlyic acid (AMP) and this reaction, catalysed by adenine phosphoribosyltransferase (APRT), does occur in mature red cells:

$$PPRP + adenine \underset{APRT}{\xrightarrow{\hspace{2cm}}} AMP + P\text{--}P$$

The reaction is part of the purine salvage pathway although its significance in mature red cells is not known. Both reactants are present in normal red cells in very low concentration (adenine, 0.6 μM; PPRP 3.4 μM) but the levels are elevated in Lesch-Nyan syndrome (Ch. 6), as is the activity of APRT. Haematologically, this syndrome presents with megaloblastic changes in the marrow and several patients have low serum folate values or anaemia; little else is known.

AMP may thus arise in red cells from the APRT reaction or from breakdown of ADP. Adenylate kinase (AK) is also present in red cells where it can regenerate ATP:

$$2ADP \underset{AK}{\xrightarrow{\hspace{2cm}}} AMP + ATP$$

AK is essential to red cells as shown by the diminished cell survival and nonspherocytic haemolytic anaemia that accompanies inherited AK deficiency (MuKusick 20160). In one report the defect coexisted with G6PD deficiency in an Arab family. Both parents and six of nine offspring had partial AK deficiency but were haematologically normal while two siblings had severe enzyme deficiency accompanied by haemolytic anaemia; the ninth child was deceased. Total adenine nucleotides (AMP+ADP+ATP) were increased only in accord with the young cell population present while ADP was somewhat raised as a proportion of total adenine nucleotide.

Adenosine deaminase (ADA) catalyses the deamination of adenosine to inosine and ADA deficiency is described in some 50 families in association with combined immunodeficiency disease which arises through disturbed purine nucleoside metabolism in T and B lymphocytes (see p. 237). A decreased ADA activity of red cells is described in two patients with severely impaired cellular immunity but red-cell survival appeared to be unimpaired. A significantly increased activity of red-cell ADA is reported in chronic renal failure although, as with AK, this could be attributed to a young cell population. A singularly marked elevation of red-cell ADA (more than 45 times normal) occurs, together with a mild hereditary haemolytic anaemia, in which red-cell ATP is only some 60% of normal.

Pyrimidine metabolism

In mature red-cells pyrimidine metabolism is little understood although its significance is clear from the haemolytic anaemia associated with pyrimidine-5'-nucleotidase (P5N) deficiency (see p. 248). A number of cases have been described with similar haematological features, in particular a mild nonspherocytic haemolytic anaemia with basophilic stippling as a prominent feature in the red cells. Basophilic stippling is a classical peculiarity of lead poisoning and P5N activity is also diminished in this disorder. It is also reduced in β-thalassaemia trait to some 60% of normal. The inherited form of the deficiency occurs as an autosomal recessive disorder and is one of the commonest of red-cell enzyme deficiencies.

Reducing capacity

The several reactions involved in protecting cells from oxidative assault are all connected with the first two steps in the PPP (Fig. 12.5).

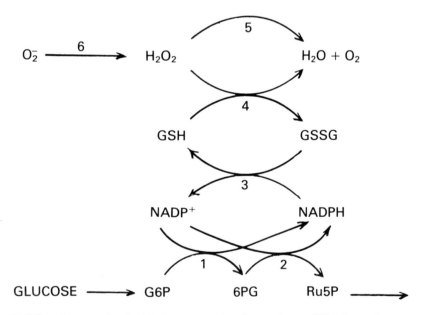

Fig. 12.5 Reactions associated with the pentose phosphate pathway. G6P, glucose 6-phosphate; 6PG, 6-phosphogluconate; GSH and GSSG, reduced and oxidised glutathione. 1, glucose-6-phosphate dehydrogenase; 2, 6-phosphogluconate dehydrogenase; 3, glutathione reductase; 4, glutathione peroxidase; 5, catalase; 6, superoxide dismutase.

Glutathione (GSH)

Red-cells contain a high concentration of GSH (approx. 2 mmol) with less than 1% of the total (GSH + GSSG) present in the oxidised and unreactive dimeric state. The primary function of GSH is protection of thiol groups of which the bulk are located on haemoglobin although membrane and enzyme-SH groups are also under protection. GSH also serves as a cofactor for glyoxalase, as a prosthetic group for glyceraldehyde-3-phosphate dehydrogenase, in the decomposition of H_2O_2 and for the detoxication of certain foreign hydrocarbons. When oxidised to the dimer form reduction back to GSH is catalysed by GSH reductase. GSH is synthesised de novo in red cells and its half life is approximately 3 days; the synthetic rate is not necessarily equivalent because GSSG is known to leak from red cells.

Abnormal GSH levels arise in several clinical conditions. High values are found in iron deficiency, in P5N deficiency, hypothyroidism and in some patients with lymphoma, myelofibrosis and acute and chronic leukaemia. Levels are also raised in the blood of normal neonates. Low levels of GSH are found notably in inherited GSH deficiency but also in G6PD and GSH reductase deficiency, renal and hepatic failure, hyperthyroidism, stomatocytosis and unstable haemoglobinopathy. An insufficiency of GSH arises either through inadequate de novo synthesis, as in hereditary GSH deficiency, or through inadequate regeneration, as in GSH reductase or G6PD deficiency. By whatever mechanism it occurs, a marked insufficiency of GSH is accompanied by haemolysis of cells. However, while stomatocytosis and unstable haemoglobinopathies are both associated with a haemolytic anaemia, low GSH is not the primary cause and in hyperthyroidism the GSH level is only mildly reduced and haemolysis does not occur.

Hereditary glutathione deficiency

GSH is synthesised in two stages:

1. L-glutamate + L-cysteine + ATP → L-γ-glutamyl-L-cysteine
$$+ \text{ADP} + P_i$$
catalysed by γ-glutamylcysteine synthetase

2. L-γ-glutamyl-L-cysteine + glycine + ATP → GSH + ADP + P_i

catalysed by GSH synthetase. Both enzymes are present in red cells but the other steps which comprise the γ-glutamyl cycle have not been reported. This cycle is described in detail in Chapter 5. Inherited GSH deficiency is a rare disorder with haemolytic anaemia and arises from defects in either of the two synthetic enzymes. The notable features of γ-glutamylcysteine synthetase deficiency (McKusick 23045) are, apart from the haemolytic anaemia, neuro-muscular degeneration and aminoaciduria. GSH synthetase deficiency appears to occur in two forms. One appears as a mild disorder (McKusick 23190) affecting red cells and the haemolytic anaemia is the only clinical feature; the enzyme is apparently adequately synthesised in other tissues. The second form of GSH synthetase deficiency is more severe and the haemolytic anaemia is accompanied by metabolic acidosis, abnormal CNS function and excessive 5-oxoprolinuria so that a number of tissues are involved (see Ch. 5).

Glutathione reductase (GR)

Deficiency of red-cell GR is well recorded but almost all reported cases were acquired and arose from low riboflavin status which depleted the enzyme of its flavin cofactor. Inherited GR deficiency (McKusick 23180) as a primary defect is rare, the mode of inheritance uncertain and the condition not associated with any haematological disorder.

GR deficiency occurring as a disorder secondary to riboflavin insufficiency is associated with a variety of haematological abnormalities for example, nonspherocytic haemolytic anaemia, pancytopenia, leukopenia, thrombocytopenia, acute leukaemia, haemophilia B, α-thalassaemia, homozygous HbC disease. It has been shown repeatedly that supplementation, either in vivo or in vitro, of riboflavin or FAD restores a low GR activity to normal, indeed elevated activity is recorded in cases of high dietary riboflavin and nicotinic acid. High levels are reported also in uraemia, cirrhosis, diabetes mellitus and gout.

Glutathione peroxidase (GSH-Px)

The decomposition of H_2O_2 in red cells is catalysed by both GSH-Px and catalase. The former route is the more important with low levels of H_2O_2 present while catalase activity increases in the presence of high H_2O_2 levels. GSH-Px is indispensable to red cells because a deficiency gives rise to haemolysis, whereas catalase deficiency is not associated with any haematological abnormalities. GSH-Px is highly specific for GSH but will reduce a number of hydroperoxides apart from H_2O_2. The enzyme is peculiar in lacking haem or flavin as a prosthetic group and in containing selenium. A direct correlation has been established between plasma selenium levels and red-cell GSH-Px activity.

Low GSH-Px activity is well recorded. Red cells of premature or full-term neonates have diminished levels which is an important cause of their undue sensitivity to oxidative assault. The deficiency is temporary and activities reach adult levels after some six months. A few cases of hereditary GSH-Px deficiency are known and these are associated with haemolytic anaemia (McKusick 23170). Several reported cases of acquired deficiency are associated with march haemoglobinuria, disseminated intravascular coagulation with red-cell fragmentation, or acanthocytosis. Low values are reported also in iron-deficiency anaemia. Ethnic differences exist in normal subjects and Jewish subjects have significantly lower values than North European non-Jews. It is this diversity of conditions for low GSH-Px activity that has made difficult the demonstration of a true inherited deficiency in association with a haemolytic anaemia. For the same reason the pattern of inheritance is not certain.

Catalase

Inherited red-cell deficiency (McKusick 20020) of catalase is a rare but well-recorded defect affecting Japanese and Swiss subjects. All evidence suggests that different mutants with low activity are present in the two groups and that neither is associated with any haematological abnormalities. The Japanese, but not the Swiss, form is associated with oral gangrene. Inheritance of the disorder amongst Japanese follows an autosomal recessive pattern, red cells of heterozygotes contain catalase which gives intermediate values of around 50% of normal while homozygotes give values of 0–3%; tissues other than red cells are implicated, namely nasal tissue, marrow and liver. In the Swiss form the mutant catalase appears less stable than the Japanese mutant. The consequence to the red cells of containing either mutant is an inability to detoxicate high levels of H_2O_2. A small increase in the rate of PPP activity has been shown with the Swiss mutant; this occurs because GSH-Px is the sole route for H_2O_2 destruction. However, this route was shown to be adequate even when acatalasic red cells were exposed to levels of primaquine which provoke a haemolytic episode in G6PD-deficient subjects.

Glucose-6-phosphate dehydrogenase (G6PD, McKusick 30590)

More than 140 variants of G6PD are known and a number partially characterised.[7] They are conveniently classified under five headings (Table 12.4). Group 1 contains variants with low activity and associated with continuous nonspherocytic haemolytic anaemia in the absence of provoking agents. In Group 2 are 37 variants which also have low activity but are not usually associated with haemolytic anaemia unless this is precipitated by oxidative agents (see later). Group 3 comprises variants with activities only mildly or moderately subnormal; this group contains the common A– or African variant and the relatively common Chinese variant G6PD Canton. In Group 4 are 19 variants including the normal B+ and common African A+ variant with activities which are normal and slightly subnormal respectively, while Group 5 comprises a single hyperactive variant. Inclusion in a group implies some degree of characterisation although for many variants basic data are lacking. Those variants with low activity tend also to be unstable, as judged by their heat lability. Although so many variants are

Table 12.4 Classification of G6PD variants

Group	Type of variant	Number of variants known	Range of activity*	Examples
1	Deficiency associated with chronic haemolytic anaemia	47	0–35, mean 9	Oklahoma, Chicago, Boston, Tokyo, Worcester
2	Deficiency usually without chronic haemolytic anaemia	37	0–10, mean 4	Mediterranean, Ferrara
3	Moderate to mild deficiency	36	7–75, mean 27	A−, Canton
4	Mild or no deficiency	19	6–105, mean 103	B+, A+, Baltimore
5	Increased activity	1	400	Hektoen

* Values are percentages of normal (100%). Further details are available.[7]

known, almost all are rare and more than 98% of affected subjects have either the African (A−) or G6PD Mediterranean (favism) variant. Our present understanding of the effects upon red cells and affected subjects of G6PD deficiency has emerged largely from biochemical and haematological studies of these two common variants.

The G6PD gene is one of a group of genes located on the X chromosome. Affected males are hemizygotes and females are heterozygotes; because of gene inactivation the latter have two red-cell populations, one normal and one deficient (see Ch. 1). The proportion of each in affected females depends upon the relative survival properties during embryonic development of normal cells and those with an inactive gene. There is a notable consistency in G6PD levels in identical twins heterozygous for the deficiency which has suggested that the inactivation process is not random.

The African variant (A−). This is the commonest variant of G6PD with around 12% males and 3% females affected. The majority of normal African males (some 70%) carry the common B+ variant while the remainder have a second variant (A+) which has a near normal activity. The A+ and B+ molecules differ in the replacement of an asparagine of the B^+ molecule by an aspartic acid in A+ and this confers a faster electrophoretic mobility towards the anode on the A+ molecule (110) compared with B+ (100). Historically it was the absence of an A+ band in haemolysates of affected African males that caused the designation A− to be used. Normal African females are also A+ or B+, but some are heterozygous for both, while affected females are heterozygous A−/A+ or A−/B+, or homozygous A−.

The enzymic activities of the B+, A+ and A− variants are 100, 90 and 8–20% respectively but their kinetic properties are similar (see Table 12.5). Thus, the Km for G6P is 50–70 μM, the Km for $NADP^+$ is 2.9–4.4 μM

Table 12.5 Characteristics of the commonest G6PD variants

Enzyme	Mobility	Activity	Heat stability	pH curve	Km G6P (μM)	Km NADP$^+$ (μM)
B+	100	100	Normal	Normal	50–70	2.9–4.4
A+	110	80–100	Normal	Normal	50–70	2.9–4.4
A–	110	8–20	Normal	Normal	50–70	2.9–4.4
Mediterranean	100	0–7	Labile	Biphasic	19–26	1.2–1.6
Canton	105	4–24	Labile	Biphasic	18–36	—

and activity with the abnormal substrate 2-deoxy G6P is the same with all three variants. The heat stability and pH optimum curves are also similar for each variant. The low activity of the A– variant is not due to impaired synthesis for activity in red-cell precursors and reticulocytes is normal; the enzyme appears to be unstable with fewer active molecules present in mature peripheral red cells.

In the absence of exogenous agents, subjects with Groups 2, 3 or 4 G6PD deficiency show no haematological symptoms despite the subnormal activity of the enzyme. The PPP activity may be slightly depressed but is adequate to maintain reducing status in the absence of oxidative stimuli, although the life span of the cells is somewhat shortened.

It is the presence in G6PD-depleted red cells of abnormal levels of oxidants which readily overwhelms their limited reducing capacity. When GSH is converted to GSSG the PPP cannot be stimulated adequately to regenerate GSH. The presence in the cells of metabolites of ingested oxidants, e.g. H_2O_2 and free radicals, none of which can be detoxicated efficiently, wreaks oxidative havoc especially in the old cohort in which the restricted protective mechanisms have additionally declined with age.

Oxidative damage to red cells can be demonstrated by the presence of Heinz bodies, methaemoglobin, sulphaemoglobin, fragmentation and all the criteria of intravascular haemolysis. The haematological changes have been carefully documented in affected male Negroes receiving 30 mg primaquine base per 24 hours. Evidence of haemolysis is apparent within three days of starting the regime. An acute haemolytic phase follows and lasts 8–12 days when the haemoglobin reaches its minimum and clinical jaundice is apparent. The urine contains excess urobilin and haemoglobinuria may be present. By the tenth day recovery is evident and a reticulocyte peak occurs at around 14 days. The haemoglobin level rises to normal or near normal at 28 or more days. With continued drug ingestion the degree of haemolysis settles to a steady state; if the drug is stopped reversion occurs to the pre-dose haematological state; if dosage is increased then haemolysis also increases and is maintained with the dose at a more severe level. This occurs because the old and more sensitive cells are preferentially destroyed and a younger cohort appears with higher enzyme levels; however, the older cells of the younger cohort become vulnerable if the drug dosage is increased.

Other haemolytic drugs differ in potency but produce a similar overall haematological picture:

★Acetanilid
Methylene blue
Nalidixic acid (Negram®, Mictral®, Uriben®)
Naphthalene (moth balls, lavatory deodorants)
Niridazole (Ambilhar®)
Nitrofurantoin (Furadantin®, Berkfurin®, Ceduran®, Furan®, Macrodantin®)
Phenylhydrazine
Primaquine
★Pamaquine
★Pentaquine
Sulphanilamide
Sulphacetamide (Albucid®, Bleph-10 Liquifilm®, Cortucid®, Isoptocetamide®, Minims®, Ocusol®, Sulfaped®, Sulphacalyre®)
Sulphapyridine (M & B 693)
Sulphamethoxazole (Gantanol®, Septrin®, Bactrim®)
★Thiazolesulphone
Toluidine blue
Trinitrotoluene
★Not marketed in UK.

Methaemoglobinaemia is less than expected because most of the methaemoglobin is contained in the old cells which are least capable of reducing it and these are the cells which are preferentially destroyed by the oxidative stress.

The levels of G6PD activity in the red cells of heterozygous females lie between the low levels of hemizygous males and normal because their blood contains a normal B or A+ and an A− population and the measured value is the resultant of the two. This is a diagnostic problem when the patient has a haemolytic episode which produces an enlarged young red-cell population containing increased G6PD activity which can mask a deficiency. The standard screening tests will not reveal the deficient group of cells but diagnosis is possible using a cytochemical technique. Alternatively, family studies may assist a diagnosis, or testing suspected blood when the haemolytic episode has stopped and the cell population has resumed its usual age distribution.

The Mediterranean variant (Favism, McKusick 13470). This is the second common G6PD variant. Favism has long been recognised in people of the Mediterranean littoral, presenting as an acute haemolytic episode which is sometimes fatal in children following ingestion of fava beans (*vicia faba*), particularly during the spring when the beans are fresh. Summated data from many surveys show that of approximately 16 000 Greek subjects tested 6.6% were G6PD deficient and of some 15 000 subjects tested in polyethnic Israel 8% were affected. Regional and ethnic differences do occur, however, in the incidence of the disorder. Thus, although rare in Central Italy, the overall incidence in Sardinia is 17%. Also, while the overall incidence in Israel is about 8%, there are widely different incidences between racial groups within the country.

The Mediterranean variant is structurally different from the A−enzyme and red-cell activity among affected males is less, 0–7%, so that they are more drug-sensitive than affected Africans. Electrophoretically, the Mediterranean and normal B enzymes are similar but have different kinetic properties (Table 12.5); the former variant is also unstable. The low activity in Mediterranean subjects may account for their sensitivity to fava beans which do not affect Africans with the A− variant. Affected Mediterranean subjects are haematologically normal in the absence of fava beans or drugs and their haemolytic crises follow a similar pattern to that of affected Africans, although more severe. Subjects with the Mediterranean variant are also sensitive to a wider range of drugs than affected Africans, for example chloramphenicol. Fava beans contain a number of redox compounds, but current studies implicate two aglycones of vicine and convicine, namely divicine and isouramil as responsible agents (Fig. 12.6). Both react with GSH and cause membrane damage in vitro. Whatever the true oxidant(s) may be, it is likely to be unstable in order to account for the decline in toxicity of the bean with storage.

A singular feature of favism is the increasing tolerance to fava beans with age of affected subjects, children are much more prone to haemolytic episodes than are adults. As with G6PDA− a haemolytic crisis in hetero-zygotes (females) is milder than in hemizygotes (males) or female homo-

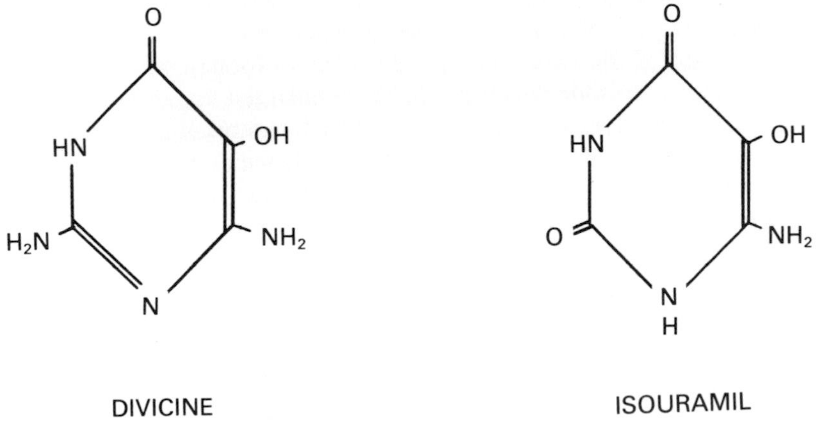

DIVICINE   ISOURAMIL

Fig. 12.6 Structures of divicine and isouramil.

zygotes. The period from ingestion of fava beans to advent of crisis varies because of factors such as type, potency and amount of bean eaten as well as gastric and intestinal transit time and activity; signs of impending crisis are present, however, within 48 hours. A further unusual and unexplained feature of this disorder is that not all subjects with the Mediterranean variant have favic crises. However, because of the indeterminable collection of variables that govern the onset of a crisis, it is difficult to be certain that a G6PD-deficient subject is not also favic.

Variants associated with chronic haemolytic anaemia. (Table 12.4 Group 1) These are rare and associated with a chronic nonspherocytic haemolytic anaemia in subjects not ingesting drugs or fava beans. Usually these variants are unstable, have low activity and abnormal kinetic properties. With some the enzyme activity is low yet greater than for red cells containing the A− variant; this is attributable in part to the young red-cell population present. It is also a consequence of the artificial conditions of enzyme assay in which maximum activity is measured with excess substrate and this does not reflect intracellular activity. The degree of anaemia is usually mild, but is worsened by administration of oxidative drugs.

Icterus neonatorum. Red-cell G6PD activity is raised in normal neonates although they remain at risk from oxidants for the first few months of life because their red cells contain low levels of GSH-Px, NADH methaemoglobin reductase, catalase and vitamin E and this sensitivity increases with prematurity. Usually however, there are no haematological problems, and the risk disappears at around three months of life when the enzyme activities reach adult levels.

With G6PD-deficient neonates the risk of oxidative haemolysis is increased and they are affected by the likelihood of neonatal jaundice, the severity of which depends upon the G6PD variant in the red cells. Thus, deficient Mediterranean, Thai and Chinese neonates have a high incidence of neonatal jaundice. Oddly, American infants with the A− variant are not unduly affected but Nigerian infants with the same variant carry a high risk.

Infection and acidosis. Haemolytic episodes in G6PD deficiency arising from infections rather than drugs are well established. A number of drugs used to treat the infections have been wrongly implicated as haemolytic because it was not clear that the infection itself was the precipitating factor. Haemolysis arising from infection tends to be mild, but can be severe, and recovery can be slow because marrow depression accompanies the infection. Haemolytic episodes from infection are common in bacterial pneumonia, viral hepatitis and typhoid fever as well as infections due to salmonella, E. coli, proteus, staphylococci, β-streptococci and rickettsiae.

Diabetic acidosis is also reported to provoke haemolytic episodes in G6PD deficiency. The PPP is not pH-sensitive although the first intermediate, glucose-6-phosphate, is also a component of the EMP whose activity falls with decreasing pH. However, glucose-6-phosphate levels rise with a fall in pH and so the mechanism of haemolytic episodes provoked by acidosis is not clear.

Cells affected other than red cells. Leucocyte G6PD activity is normal in Africans with the A− variant but low in affected subjects of Mediterranean and Chinese origin. It is also low or absent in subjects with G6PD deficiency associated with chronic haemolytic anaemia in whom other tissues reported deficient are eye lens, saliva, liver, kidney, platelets and sperm. Eye lens cells and platelets have no nucleus and like red cells tend to have lower activities than nucleated cells in which enzyme synthesis occurs. Eye lens cells have a similar metabolism to red cells and it is noteworthy that only occasionally has cataract been reported in G6PD deficiency.

DISORDERS OF HAEMOGLOBIN

Abnormalities of haem synthesis are described in Chapter 7; in the present chapter red-cell disorders are considered which are a result either of structurally abnormal globins (haemoglobinopathies) or of a reduced rate of synthesis of normal globin (thalassaemia syndromes).

Haemoglobinopathies (McKusick 14190)

There are many variants of normal haemoglobin (HbA), but few are associated with haematological disorders; these are HbS, homozygous HbC and HbE, the HbM group, unstable haemoglobinopathies and haemoglobins with abnormal oxygen affinity. The structure and function of normal haemoglobin are considered in numerous publications (see ref. 8 for example) and are not dealt with here.

Sickle-cells (HbS)

The primary defect in HbS is the replacement of glutamic acid by valine in the sixth amino acid of the β-chain; this confers a different electric charge on the molecule and a slower electrophoretic mobility, by which it can be identified. The abnormality is genetically determined; in the homozygous form, sickle cell disease, an abnormal gene is inherited from each parent whereas in the mild heterozygous form, sickle cell trait, only one abnormal gene is inherited. The disorder is present mainly within the Negro population but there is also a low incidence in the Mediterranean area, Southern Arabia and India. HbS does not appear at birth, nor for a few months. It becomes apparent when the abnormal β-chains are synthesised and HbS and HbA begin to replace HbF. The presence of HbS provides some benefit, by giving protection against malaria. Affected red cells invaded by the parasites undergo sickling and are destroyed in the spleen, which interrupts the parasites' normal life cycle.

In sickle-cell disease the degree of anaemia is usually severe and variable haemolysis is present. Reticulocyte counts vary from 10–20% with notable polychromasia and some punctate basophilia. Howell-Jolly bodies and siderocytes can occur, with normoblasts in severe cases. The tendency of red cells to sickle in vivo can produce a range of clinical symptoms and painful crises; abdominal, bone or joint pain, leg ulcers, haemolytic crises, retinal and pulmonary lesions, priapism, hepatic damage or renal involvement which may provoke haematuria. The local conditions which inititate sickling are unknown but a sequence of events is set up of sickling, red-cell aggregation, increased blood viscosity, stagnation and anoxia with further sickling and the formation of thrombus-like clumps. This process can occur anywhere in the body, and so gives rise to the diversity of symptoms. Sickled cells are sufficiently abnormal in shape to be sequestered by the spleen and the adverse environment within the splenic vessels enhances the sickling process. Eventually blockage of the vessels occurs and this, together with thrombus formation, produces, in later life, a shrunken and fibrosed organ. Skeletal changes also occur with periosteal thickening of bones in hands and feet in infancy, widening of the diploe in the skull and osteomyelitis arising from earlier thromboses in bones and joints.

Sickle-cell trait does not give rise to anaemia, nor are there usually any clinical or haematological abnormalities. Red cells contain 20–45% HbS and sickle only at unphysiologically low O_2 tension.

The sickling process is initiated only at low O_2 tension and results in the aggregation of deoxyHbS into long, straight fibres which form parallel bundles and force the cell to deform. A sickle fibre comprises seven filaments plaited together and each filament is made of two linear threads of molecules. Polymerisation takes place only if a cell contains more than a certain minimum of deoxyHbS. In the homozygous condition the HbS content is high, and can be 80–100%; such cells sickle within the normal range of O_2 tension. The HbS component of blood is not, however, spread uniformly throughout the cell population and the degree of sickling varies within patients. Any haemoglobin in the oxy-form is not involved in the polymerisation process and (of relevance to infants) HbF is more effective than HbA in inhibiting sickling. Thus, a red-cell population containing HbF and HbS gives a milder disorder than one with HbA and S. HbF is also distributed non-uniformly among red cells and those with a higher content will survive longer.

Sickling in vivo occurs mainly in the venous circulation with reversal of sickling in the arterial circulation. Cells which remain sickled cannot negotiate the capillaries and are destroyed. This is one cause of the haemolytic process. Sickled cells contain rigid spicules which can break off; this also may cause the cell to be lost or its membrane to be affected, as shown by an increased mechanical fragility of the cells. Cell-membrane damage also occurs by precipitation of HbS on the inner surface. Repeated sickling-unsickling further damages the membrane and produces stiffening which eventually gives irreversibly sickled cells (ISC). Such cells do not survive long and are a major cause of haemolysis, especially where the spleen continues to function. Further evidence of a defective membrane in sickled cells is the increased Na^+ and K^+ flux with net loss of K^+ over Na^+ and cell dehydration. Lactate production is increased in vitro with a rise in intracellular pH. Red cells in sickle-cell disease have an increased Ca^{2+} content and an increased Ca^{2+} permeability on sickling and this may contribute to their increased stiffness.

Homozygous HbC and E

Only the homozygous forms of HbC and HbE are of clinical importance; both are associated with a mild anaemia which is haemolytic in HbC. HbE is the second commonest abnormal haemoglobin and occurs in South-East Asia while HbC is relatively common in West Africa.

Methaemoglobin and HbM

The loss of an electron from haem Fe (II) to give haem Fe (III) converts Hb into methaemoglobin (MetHb) which has no oxygen-carrying capacity. MetHb is formed continuously in vivo at a slow rate but the level in whole blood is maintained at less than 1% by the several reducing systems in the cell, notably NADH-linked MetHb reductase (diaphorase). Abnormally high levels of MetHb arise in one of three ways: induction by chemical agents including drugs, inherited diaphorase deficiency or the presence of a HbM variant.

MetHb is not haemolytic and the main symptom of methaemoglobinaemia is cyanosis; this is present when MetHb reaches 10–25% of the total haemoglobin, although this level can be tolerated without ill effects. At around 40%, fatigue, dizziness, headaches, exertional dyspnoea, and tachycardia may be present and at approximately 60% stupor occurs; above 70% is lethal.

When MetHb arises through assault by chemical agents or drugs there is usually concomitant oxidative damage to cell constituents e.g. conversion of -SH to -S-S- groups in the membrane, globin and enzyme systems. Dependent upon the severity of this damage haemolysis may accompany the methaemoglobinaemia. An exception is nitrite which, at a level that causes methaemoglobinaemia, appears to exert no other damage and no haemolysis. In diaphorase deficiency MetHb accumulates at a rate of up to 5% per day because the primary reducing system has a low activity. Apart from methaemoglobinaemia and its clinical consequences there are no other manifestations of the abnormality. Diaphorase deficiency (McKusick 25080) is one of two inherited red-cell disorders, the other is hereditary spherocytosis (see earlier), which can be treated. Either ascorbate (500 mg/24h orally) or, more effectively, methylene blue (100–300 mg/24h orally), will maintain MetHb at a normal level.

The HbM group comprises five variants (HbM Boston,Hyde Park, Milwaukee, Saskatoon and Iwate) in each of which an amino acid replacement affects the normal binding of haem Fe (II) with histidine. In four of the variants histidine itself is replaced by tyrosine while in HbM Milwaukee a substitution of glutamate for valine in the β-chain haem pocket results in bonding of the glutamate γ-COOH group with Fe (III). As a consequece the iron in these haemoglobins is locked in the Fe (III) state and cannot be reduced by any of the systems which convert MetHb to Hb. Other HbM variants are described but not presently fully characterised. In some the red-cell life span is shortened but no other abnormalities are described and the only clinical symptom is cyanosis. Affected subjects are heterozygotes with 10–25% of their haemoglobin in the fixed Fe (III) state.

The distinction between MetHb and HbM is easily made. MetHb is detectable by a characteristic absorption peak at 630 nm while a HbM has an identifiable peak at wavelengths lower than 630 nm. In addition, some variants display differences in the 500–600 nm region. HbM can also be determined electrophoretically.

The unstable haemoglobins

This rather rare group of inherited blood disorders has in common an intrinsic instability of the haemoglobin molecule, which results in spontaneous intracellular degradation to give inclusion bodies. These are seen in appropriately stained fresh cells only from splenectomised patients because the spleen can extract intracellular particles without sequestering the cells. Affected subjects have a nonspherocytic haemolytic anaemia because red cells containing insoluble haemoglobin breakdown products undergo irreversible damage.

Detection of these haemoglobins can be effected by electrophoresis or by exploiting their instability. Electrophoresis on paper is not satisfactory but media such as acrylamide or starch gel can be used. Tests which depend upon the lability of the haemoglobin involve warming buffered haemolysates at 50°C, or at 37°C in the presence of isopropanol, and noting any precipitated haemoglobin or incubating fresh red cells for 24 hours and detecting inclusion bodies and MetHb in the incubated cells. Variants differ both in their stability and intracellular concentration, and this is reflected in the severity of their haemolytic anaemia which varies between patients from mild to severe. Blood films show anisocytosis, polychromasia, hypochromia and sometimes punctate basophilia. The oxygen affinity differs among variants as does the degree of methaemoglobinaemia and some variants give rise to darkened urine through excretion of dipyrrolic metabolites of haemoglobin.

The haemoglobin molecule becomes unstable in several ways.[8] Loss of haem groups will destabilise the globin moiety which becomes insoluble; dissociation of the molecule into separate α and β chains can occur and finally a sub-unit can be weakened by distortion. Depending upon the variant, some or all of these defects may be present. Breakdown of unstable haemoglobin is accompanied by increased MetHb and hemichrome (dimer) formation and -SH groups become inactive through mixed disulphide formation with GSH. This loss of some GSH, but especially the production of insoluble, degraded material which becomes attached to the cytoplasmic membrane surface, damages the cell and shortens its life span. A further hazard is the sensitivity of unstable haemoglobins to those drugs which are haemolytic in G6PD deficiency.

The thalassaemia syndromes (McKusick 14180, 14185, 14190 and 27350)

The common feature or this group of disorders is an inherited abnormality in the rate of globin synthesis. This is manifested by a diversity of haematological symptoms which includes haemolysis, ineffective erythropoiesis and a variable degree of anaemia. Additionally, thalassaemia may occur simultaneously with certain haemoglobin variants, which may be found in high frequency in the same populations; the presence of two genetic defects within one subject increases the diversity of disorders. The collective term *thalassaemia syndromes* is used for this whole group of disorders; they are complex, and understanding of them is rapidly increasing. They are described elsewhere[9] with the necessary detail not possible in the present chapter.

The primary defect in thalassaemia is in the DNA sequence but it can be expressed at any stage of protein biosynthesis. The consequence is a disruption of normal α- and β-chain production, as shown by an abnormal α/β ratio; red cells are consequently inadequately haemoglobinised. The unaffected α- or β-chain is produced normally, and in the homozygous condition the presence of excess free chains may affect cell maturation and function, resulting in a shortened cell life. The primary classification of the thalassaemias into α- and β-thalassaemia indicates the affected chain.

In α-*thalassaemia*, defective production of α-chains is usually due to gene deletion and affects both HbA ($\alpha_2\beta_2$) and HbF ($\alpha_2\gamma_2$) levels. Fetal synthesis of excess γ-chains can lead to γ_4 tetramers (Hb Barts) and in adults to β_4 tetramers (HbH). The clinical expression of α-thalassaemia depends on the fact that the structural gene coding for α-chains is duplicated on each of a pair of homologous chromosomes, so that the genome contains four α-chain genes. Gene deletion may affect one or both genes on either or both chromosomes, so that four degrees of severity of α-thalassaemia can exist, depending on how many genes are deleted.

Deletion of one of the four genes results in a silent condition, undetectable except at birth, when approximately three times the normal level (0.5%) of Hb Barts is present. Deletion of two genes results in α-*thalassaemia trait*, which is also usually asymptomatic; some 5% Hb Barts is present at birth, and other features include persistent hypochromia, microcytosis, poikilocytosis, target cells and occasional inclusions. Anaemia, if it occurs, is very mild. Deletion of three of the four genes results in *HbH disease*; here there may be up to 40% HbH present in the cells, with a small amount of Hb Barts and a low level of Hb A_2 ($\alpha_2\delta_2$; normally approximately 2.5%). This condition is accompanied by a haemolytic anaemia. Deletion of all four α-chain genes is a lethal condition, giving rise to *hydrops fetalis*. The red cells contain no α-chains; some 80% of the haemoglobin is Hb Barts, with small amounts of HbH and Hb Portland (an embryonic haemoglobin, $\zeta_2\gamma_2$). This form of thalassaemia results in miscarriage in late pregnancy.

In β-*thalassaemia*, the synthesis of β-chains by the affected chromosome may be reduced (β^+) or absent (β^o). In most cases the genetic defect does not involve deletion of the structural gene for the β-chain, but involves later steps in gene transcription. In the homozygous state (β-*thalassaemia major*), the symptoms of severe anaemia develop some two months after birth, when β-chain production should be taking place. The blood film shows hypochromia, anisocytosis, poikilocytosis, misshapen microcytes, target cells, erythroblasts and elliptocytes; after splenectomy there are also red cells with irregular inclusions. The lifespan of red cells is shortened, with some extremely shortlived cells, and the reticulocyte count is raised. Excess α-chains are present in precursor cells and some cells may be retained in the marrow; others enter the circulation where inclusions are removed by the spleen. The HbA_2 level is raised while HbF is normal or slightly raised. β-*Thalassaemia intermedia* comprises a diversity of genetic abnormalities affecting the rate of β-chain production, resulting in anaemia, jaundice and splenomegaly. In β-*thalassaemia minor*, the common heterozygous form of the condition, the HbA_2 level is raised (4–6%) and HbF is normal or slightly raised; if anaemia is present it is generally mild. β-*Thalassaemia minima* is the mildest heterozygous form of this disorder, with a so-called silent thalassaemia gene. Both the MCV and MCH of the red cells are decreased, but HbH_2 and HbF are normal.

Other variants of α- and β-thalassaemia exist. In δβ-*thalassaemia*, both δ- and β-chain synthesis is diminished; in homozygotes the synthesis of both these chains is absent, and haemoglobin is entirely HbF. There is an associated variable anaemia and a typically thalassaemic blood film. Heterozygotes for the condition have 5–20% HbF and essentially normal HbA_2 values, with the clinical and haematological abnormalities seen in heterozygous β-thalassaemia. A β-thalassaemia syndrome may also be caused by the presence of Hb Lepore, a variant with normal α chains and a pair of δβ chains fused at specific sides. Individuals doubly heterozygous for β-thalassaemia and a β-chain variant such as Hb Sv, C or E show a variety of clinical pictures due to interaction of the two abnormal genes. Lastly, there occurs a syndrome of *hereditary persistence of fetal haemoglobin* (HPFH), without associated thalassaemic features. HPFH shows racial differences in respect of the amount of HbF in the red cells, and its distribution among a few of the cells (e.g. Swiss type) or all cells (e.g. Greek type).

The pathophysiology of the red cells in thalassaemia is ill-understood. Where the red-cell lifespan is shortened, the membrane is likely to have been damaged by intracellular inclusions of excess α- or β-chains, either in the marrow or later on in the circulation. If these inclusions are large then the cells may never emerge from the marrow, and indeed ineffective erythropoiesis is more important than extramedullary haemolysis in β-thalassaemia. In HbH disease, cation permeability of peripheral red cells is increased, a sign of membrane abnormality; and in older cells containing inclusions GSH is lower and PPP activity high. It is likely too, that any red cell which has experienced inclusions will have a damaged membrane that has been further harmed by removal of the inclusions in the spleen.

REFERENCES

1 Lux S E 1983 Disorders of the red cell skeleton: hereditary spherocytosis and hereditary elliptocytosis. In: Stanbury J B, Wyngaarden J B, Fredrickson D S, Goldstein J L, Brown M S (eds) The metabolic basis of inherited disease, 5th edn. McGraw-Hill, New York, ch 72, p 1573–1605
2 Fairbanks G, Steck T L, Wallach D F H 1971 Electrophoretic analysis of the major polypeptides of the human erythrocyte membrane. Biochemistry 10: 2606–2617
3 Steck T L 1974 The organisation of proteins in the human red blood cell membrane. Journal of Cell Biology 62: 1–19
4 Beutler E, Blume K G, Kaplan J C, Löhr G W, Ramot B, Valentine W N 1977 International Committee for Standardisation in Haematology: recommended methods for red-cell enzyme analysis. British Journal of Haematology 35: 331–340
5 Boulard-Heitzmann P, Boulard M, Tallineau C et al 1984 Decreased red cell enolase activity in a 40-year-old woman with compensated haemolysis. Scandinavian Journal of Haematology 33: 401–404
6 Valentine W N, Tanaka K R, Paglia D E 1983 Pyruvate kinase and other enzyme deficiency disorders of the erythrocyte. In: Stanbury J B, Wyngaarden J B, Fredrickson D S, Goldstein J L, Brown M S (eds) The metabolic basis of inherited disease, 5th edn. McGraw-Hill, New York, ch 73, p 1606–1628
7 Beutler E 1978 Glucose-6-phosphate dehydrogenase deficiency. In: Hemolytic anemia in disorders of red cell metabolism. Plenum Medical, ch 2, p 23–167
8 Huehns E R 1982 The structure and function of haemoglobin: clinical disorders due to abnormal haemoglobin structure. In: Hardisty R M, Weatherall D J (eds) Blood and its disorders, 2nd edn. Blackwell Scientific Publications, Oxford, ch 8 p 323–400
9 Weatherall D J, Clegg J B 1982 The molecular genetics of haemoglobin: the thalassaemia syndromes. In: Hardisty R M, Weatherall D J (eds) Blood and its disorders, 2nd edn. Blackwell Scientific Publications, Oxford, ch 9, p 401–452

INDEX

Index